Perinatal Interventions to Improve Neonatal Outcomes

Editors

RAVI MANGAL PATEL
TRACY A. MANUCK

CLINICS IN PERINATOLOGY

www.perinatology.theclinics.com

Consulting Editor
LUCKY JAIN

June 2018 • Volume 45 • Number 2

ELSEVIER

1600 John F. Kennedy Boulevard • Suite 1800 • Philadelphia, Pennsylvania, 19103-2899

http://www.theclinics.com

CLINICS IN PERINATOLOGY Volume 45, Number 2
June 2018 ISSN 0095-5108, ISBN-13: 978-0-323-58413-5

Editor: Kerry Holland
Developmental Editor: Casey Potter

Clinics in Perinatology (ISSN 0095-5108) is published quarterly by Elsevier Inc., 360 Park Avenue South, New York, NY 10010-1710. Months of issue are March, June, September, and December. Business and Editorial Offices: 1600 John F. Kennedy Blvd., Ste. 1800, Philadelphia, PA 19103-2899. Customer Service Office: 3251 Riverport Lane, Maryland Heights, MO 63043. Periodicals postage paid at New York, NY and additional mailing offices. Subscription prices are $299.00 per year (US individuals), $548.00 per year (US institutions), $351.00 per year (Canadian individuals), $670.00 per year (Canadian institutions), $433.00 per year (international individuals), $670.00 per year (international institutions), $100.00 per year (US students), and $195.00 per year (Canadian and international students). International air speed delivery is included in all Clinics subscription prices. All prices are subject to change without notice. **POSTMASTER:** Send address changes to *Clinics in Perinatology*, Elsevier Health Sciences Division, Subscription Customer Service, 3251 Riverport Lane, Maryland Heights, MO 63043. **Customer Service: Telephone: 1-800-654-2452** (U.S. and Canada); **1-314-447-8871** (outside U.S. and Canada). **Fax: 1-314-447-8029. E-mail: journalscustomerservice-usa@elsevier.com** (for print support); **journalsonlinesupport-usa@elsevier.com** (for online support).

Reprints. For copies of 100 or more, of articles in this publication, please contact the Commercial Reprints Department, Elsevier Inc., 360 Park Avenue South, New York, NY 10010-1710. Tel. 212-633-3874; Fax: 212-633-3820; E-mail: reprints@elsevier.com.

Clinics in Perinatology is also publilshed in Spanish by McGraw-Hill Interamericana Editores S.A., P.O. Box 5-237, 06500 Mexico D.F., Mexico.

Clinics in Perinatology is covered in *MEDLINE/PubMed (Index Medicus) Current Contents, Excepta Medica, BIOSIS and ISI/BIOMED.*

Contributors

CONSULTING EDITOR

LUCKY JAIN, MD, MBA
George W. Brumley Jr Professor and Chair, Emory University School of Medicine, Department of Pediatrics, Chief Academic Officer, Children's Healthcare of Atlanta, Atlanta, Georgia, USA

EDITORS

RAVI MANGAL PATEL, MD, MSc
Associate Professor, Department of Pediatrics, Division of Neonatal-Perinatal Medicine, Emory University School of Medicine, Children's Healthcare of Atlanta, Atlanta, Georgia, USA

TRACY A. MANUCK, MD, MS
Associate Professor, Department of Obstetrics and Gynecology, Division of Maternal-Fetal Medicine, University of North Carolina at Chapel Hill School of Medicine, Medical Director, UNC Prematurity Prevention Program, Chapel Hill, North Carolina, USA

AUTHORS

KJERSTI M. AAGAARD, MD, PhD, FACOG
Professor and Vice Chair of Research, Henry and Emma Meyer Chair, Department of Obstetrics and Gynecology, Division of Maternal-Fetal Medicine, Translational Biology and Molecular Medicine, Medical Scientist Training Program, Alkek Center for Metagenomics and Microbiome Research, Departments of Molecular and Human Genetics, and Molecular and Cell Biology, Baylor College of Medicine, Houston, Texas, USA

MARTINA L. BADELL, MD
Department of Gynecology and Obstetrics, Emory University, Emory University Hospital, Midtown Perinatal Center, Atlanta, Georgia, USA

WHITNEY A. BOOKER, MD
Division of Maternal-Fetal Medicine, Department of Obstetrics and Gynecology, Columbia University College of Physicians and Surgeons, Columbia University Irving Medical Center, New York, New York, USA

IRINA BURD, MD, PhD
Associate Professor, Maternal-Fetal Medicine Fellowship Director, Department of Gynecology and Obstetrics, Division of Maternal-Fetal Medicine, Integrated Research Center for Fetal Medicine, Neuroscience Intensive Care Nursery Program, Department of Neurology, Johns Hopkins University School of Medicine, Baltimore, Maryland, USA

DERRICK M. CHU, BSc
Department of Obstetrics and Gynecology, Division of Maternal-Fetal Medicine, Translational Biology and Molecular Medicine, Medical Scientist Training Program, Baylor College of Medicine, Houston, Texas, USA

REBECCA C. FRY, PhD, MS
Carol Remmer Angle Distinguished Professor and Associate Chair, Department of Environmental Sciences and Engineering, UNC Gillings School of Global Public Health, University of North Carolina at Chapel Hill, Chapel Hill, North Carolina, USA

CYNTHIA GYAMFI-BANNERMAN, MD, MSc
Division of Maternal-Fetal Medicine, Department of Obstetrics and Gynecology, Columbia University College of Physicians and Surgeons, Columbia University Irving Medical Center, New York, New York, USA

BRENNA L. HUGHES, MD
Associate Professor, Division of Maternal Fetal Medicine, Department of Obstetrics and Gynecology, Duke University Medical Center, Durham, North Carolina, USA

VISHAL KAPADIA, MD, MSCS
Assistant Professor, Department of Pediatrics, Division of Neonatal-Perinatal Medicine, University of Texas Southwestern Medical Center, Dallas, Texas, USA

SARAH KEENE, MD
Assistant Professor of Pediatrics, Division of Neonatal Medicine, Emory University School of Medicine, Atlanta, Georgia, USA

ABBOT LAPTOOK, MD
Department of Pediatrics, Division of Neonatology, Women and Infants Hospital of Rhode Island, Brown University, Providence, Rhode Island, USA

HENRY C. LEE, MD
Division of Neonatal and Developmental Medicine, Department of Pediatrics, Stanford School of Medicine, California Perinatal Quality Care Collaborative, Stanford, California, USA

TRACY A. MANUCK, MD, MS
Associate Professor, Department of Obstetrics and Gynecology, Division of Maternal-Fetal Medicine, University of North Carolina at Chapel Hill School of Medicine, Medical Director, UNC Prematurity Prevention Program, Chapel Hill, North Carolina, USA

BARBARA L. McFARLIN, PhD, CNM, RDMS
Professor and Head, Department of Women, Children, and Family Health Science, College of Nursing, University of Illinois at Chicago, Chicago, Illinois, USA

GIRIJA NATARAJAN, MD
Department of Pediatrics, Division of Neonatology, Wayne State University, Children's Hospital of Michigan, Hutzel Women's Hospital, Detroit, Michigan, USA

CHRISTOPHER M. NOVAK, MD
Maternal-Fetal Medicine Fellow, Department of Gynecology and Obstetrics, Division of Maternal-Fetal Medicine, Johns Hopkins University School of Medicine, Baltimore, Maryland, USA

MAIDE OZEN, MD
Assistant Professor (Part-time), Department of Pediatrics, Division of Neonatal-Perinatal Medicine, Integrated Research Center for Fetal Medicine, Johns Hopkins University School of Medicine, Baltimore, Maryland, USA

VIDYA V. PAI, MD
Division of Neonatal and Developmental Medicine, Department of Pediatrics, Stanford School of Medicine, Stanford, California, USA

MITALI ATUL PAKVASA, MD
Assistant Professor, Department of Pediatrics, Division of Neonatal-Perinatal Medicine, Emory University School of Medicine, Children's Healthcare of Atlanta, Atlanta, Georgia, USA

RAVI MANGAL PATEL, MD, MSc
Associate Professor, Department of Pediatrics, Division of Neonatal-Perinatal Medicine, Emory University School of Medicine, Children's Healthcare of Atlanta, Atlanta, Georgia, USA

RICHARD A. POLIN, MD
William T. Speck Professor and Vice Chair for Academic and Clinical Affairs, Department of Pediatrics, Director, Division of Neonatology, Columbia University College of Physicians and Surgeons, NewYork-Presbyterian Morgan Stanley Children's Hospital, New York, New York, USA

JOCHEN PROFIT, MD, MPH
Division of Neonatal and Developmental Medicine, Department of Pediatrics, Stanford School of Medicine, California Perinatal Quality Care Collaborative, Stanford, California, USA

MATTHEW A. RYSAVY, MD, PhD
Resident Physician, Department of Pediatrics, University of Iowa Stead Family Children's Hospital, Iowa City, Iowa, USA

RAKESH SAHNI, MD
Professor, Department of Pediatrics, Medical Director, NICU, Columbia University College of Physicians and Surgeons, NewYork-Presbyterian Morgan Stanley Children's Hospital, Columbia University Medical Center, New York, New York, USA

VIVEK SAROHA, MD, PhD
Fellow, Department of Pediatrics, Division of Neonatal-Perinatal Medicine, Emory University School of Medicine, Children's Healthcare of Atlanta, Atlanta, Georgia, USA

ELIZABETH K. SEWELL, MD, MPH
Assistant Professor of Pediatrics, Division of Neonatal Medicine, Emory University School of Medicine, Atlanta, Georgia, USA

SEETHA SHANKARAN, MD
Department of Pediatrics, Division of Neonatology, Wayne State University, Children's Hospital of Michigan, Hutzel Women's Hospital, Detroit, Michigan, USA

LAURIE G. SHERLOCK, MD
Fellow, Neonatal Perinatal Medicine, Section of Neonatology, Department of Pediatrics, University of Colorado School of Medicine, Children's Hospital Colorado, Perinatal Research Center, Aurora, Colorado, USA

CHRISTOPHER J. STEWART, PhD
Alkek Center for Metagenomics and Microbiome Research, Baylor College of Medicine, Houston, Texas, USA

JIM G. THORNTON, MD, FRCOG
Professor of Obstetrics and Gynaecology, Division of Child Health, Obstetrics and Gynaecology, Maternity Department, School of Medicine, University of Nottingham, Nottingham City Hospital, Nottingham University Hospitals NHS Trust, Nottingham, United Kingdom

GREGORY VALENTINE, MD
Department of Pediatrics, Baylor College of Medicine, Division of Neonatology, Texas Children's Hospital, Houston, Texas, USA

KATE F. WALKER, PhD, MRCOG
Clinical Assistant Professor of Obstetrics and Gynaecology, Division of Child Health, Obstetrics and Gynaecology, Maternity Department, School of Medicine, University of Nottingham, Nottingham City Hospital, Nottingham University Hospitals NHS Trust, Nottingham, United Kingdom

AMBER M. WOOD, MD
Fellow, Division of Maternal Fetal Medicine, Department of Obstetrics and Gynecology, Duke University Medical Center, Durham, North Carolina, USA

CLYDE J. WRIGHT, MD
Associate Professor, Section of Neonatology, Department of Pediatrics, University of Colorado School of Medicine, Children's Hospital Colorado, Perinatal Research Center, Aurora, Colorado, USA

MYRA H. WYCKOFF, MD
Professor, Department of Pediatrics, Division of Neonatal-Perinatal Medicine, University of Texas Southwestern Medical Center, Dallas, Texas, USA

LEILAH ZAHEDI-SPUNG, MD
Department of Gynecology and Obstetrics, Emory University, Atlanta, Georgia, USA

Contents

Billions of dollars are spent yearly in perinatal medicine on studies designed to improve outcomes for mothers and their neonates. However, implementing research findings is challenging and imperfect. Strategies for implementation must be multifaceted and comprehensive. These implementation challenges extend to, and are often greater in, translational and basic science research. This article discusses current challenges in the provision of quality perinatal and neonatal medical care, particularly those related to preterm birth, and provides examples of prematurity-related perinatal quality collaborative initiatives. Finally, the authors review considerations in implementing both clinical and translational/basic science prematurity research.

Regional and statewide quality improvement collaboratives have been instrumental in implementing evidence-based practices and facilitating quality improvement initiatives within neonatology. Statewide collaboratives emerged from larger collaborative organizations, such as the Vermont Oxford Network, and play an increasing role in collecting and interpreting data, setting priorities for improvement, disseminating evidence-based clinical practice guidelines, and creating regional networks for synergistic learning. In this article, the authors highlight examples of successful statewide collaborative initiatives, as well as challenges that exist in initiating and sustaining collaborative efforts.

Antenatal corticosteroids remain one of the crucial interventions in those at risk for imminent preterm birth. Therapeutic benefits include reducing major complications of prematurity, such as respiratory distress syndrome, intraventricular hemorrhage, and necrotizing enterocolitis, as well as an overall decrease in neonatal deaths. Optimal reductions in neonatal morbidity and mortality require a thoughtful review of the timing of administration. In addition, a thorough understanding is required of which patients maximally benefit from this intervention in the management and counseling of those at risk for preterm birth.

There is growing evidence from randomized trials that induction of labor at or near term does not increase cesarean delivery; observational data show that the optimal gestation for spontaneous delivery for the baby is 39 weeks. Elective cesarean at these gestations is also sometimes considered, but evaluating the associated risks is complex. For the baby, although cesarean obviates the risks of labor, it carries a risk of respiratory problems, which may be severe. For the mother, cesarean is more dangerous than vaginal and emergency cesarean is more dangerous than elective. The authors consider the evidence base for near-term induction of labor and cesarean for a range of scenarios.

Prenatal diagnosis has changed perinatal medicine dramatically, allowing for additional fetal monitoring, referral and counseling, delivery planning, the option of fetal intervention, and targeted postnatal management. Teams participating in the delivery room care of infants with known anomalies should be not only knowledgeable about specific needs and expectations but also ready for unexpected complications. A small number of neonates need rapid access to postnatal interventions, such as surgery, but most can be stabilized with appropriate neonatal care. These targeted perinatal interventions have been shown to improve outcome in selected diagnoses.

This article elaborates on how neonatologists and perinatologists might conceive of prognosis as an intervention with outcomes relevant to patients, families, and society at large and highlights aspects of this important area of practice requiring further study.

Neonatal hypoxic-ischemic encephalopathy remains associated with considerable death and disability. In multiple randomized controlled trials, therapeutic hypothermia for neonatal moderate or severe hypoxic-ischemic encephalopathy among term infants has been shown to be safe and effective in reducing death and disability in survivors. In this article, the current status of infant and childhood outcomes following this therapy is reviewed. The clinical approaches that may help to optimize this innovative neuroprotective therapy are presented.

Routine use of continuous positive airway pressure (CPAP) to support preterm infants with respiratory distress is an evidenced-based strategy to decrease the incidence of bronchopulmonary dysplasia. However, rates of CPAP failure remain unacceptably high in very premature neonates, who are at high risk for developing bronchopulmonary dysplasia. Using the GRADE framework to assess the quality of available evidence, this article reviews strategies aimed at decreasing CPAP failure, starting with delivery room interventions and followed through to system-based efforts in the neonatal intensive care unit. Despite best efforts, some very premature neonates fail CPAP. Also reviewed are predictors of CPAP failure in this vulnerable population.

Caffeine reduces the risk of bronchopulmonary dysplasia (BPD). Optimizing caffeine use could increase therapeutic benefit. The authors performed a systematic review and random-effects meta-analysis of studies comparing different timing of initiation and dose of caffeine on the risk of BPD. Earlier initiation, compared with later, was associated with a decreased risk of BPD (5 observational studies; n = 63,049; adjusted OR, 0.69; 95% CI, 0.64–0.75; GRADE, low quality). High-dose caffeine, compared with standard dose, was associated with a decreased risk of BPD (3 randomized trials; n = 432; OR, 0.65; 95% CI, 0.43–0.97; GRADE, low quality). Higher-quality evidence is needed to guide optimal caffeine use.

Oxygen is the most common medicine used during neonatal resuscitation in the delivery room. Oxygen therapy in the delivery room should be used judiciously to avoid oxygen toxicity while delivering sufficient oxygen to prevent hypoxia. Measurement of appropriate oxygenation relies on pulse oximetry, but adequate ventilation and perfusion are equally important for oxygen delivery. In this article, the authors review oxygenation while transitioning from fetal to neonatal life, the importance of appropriate oxygen therapy, its measurement in the delivery room, and current recommendations for oxygen therapy and its limitations.

Congenital cytomegalovirus is the most common viral congenital infection and affects up to 2% of neonates. Significant sequelae may develop after congenital cytomegalovirus, including hearing loss, cognitive defects, seizures, and death. Zika virus is an emerging virus with perinatal implications; a congenital Zika virus syndrome has been identified and includes findings such as microcephaly, fetal nervous system abnormalities, and neurologic sequelae after birth. Screening, diagnosis, prevention, and treatment of these perinatal infections are reviewed in this article.

The World Health Organization's Millennium Development Goal 6 includes eliminating human immunodeficiency virus (HIV) in children as a top priority. Many states in the United States report maternal-to-child transmission rates less than 1% using the current recommendations for the management of HIV-infected pregnant women. This article summarizes the most current management guidelines in caring for HIV-infected women and their infants to prevent maternal-to-child transmission.

The human microbiome acquires its vastness and diversity over a relatively short time period during development. Much is unknown, however, about the precise prenatal versus postnatal timing or its sources and determinants. Given early evidence of a role for influences during pregnancy and early neonatal and infant life on the microbiome and subsequent metabolic health, research investigating the development and shaping of the microbiome in the fetus and neonate is an important arena for study. This article reviews the relevant available literature and future questions on what shapes the microbiome during early development and mechanisms for doing so.

Perinatal brain injury may lead to long-term morbidity and neurodevelopmental impairment. Improvements in perinatal care have resulted in the survival of more infants with perinatal brain injury. The effects of hypoxia-ischemia, inflammation, and infection during critical periods of development can lead to a common pathway of perinatal brain injury marked by neuronal excitotoxicity, cellular apoptosis, and microglial activation. Various interventions can prevent or improve the outcomes of different types of perinatal brain injury. This article reviews the mechanisms of perinatal brain injury, approaches to prevention, and outcomes among children with perinatal brain injury.

PROGRAM OBJECTIVE

The goal of *Clinics in Perinatology* is to keep practicing perinatologists, neonatologists, obstetricians, practicing physicians and residents up to date with current clinical practice in perinatology by providing timely articles reviewing the state of the art in patient care.

TARGET AUDIENCE

Perinatologists, neonatologists, obstetricians, practicing physicians, residents and healthcare professionals who provide patient care utilizing findings from *Clinics in Perinatology.*

LEARNING OBJECTIVES

Upon completion of this activity, participants will be able to:
1. Review perinatal care of infants with congenital birth defects
2. Discuss quality improvement strategies and interventions in perinatal medicine.
3. Recognize current prevention strategies for maternal-to-child transmission of HIV and perinatal infections.

ACCREDITATION

The Elsevier Office of Continuing Medical Education (EOCME) is accredited by the Accreditation Council for Continuing Medical Education (ACCME) to provide continuing medical education for physicians.

The EOCME designates this enduring material for a maximum of 15 *AMA PRA Category 1 Credit*(s)™. Physicians should claim only the credit commensurate with the extent of their participation in the activity.

All other health care professionals requesting continuing education credit for this enduring material will be issued a certificate of participation.

DISCLOSURE OF CONFLICTS OF INTEREST

The EOCME assesses conflict of interest with its instructors, faculty, planners, and other individuals who are in a position to control the content of CME activities. All relevant conflicts of interest that are identified are thoroughly vetted by EOCME for fair balance, scientific objectivity, and patient care recommendations. EOCME is committed to providing its learners with CME activities that promote improvements or quality in healthcare and not a specific proprietary business or a commercial interest.

The planning committee, staff, authors and editors listed below have identified no financial relationships or relationships to products or devices they or their spouse/life partner have with commercial interest related to the content of this CME activity:

Kjersti M. Aagaard, MD, PhD, FACOG; Martina L. Badell, MD; Whitney A. Booker, MD; Irina Burd, MD, PhD; Derrick M. Chu, BSc; Rebecca C. Fry, PhD, MS; Cynthia Gyamfi-Bannerman, MD, MSc; Kerry Holland; Brenna L. Hughes, MD; Lucky Jain, MD, MBA; Vishal Kapadia, MD, MSCS; Sarah Keene, MD; Alison Kemp; Abbot Laptook, MD; Henry C. Lee, MD; Tracy A. Manuck, MD, MS; Barbara L. McFarlin, PhD, CNM, RDMS; Girija Natarajan, MD; Christopher M. Novak, MD; Maide Ozen, MD; Vidya V. Pai, MD; Mitali Atul Pakvasa, MD; Ravi Mangal Patel, MD, MSc; Richard A. Polin, MD; Jochen Profit, MD, MPH; Matthew A. Rysavy, MD, PhD; Rakesh Sahni, MD; Vivek Saroha, MD, PhD; Elizabeth K. Sewell, MD, MPH; Seetha Shankaran, MD; Laurie G. Sherlock, MD; Christopher J. Stewart, PhD; Jim G. Thornton, MD, FRCOG; Subhalakshmi Vaidyanathan; Gregory Valentine, MD; Kate F. Walker, PhD, MRCOG; Amber M. Wood, MD; Clyde J. Wright, MD; Myra H. Wyckoff, MD; Leilah Zahedi-Spung, MD.

UNAPPROVED/OFF-LABEL USE DISCLOSURE

The EOCME requires CME faculty to disclose to the participants:
1. When products or procedures being discussed are off-label, unlabelled, experimental, and/or investigational (not US Food and Drug Administration [FDA] approved); and
2. Any limitations on the information presented, such as data that are preliminary or that represent ongoing research, interim analyses, and/or unsupported opinions. Faculty may discuss information about pharmaceutical agents that is outside of FDA-approved labelling. This information is intended solely for CME and is not intended to promote off-label use of these medications. If you have any questions, contact the medical affairs department of the manufacturer for the most recent prescribing information.

TO ENROLL

To enroll in the *Clinics in Perinatology* Continuing Medical Education program, call customer service at 1-800-654-2452 or sign up online at http://www.theclinics.com/home/cme. The CME program is available to subscribers for an additional annual fee of 244.40 USD.

METHOD OF PARTICIPATION

In order to claim credit, participants must complete the following:

1. Complete enrolment as indicated above.
2. Read the activity.
3. Complete the CME Test and Evaluation. Participants must achieve a score of 70% on the test. All CME Tests and Evaluations must be completed online.

CME INQUIRIES/SPECIAL NEEDS

For all CME inquiries or special needs, please contact elsevierCME@elsevier.com.

CLINICS IN PERINATOLOGY

Foreword

Unfinished Business: Prematurity, Birth Asphyxia, and Stillbirths

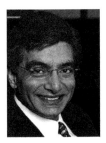

Lucky Jain, MD, MBA
Consulting Editor

Obstetricians and neonatologists everywhere ought to be proud of the tremendous progress we have collectively made in making childbirth safer. No matter where the starting point was twenty or thirty years ago, or the availability of resources, perinatal mortality has declined significantly. Better management of pregnancy and delivery has played a big role in achieving these targets, just as advances in neonatal care have. In particular, much credit goes to early recognition and management of high-risk pregnancies since undiagnosed maternal or fetal jeopardy carries exceedingly high morbidity and mortality.

No good deed goes unpunished, however. As perinatal interventions to salvage at-risk pregnancies grew, a new set of problems arose. Medically indicated preterm and early term births, inductions, and cesarean sections rose dramatically, and all had their own set of unanticipated side effects. Many of these interventions were based on empirical evidence alone. A natural tug of war ensued between medically indicated early births and ill effects of loss of term gestation. One approach to reconcile this dilemma is to use the "fetus-at-risk" approach advanced by Joseph and colleagues[1,2] (**Fig. 1**). Such a model better addresses the coherence in pregnancy complications and perinatal interventions used to address them.

Perinatal interventions, neonatal morbidity and mortality, and the "fetus-at-risk" approach also allow us to focus more closely on the unacceptably high global

Clin Perinatol 45 (2018) xv–xviii
https://doi.org/10.1016/j.clp.2018.03.001
0095-5108/18/© 2018 Published by Elsevier Inc.

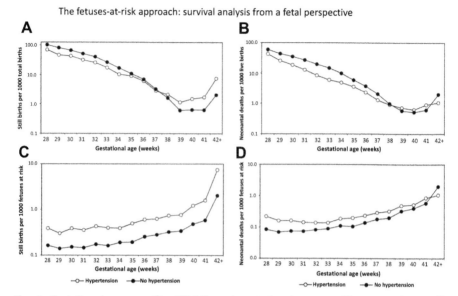

The fetuses-at-risk approach: survival analysis from a fetal perspective

Fig. 1. Gestational age-specific stillbirth and gestational age-specific neonatal mortality rates among women with and without hypertensive disorders of pregnancy with rates calculated using the traditional perinatal formulation (per 1000 total births; [A] and [B], respectively) and rates calculated using the fetuses-at-risk approach (per 1000 fetuses at risk; [C] and [D], respectively), USA, 2011 to 2013. (*Adapted from* Joseph KS, Kramer MS. The fetuses-at-risk approach: survival analysis from a fetal perspective. Acta Obstet Gynecol Scand 2018;97(4):457; with permission.)

stillbirth rate. Estimated at 18.4 per 1000 births for ≥28 weeks' gestation, this tragedy strikes 2.6 million fetuses each year.[3] Global health organizations have an ambitious agenda of reducing this rate to 12 per 1000 births over the next decade. A quick glance at the causes of stillbirths helps explain why progress has been slow (**Fig. 2**).[3] Add to this the global burden of birth asphyxia and perinatal infections; meaningful improvements that stick will require a coordinated public health approach that brings to bear all of the resources at our disposal, but most of all, political will to get rid of this blight.

This issue of the *Clinics in Perinatology* addresses many of the interventions that can help us move in the right direction. Drs Patel and Manuck are to be congratulated for putting together a comprehensive set of articles written by experts in the field. As always, I am grateful to the authors for their valuable contributions and to my publishing partners at Elsevier (Kerry Holland and Casey Potter) for their help in bringing this amazing resource to you.

Lucky Jain, MD, MBA
Department of Pediatrics
Emory University School of Medicine
Children's Healthcare of Atlanta
1760 Haygood Drive
Atlanta, GA 30322, USA

E-mail address:
ljain@emory.edu

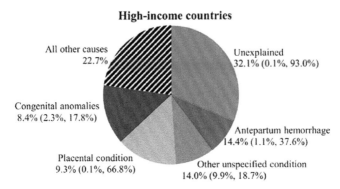

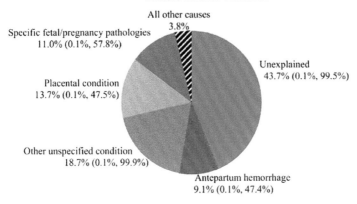

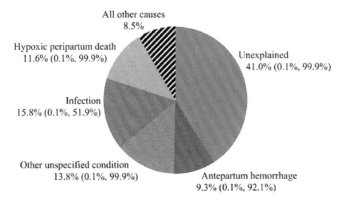

Fig. 2. Making stillbirths visible: a systematic review of globally reported causes of still-birth. (*Adapted with* Reinebrant HE, Leisher SH, Coory M, et al. Making stillbirths visible: a systematic review of globally reported causes of stillbirth. BJOG 2017;125:218; with permission).

REFERENCES

1. Joseph KS. Theory of obstetrics: an epidemiologic framework for justifying medically indicated early delivery. BMC Pregnancy Childbirth 2007;7(4):1–15.

2. Joseph KS, Kramer MS. The fetuses-at-risk approach: survival analysis from a fetal perspective. Acta Obstet Gynecol Scand 2018;97(4):454–65.
3. Reinebrant HE, Leisher SH, Coory M, et al. Making stillbirths visible: a systematic review of globally reported causes of stillbirth. BJOG 2018;125:212–24.

Preface

Collaboratively Understanding and Improving Outcomes for the Mother, Fetus, and Infant

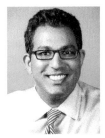 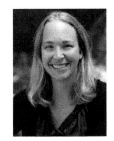

Ravi Mangal Patel, MD, MSc   Tracy A. Manuck, MD, MS
Editors

Birth is an incredibly exciting and yet potentially dangerous period for a woman and her fetus, who attempts to navigate the complex transition to neonatal life. Many events during this period establish or disrupt long-lasting health for both the mother and her infant. The challenges during this period are too numerous to quantify, but yield opportunities for prevention and treatment strategies to improve perinatal care and neonatal outcomes. In this issue of *Clinics of Perinatology*, we highlight these opportunities by including articles that span across obstetrics and neonatology. We believe coordinated efforts across the spectrum of care are essential to yield the best possible outcomes. Toward that goal, Tracy A. Manuck and colleagues' article, "Quality Improvement in Perinatal Medicine and Translation of Preterm Birth Research Findings into Clinical Care," and Vidya V. Pai and colleagues' article, "Improving Uptake of Key Perinatal Interventions Using Statewide Quality Collaboratives," provide a context for improving perinatal care, with a focus on quality improvement and coordinated efforts by statewide collaboratives that have had marked success in improving perinatal care.[1] Several topics provide the latest guidance and considerations on the "personalization" of common perinatal interventions, including the use of antenatal corticosteroids (See Whitney A. Booker and Cynthia Gyamfi-Bannerman's article, "Antenatal Corticosteroids: Who Should We Be Treating?"), methods of delivery (See Kate F. Walker and Jim G. Thornton's article, "Delivery at Term: When, How, and Why"), care of infants with specific birth defects (See Elizabeth K. Sewell and Sarah Keene's article, "Perinatal Care of Infants with Congenital Birth Defects"), and counseling at periviable gestational ages (See Matthew A. Rysavy's article, "Prognosis as an Intervention"). We also discuss optimization of commonly used or highly effective neonatal therapies started in the early postnatal period, including therapeutic

Clin Perinatol 45 (2018) xix–xx
https://doi.org/10.1016/j.clp.2018.01.016
0095-5108/18/© 2018 Published by Elsevier Inc.

hypothermia (See Girija Natarjan and colleagues' article, "Therapeutic Hypothermia: How Can We Optimize This Therapy to Further Improve Outcomes"), continuous positive airway pressure (See Clyde J. Wright and colleagues' article, "Continuous Positive Airway Pressure Failure: Evidence-Based and Physiologically Sound Practices from Delivery Room to the Neonatal Intensive Care Unit"), caffeine therapy (See Mitali Atul Pakvasa and colleagues' article, "Optimizing Caffeine Use and Risk of Bronchopulmonary Dysplasia in Preterm Infants: A Systematic Review, Meta-analysis and Application of Grading of Recommendations Assessment, Development, and Evaluation Methodology"), and oxygen administration (See Vishal Kapadia and Myra H. Wyckoff's article, "Oxygen Therapy in the Delivery Room: What Is the Right Dose?"). Our series also touches on perinatal infections, including new threats by Zika virus (See Amber M. Wood and Brenna L. Hughes' article, "Detection and Prevention of Perinatal Infection: Cytomegalovirus and ZIKA Virus") and established threats by HIV (See Leilah Zahedi-Spung and Martina L. Badell's article, "Current Strategies to Prevent Maternal-to-Child Transmission of Human Immunodeficiency Virus"). The perinatal period also sets in motion critical events shaping an infant's gut and brain health, and two articles review the latest on the maternal-infant microbiome (See Gregory Valentine and colleagues' article, "Relationship Between Perinatal Interventions, Maternal-Infant Microbiome and Neonatal Outcomes") and perinatal brain injury (See Christopher M. Novak and colleagues' article, "Perinatal Brain Injury: Mechanisms, Prevention and Outcomes").

We hope the readers of *Clinics in Perinatology* find these topics timely and of interest. We would like to thank and acknowledge the contributions of pediatricians, neonatologists, obstetricians, and maternal-fetal medicine specialists who have provided their expertise to guide perinatal interventions to improve neonatal outcomes.

Ravi Mangal Patel, MD, MSc
Division of Neonatology
Emory University School of Medicine and
Children's Healthcare of Atlanta
2015 Uppergate Drive Northeast, 3rd Floor
Atlanta, GA 30322, USA

Tracy A. Manuck, MD, MS
University of North Carolina-Chapel Hill
Division of Maternal Fetal Medicine
UNC Prematurity Prevention Program
3010 Old Clinic Building CB#7516
Chapel Hill, NC 27599-7516, USA

E-mail addresses:
rmpatel@emory.edu (R.M. Patel)
tmanuck@med.unc.edu (T.A. Manuck)

REFERENCE

1. Wirtschafter DD, Danielsen BH, Main EK, et al, California Perinatal Quality Care Collaborative. Promoting antenatal steroid use for fetal maturation: results from the California Perinatal Quality Care Collaborative. J Pediatr 2006;148(5):606–12.

Quality Improvement in Perinatal Medicine and Translation of Preterm Birth Research Findings into Clinical Care

Tracy A. Manuck, MD, MS[a],*, Rebecca C. Fry, PhD, MS[b],
Barbara L. McFarlin, PhD, CNM, RDMS[c]

KEYWORDS

- Spontaneous preterm birth • Translational research implementation
- Perinatal quality collaboratives

KEY POINTS

- Implementation of clinical and translational research studies into clinical practice is challenging and imperfect.
- The process of implementation occurs over years to decades but may be facilitated by multicenter networks and perinatal quality collaboratives.
- Strategies for implementation of prematurity research must be multifaceted and comprehensive.

INTRODUCTION

Billions of dollars of research money are spent each year within the fields of obstetrics and neonatology focusing on prevention or management strategies designed to improve outcomes for mothers and their neonates. However, the process of

Disclosure Statement: The authors report no conflict of interest.
Financial Support: Funded by NIH/NIMHD, R01-MD011609 (Dr T.A. Manuck) and NIH/NICHD, R01-HD089935 (Dr B.L. McFarlin).
[a] Division of Maternal-Fetal Medicine, Department of Obstetrics and Gynecology, University of North Carolina School of Medicine, 3010 Old Clinic Building, CB#7516, Chapel Hill, NC 27599-7516, USA; [b] Department of Environmental Sciences and Engineering, Gillings School of Global Public Health, University of North Carolina School, 140 Rosenau Hall, CB #7431, Chapel Hill, NC 27599, USA; [c] Department of Women, Children, and Family Health Science, College of Nursing, University of Illinois-Chicago, 845 S. Damen Avenue, Chicago, IL 60612, USA
* Corresponding author.
E-mail address: tmanuck@med.unc.edu

implementing research findings is challenging and imperfect. Appropriate and timely implementation may improve both maternal and neonatal morbidity and mortality. Conversely, premature adoption of studies without adequate scientific backing may produce inadvertent harm. For example, a trial demonstrating that intrapartum exposure to a medication reduces the risk of neonatal intraventricular hemorrhage is the first step necessary to change clinical practice. The actual real-world implementation of that medication is challenging and requires multiple steps, including necessary provider education, consideration of the logistics of making the medication available, and development of appropriate methods for ensuring appropriate use. Strategies for implementation must be multifaceted and consider the audience; for example, a comprehensive program would provide patient education, clinician guidelines, and national policymaker messages. These implementation challenges extend to, and are often greater in, "translational" and basic science research. This review discusses current challenges related to the provision of quality care in perinatal and neonatal medicine, particularly as they relate to preterm birth. Furthermore, the authors provide examples of perinatal quality collaborative initiatives within the field of prematurity. Finally, the authors review considerations in implementing both clinical and translational/basic science research within the field of prematurity.

PROVISION OF QUALITY MEDICAL CARE

Over the past 2 decades, significant emphasis has been placed on not only the provision of medical care but also the provision of "quality" medical care. This work was spurred by the Institute of Medicine's influential report, published in 2001, entitled "Crossing the Quality Chasm."[1] Initiatives in specific areas of health care, reaching across different fields of medicine, have caught the attention of policymakers, health care leaders, and payers. Increasingly, health care systems have realized the importance of integrated quality improvement approaches, in-person learning solutions, and ongoing support following these initial improvement efforts. In order to appropriately discuss and evaluate the use of quality improvement initiatives and preterm birth research, it is essential to understand the critical components of quality improvement collaboratives. Quality improvement initiatives should identify a target for improvement, the study sample (which may involve several different organizations, hospitals, or providers within a hospital system), and measurable outcomes. Typically, these outcomes are patient, provider, and health care system specific. Initiatives may include "bundles," which are often aimed at providing a specific set of algorithms or checklists for practicing providers, to ensure that national society guidelines and recommendations are followed. Theoretically, quality improvement collaboratives allow for change at multiple levels within the structure of an organization or across organizations.[2]

In February 2016, the Society for Maternal-Fetal Medicine, National Institute of Child Health and Human Development, and American College of Obstetricians and Gynecologists convened a "Quality Measures in High-Risk Pregnancies Workshop" to review topics specifically related to quality medical care in obstetrics.[3] Preterm birth was identified as a major topic at the workshop, and several measures were proposed by the workshop participants as quality measures (**Table 1**).[3]

Preterm birth has been a focus of multiple local- and state-level quality collaborative initiatives across the United States. Preterm birth has modifiable risk factors, and the risk of prematurity may be reduced with adequate interconception care, routine

Table 1
Quality measures in preterm birth

Quality Measure	Role in Prevention	Role in Treatment
Transvaginal ultrasound cervical length screening	Identification of women with short cervix provides opportunity for treatment	Presence of long cervix is helpful in determining who is not at risk for preterm birth among women with symptoms of preterm labor
Vaginal progesterone for cervical shortening	Studies suggest treatment is associated with reduction in preterm birth and is supported by ACOG and SMFM	No current evidence to support vaginal progesterone use for treatment of acute preterm labor
Intramuscular 17P for women with a history of spontaneous preterm birth	History of spontaneous preterm birth is a significant risk factor for recurrence; prophylaxis with 17P is associated with reduced risk of recurrence and is supported by ACOG and SMFM	No current evidence to support treatment with 17P for treatment of acute spontaneous preterm labor
Cerclage for women with a prior spontaneous preterm birth and cervical shortening	Ultrasound-indicated cerclage in women with a prior spontaneous preterm birth reduces risk of recurrent preterm birth	Cerclage is not indicated as a treatment of acute preterm labor
Antenatal corticosteroids	Use of antenatal corticosteroids is associated with reduced neonatal morbidity and mortality. Use is recommended by ACOG and SMFM	Not applicable
Magnesium sulfate for neuroprotection	Meta-analyses demonstrate decreased moderate-severe cerebral palsy or death; current use for women at risk of imminent preterm birth between 24 and 32 wk gestation is standard of care per ACOG and SMFM	Not applicable
Antenatal use of low-dose aspirin	Evidence suggests reduction in adverse outcomes and reduction in risk of preeclampsia in high-risk women	Not applicable

Abbreviations: ACOG, American College of Obstetricians and Gynecologists; SMFM, Society for Maternal-Fetal Medicine.

prenatal care, and specialty prenatal care as appropriate. Delivery gestational age is an objective measure that is easy to track and generally not subject to bias. Therefore, many studies and initiatives focusing on perinatal quality include preterm birth as a key outcome measure. For example, several maternal safety bundles that are the focus of the Council for Patient Safety in Women's Healthcare's Alliance for Innovation on Maternal Health have medically indicated preterm birth as key outcomes (http://safehealthcareforeverywoman.org/aim-program/). The following provide examples of long-standing population-based approaches to preterm birth provider education, consistent medical care, and risk reduction.

The Ohio Perinatal Quality Collaborative

The Ohio Perinatal Quality Collaborative is an established statewide quality improvement project initially formed in response to a request from the Ohio Department of Medicaid in the Ohio Department of Health. It was designed broadly to improve perinatal health outcomes. Several key initiatives and studies have been produced from this collaborative. In 2011, Kaplan and colleagues[4] used the Institute for Healthcare Improvement Breakthrough Series quality improvement model to modify the implementation procedures regarding indwelling catheters in the neonatal intensive care unit and studied whether use of this initiative influenced the rate of late-onset sepsis among preterm infants. They reported excellent compliance with the education initiative, with greater than 90% compliance 7 months after the study began. Notably, although most infections were related to indwelling catheters during the study period (69%), there was a 20% reduction in the incidence of late-onset infection after the intervention.[4]

More recently, the Ohio Perinatal Quality Collaborative instituted a program to enact system-level changes to increase the use of 17-alpha hydroxyprogesterone (17P) caproate among women with a prior singleton spontaneous preterm birth. The program tracked 2562 women who were eligible for treatment with 17P between January 1, 2014 and November 30, 2015.[5] Reductions in preterm birth were seen in all hospitals participating in the initiative, and in individuals at highest risk, including African Americans and those receiving Medicaid. After adjusting for risk factors and birth clustering, institution of the progesterone program was associated with a reduction in the rate of preterm birth before 32 weeks' gestation of 13%.[5] Importantly, this reduction was sustained over the study period. This finding is particularly notable because preterm birth less than 32 weeks is notoriously difficult to prevent, and recent nationwide improvements in the rate of preterm birth have been seen mainly among preterm deliveries at 34 to 36 weeks, but not at earlier gestational ages.[6]

The Vermont Oxford Network

The Vermont Oxford Network is a nonprofit, voluntary collaboration of health care professionals focused on primarily postnatal prematurity care and neonatology with a long-standing attention to quality improvement collaboratives. The quality improvement collaboratives through the Vermont Oxford Network use the Network's existing data infrastructure in order to identify need, incorporate group training, set benchmarks for improvement, and assess change.

One key study conducted in 10 self-selected studies in the Vermont Oxford Network evaluated whether the formation of multidisciplinary teams improved outcomes, focusing on either chronic lung disease (n = 4 neonatal intensive care units) or infection (n = 6 neonatal intensive care units). These teams met regularly over a 3-year period, analyzed care processes, reviewed performance data, and implemented "better practices" based on the literature and the work of the team. Rates of these complications in the intervention neonatal intensive care units were compared with 66 other neonatal intensive care units that had not undergone this intervention. They found that the rate of oxygen use decreased from 43.5% to 31.5% at the neonatal intensive care units in the chronic lung disease multidisciplinary team group, and similarly, rates of coagulase-negative staphylococcus infection were reduced at the neonatal intensive care units in the infection team group from 22.0% to 16.6%.[7] A companion study evaluating whether this intervention was cost-effective found that the average savings per hospital in patient care costs for very low-birth-weight infants in the infection group was $2.3 million in the first year after intervention (1996); this is equivalent to $3.6 million in 2017.[8]

Recent work published by the Vermont Oxford Network in the area of perinatal quality has examined disparities in nursing care provided in the neonatal intensive care unit,[9] influence of quality indicators versus admission volumes on risk of neonatal mortality in preterm infants,[10] and disparities in perinatal quality outcomes among very low-birth-weight infants receiving neonatal intensive care.[11]

The Society for Maternal Fetal Medicine Prematurity Bundle

In 2016, the Society for Maternal Fetal Medicine released a "Preterm Birth Toolkit," providing a comprehensive set of protocols and algorithms for clinical use when caring for women at risk for preterm birth, women diagnosed with acute preterm labor, or those who have just had a preterm birth. The toolkit provides expert opinions in areas where evidence is less clear or literature is lacking, with the goal of striking "a balance between standardization and clinical discretion." Furthermore, specific instruments designed to assess barriers and aid in the execution of the strategies outlined in the toolkit are included. The toolkit is available online (www.smfm.org/publications/231-smfm-preterm-birth-toolkit).

WHEN IS RESEARCH READY FOR IMPLEMENTATION?

Modern clinical practice frequently cites one pivotal study as rationale for practice management. However, although a single study may at times serve as a "tipping point" by which national organizations base their decision to make specific changes in management recommendations, individual studies are rarely sufficient, in isolation, to effect large-scale changes. When an apparent "landmark" study is published, decisions regarding whether to proceed with changes to policies must also consider the strength of the preliminary data used as the justification for the study in addition to other evidence to support the particular test or intervention. In studies evaluating the evolution of health care evidence, the first published study on a scientific question may find the most dramatic effect sizes; this is true for both clinical and basic science studies.[12] Subsequent validation studies following widespread implementation may fail to reproduce initial apparently dramatic effects, because the heterogeneity of the studied population increases and more evidence is accumulated.[13]

Levels of evidence in medical research studies were first used in 1979 in a report by the Canadian Task Force on the Periodic Health Examination to "grade the effectiveness of an intervention according to the quality of evidence obtained." At that time, there were only 3 levels of evidence, which were simple: level I included evidence from at least one randomized controlled trial; level II-1 from at least one well designed cohort or case-control study and II-2 from comparisons of times and places with or without the intervention; and level III was based on expert opinion or descriptive studies.[14] The first guidelines specific to the United States were released in 1988 by the United States Preventive Task Force. The same 3 levels were used, but level II was further divided into II-3, which was evidence obtained from multiple time series designs with or without the intervention.[15] In 2013, the Society for Maternal Fetal Medicine adopted the Grading of Recommendations Assessment, Development, and Evaluation system, which provides further guidance as follows: A = high quality evidence, based on several high-quality studies with consistent results or one large, high-quality multicenter trial and further research is unlikely to change confidence in the estimate of effect; B = moderate-quality evidence, based on one high-quality study or several studies with some limitations, and further research is likely to have an important impact on the confidence in the estimate of effect and may change the estimate; C = low-quality evidence, based on one or more studies with severe limitations, and further research is very likely to have an important impact on the confidence in the estimate of effect and is likely to change the estimate; D = very low-quality evidence, based on expert opinion, no direct research evidence, or one or more studies with very severe limitations, and any estimate of effect is very uncertain.[16] The level of evidence can be used by individual clinicians as a guide to interpret the relative quality of the research. Furthermore, it can be used to help judge the appropriateness for inclusion of a study in a meta-analysis or larger review such as a *Cochrane Review*.[17]

SPECIFIC CONSIDERATIONS FOR IMPLEMENTING PREMATURITY RESEARCH

In all situations, the research population must be considered when determining the generalizability to practice and the real-world effects of a diagnostic test or therapeutic intervention. Particularly in obstetrics, significant racial and ethnic disparities are present. The rate of prematurity is nearly 2-fold higher in black infants in the United States compared with white infants.[18,19] The reasons for these disparities are poorly understood. Neither social nor genetic factors can entirely explain these differences in prematurity outcomes; it is likely that a combination of both social and genetic factors is responsible for the observed differences. Nevertheless, multiple measures of the quality of prenatal care, including the gestational age at the initiation of care and number of prenatal visits, are known to differ by maternal race and ethnicity. These factors affect the a priori risk of preterm birth in the population and may, therefore, also impact the results of any study involving black women and infants. Likewise, a study demonstrating a positive effect in a primarily white or Hispanic population may not show similar effects in a primarily black population. Multicenter studies enrolling broadly across the United States comprised women who have socioeconomic status, race and ethnicity, and previous pregnancy history representative of a general obstetric population are the most generalizable.

TRANSLATIONAL RESEARCH

The application of basic biomedical research into clinical practice is essential to move new bench knowledge beyond the laboratory and deliver it to patients. Particularly when genetic studies are considered, thousands of samples are needed to adequately estimate genetic associations and disease.[20] In all cases, an adequate sample size and power with a sufficient replication cohort are essential. Caution is needed when interpreting and implementing genetic study data in the setting of admixed populations and is particularly prudent. Several large-scale, consortium-based sequencing projects have shown that admixed populations have significant genetic diversity compared with those with traditional African ancestry. For example, the 1000 genomes project demonstrated increased linkage disequilibrium (shared chromosomal segments inherited together), and a higher frequency of rare variants in those with African compared with European ancestry.[21] Furthermore, patterns of rare and common variants are specific to each ancestry group.[21]

It is imperative that there are clear, biologically plausible mechanisms linking translational and basic science research with clinical disease. For example, although the underlying mechanisms behind preterm birth are poorly elucidated, recent research supports that epigenetic modifications (such as DNA methylation at cytosine-guanine dinucleotide sites, or CpG sites) may influence gene expression and the risk for adverse outcomes. Evaluation of site-specific CpG methylation and/or gene expression in maternal blood in early pregnancy holds significant promise in efforts to find biomarkers that can be used to screen for preterm birth. Several small studies report CpG methylation differences are associated with delivery gestational age.[22] Still other studies suggest a potential role for evaluation of CpG methylation differences in predicting neonatal infectious morbidity, because specific methylation changes in the calcitonin-related polypeptide alpha (*CALCA*) gene were implicated in the diagnosis of both early- and late-onset sepsis.[23] However, no CpG methylation tests currently have sufficient evidence to support commercial use by providers to predict preterm birth or outcomes related to prematurity.

The term "pharmacogenetics" was first coined in 1957 and was used to describe the variability in the response to a standard dose of drugs attributable to one or more single nucleotide polymorphisms. In modern times, the term pharmacogenomics is more commonly used, because this encompasses the effect of the entire genome (rather than an individual gene or genes) on drug response. Robust pharmacogenetics data from other medical fields demonstrate variable drug response in individuals by racial and ethnic subgroups, which is attributed to the underlying minor allele frequency of a particular single nucleotide polymorphism. For example, β-blocker drugs may be less effective in individuals with specific functional variants in the G protein-coupled pathway of the β-1 adrenergic receptor (*ADRB1*) and G protein receptor kinase 5 (*GRK5*) genes; these variants are more common in individuals with African ancestry.[24] It is not unreasonable to hypothesize that these variants may also influence response to β-blockers for the treatment of chronic hypertension during pregnancy, although this has not been studied. The best example of pharmacogenomics research applied to obstetric and neonatal medicine is related to the use of codeine in breastfeeding mothers. Maternal carriage of the cytochrome CYP2D6*N allele results in ultrarapid metabolism of codeine to morphine, which may produce codeine-related sedation, respiratory depression, and neonatal death. In this instance, because testing for CYP2D6 genotype is not widely available and there are suitable alternatives for after-delivery pain control, simple practice recommendations have been made to use other narcotic medications when indicated. Furthermore, placement of a "black box" warning regarding CYP2D6 use in nursing mothers resulted in significant press attention, aiding in quickly disseminating the information to prescribers and caregivers.

THE FUTURE OF IMPLEMENTATION SCIENCE AND THE PROVISION OF QUALITY CARE

Comprehensive computer science models are being developed to improve the synthesis and interpretation of evidence and then measure the uptake of this information. Global implementation science is a priority of the National Institutes of Health; several initiatives are underway in other fields, including online discussions, cyber seminars, and webinars. These initiatives include the "Research to Reality" online community of practice, designed to link cancer control practitioners and researchers to move evidence-based programs into practice. In obstetrics, initiatives to translate research "from bench to bedside" are the focus of several national conferences. For example, the planned meeting theme for the 2019 Annual Scientific Meeting for the Society for Reproductive Investigation is "From Innovation to Impact."

SUMMARY

It is estimated that it takes a minimum of 17 years or more to translate research into clinical practice.[25] Although rapid translation could bring new effective life-saving interventions into clinical practice, the inappropriate translation of research into clinical practice ultimately results in suboptimal care at the level of the individual patient, whether from failure to incorporate knowledge of diagnostics or therapeutics with adequate knowledge or from exposure to unnecessary iatrogenic harms. Every effort should be made by researchers and stakeholders to facilitate dissemination of research knowledge to expedite implementation, while monitoring "real-world" outcomes.

REFERENCES

1. Schiff GD, Young QD. You can't leap a chasm in two jumps: the Institute of Medicine health care quality report. Public Health Rep 2001;116:396–403.
2. Plsek PE. Collaborating across organizational boundaries to improve the quality of care. Am J Infect Control 1997;25:85–95.
3. Iriye BK, Gregory KD, Saade GR, et al. Quality measures in high-risk pregnancies: executive summary of a cooperative workshop of the Society for Maternal-Fetal Medicine, National Institute of Child Health and Human Development, and the American College of Obstetricians and Gynecologists. Am J Obstet Gynecol 2017;217:B2–25.
4. Kaplan HC, Lannon C, Walsh MC, et al, Ohio Perinatal Quality Collaborative. Ohio statewide quality-improvement collaborative to reduce late-onset sepsis in preterm infants. Pediatrics 2011;127:427–35.
5. Iams JD, Applegate MS, Marcotte MP, et al. A statewide progestogen promotion program in Ohio. Obstet Gynecol 2017;129:337–46.
6. Martin JA, Hamilton BE, Osterman MJ, et al. Births: final data for 2015. Natl Vital Stat Rep 2017;66:1.
7. Horbar JD, Rogowski J, Plsek PE, et al. Collaborative quality improvement for neonatal intensive care. NIC/Q project investigators of the Vermont Oxford Network. Pediatrics 2001;107:14–22.
8. Rogowski JA, Horbar JD, Plsek PE, et al. Economic implications of neonatal intensive care unit collaborative quality improvement. Pediatrics 2001;107:23–9.
9. Lake ET, Staiger D, Edwards EM, et al. Nursing care disparities in neonatal intensive care units. Health Serv Res 2017. [Epub ahead of print].
10. Rochow N, Landau-Crangle E, Lee S, et al. Quality indicators but not admission volumes of neonatal intensive care units are effective in reducing mortality rates of preterm infants. PLoS One 2016;11:e0161030.
11. Lake ET, Staiger D, Horbar J, et al. Disparities in perinatal quality outcomes for very low birth weight infants in neonatal intensive care. Health Serv Res 2015; 50:374–97.
12. Ioannidis JP. Evolution and translation of research findings: from bench to where? PLoS Clin Trials 2006;1:e36.
13. Ioannidis JP. Contradicted and initially stronger effects in highly cited clinical research. JAMA 2005;294:218–28.
14. The periodic health examination: 2. 1987 update. Canadian Task Force on the periodic health examination. CMAJ 1988;138:618–26.
15. Pels RJ, Bor DH, Lawrence RS. Decision making for introducing clinical preventive services. Annu Rev Public Health 1989;10:363–83.
16. Society for Maternal-Fetal Medicine (SMFM), Chauhan SP, Blackwell SC. SMFM adopts GRADE (grading of recommendations assessment, development, and evaluation) for clinical guidelines. Am J Obstet Gynecol 2013;209:163–5.
17. GRADE approach to evaluating the quality of evidence: a pathway. 2017. Available at: http://training.cochrane.org/path/grade-approach-evaluating-quality-evidence-pathway. Accessed December 11, 2017.

18. Hamilton BE, Martin JA, Osterman MJ, et al. Births: final data for 2014. Natl Vital Stat Rep 2015;64:1–64.

19. DeFranco EA, Hall ES, Muglia LJ. Racial disparity in previable birth. Am J Obstet Gynecol 2016;214:394.e1-7.

20. Ioannidis JP, Ntzani EE, Trikalinos TA, et al. Replication validity of genetic association studies. Nat Genet 2001;29:306–9.

21. Genomes Project C, Abecasis GR, Auton A, et al. An integrated map of genetic variation from 1,092 human genomes. Nature 2012;491:56–65.

22. Burris HH, Rifas-Shiman SL, Baccarelli A, et al. Associations of LINE-1 DNA methylation with preterm birth in a prospective cohort study. J Dev Orig Health Dis 2012;3:173–81.

23. Tendl KA, Schulz SM, Mechtler TP, et al. DNA methylation pattern of CALCA in preterm neonates with bacterial sepsis as a putative epigenetic biomarker. Epigenetics 2013;8:1261–7.

24. Liggett SB, Cresci S, Kelly RJ, et al. A GRK5 polymorphism that inhibits beta-adrenergic receptor signaling is protective in heart failure. Nat Med 2008;14: 510–7.

25. Morris ZS, Wooding S, Grant J. The answer is 17 years, what is the question: understanding time lags in translational research. J R Soc Med 2011;104:510–20.

Improving Uptake of Key Perinatal Interventions Using Statewide Quality Collaboratives

Vidya V. Pai, MD[a], Henry C. Lee, MD[a,b,*], Jochen Profit, MD, MPH[a,b]

KEYWORDS

- Quality improvement • Evidence-based practice • Statewide quality collaboratives
- Neonatal medicine

KEY POINTS

- Statewide collaboratives foster a community that can facilitate strategies for adoption of evidence-based practices.
- Statewide collaboratives use a variety of strategies to facilitate both multicenter and individual hospital-level quality improvement initiatives.
- Further development of state collaboratives may help to address the gaps and challenges to efficient and effective dissemination and implementation of evidence-based practices.

INTRODUCTION

For two decades, the application of quality improvement methods to spread evidence-based practices and reduce variation in health care delivery has been a health policy priority.[1,2] This measure has been motivated primarily by the desire to provide quality and high-value health care and improve outcomes for the general population, while minimizing costs and unnecessary variation in clinical practice. We receive numerous reminders of how increased spending and advances in medical treatments and technology do not automatically translate to improved quality of care for patients. The United States lags in many quality indicators compared with other countries, despite spending a disproportionately large amount on health care.[3–5] There is also a

Conflicts of Interest: None.
Funding Source for This Article: None.
[a] Division of Neonatal and Developmental Medicine, Department of Pediatrics, Stanford School of Medicine, 750 Welch Road Suite #315, Stanford, CA 94305, USA; [b] California Perinatal Quality Care Collaborative, 1265 Welch Road, Stanford, CA 94305, USA
* Corresponding author. Division of Neonatal and Developmental Medicine, Department of Pediatrics, Stanford School of Medicine, 750 Welch Road Suite #315, Stanford, CA 94305.
E-mail address: hclee@stanford.edu

Clin Perinatol 45 (2018) 165–180
https://doi.org/10.1016/j.clp.2018.01.013
0095-5108/18/© 2018 Elsevier Inc. All rights reserved.

significant delay in uptake of evidence-based recommendations. Actual clinical practice often lags evidence-based science by an average of 17 years, although this varies by intervention and measurement methods.[6] An example is antenatal corticosteroids for preterm delivery, an evidence-based therapy that has ultimately taken many years to fully adopt, despite proceeding along a successful biomedical research pathway.[7] Wide variation exists in practices and outcomes that is not easily explained by patient case mix, with ample examples in perinatal care.[8–12] Comprehensive reports have documented large gaps in safety and quality for many health care systems.[2,13]

In that context, quality improvement has gained exposure and attention across all medical disciplines. In many respects, neonatology has been at the forefront of the discipline of quality improvement, with statewide collaboratives playing a large role in that leadership. In this review of statewide collaborative efforts, we highlight their critical role in disseminating and implementing evidence-based practices at scale, an overview of their history, and examples of successes in statewide quality improvement. We also describe some of the lessons learned by the experiences of statewide collaboratives and list some challenges as we move forward to tackle more difficult areas of perinatal quality improvement.

BARRIERS TO THE IMPLEMENTATION OF EVIDENCE-BASED PRACTICE AND THE ROLE OF STATE COLLABORATIVES

It has been noted that the path of evidence-based science leading to changes in clinical care and improved outcomes takes longer than expected, often getting "lost in translation."[14] One reason for this delay may be that a history of applying interventions and therapies that later are found to be unnecessary or even harmful has led to well-intentioned conservatism on the part of the medical community. A prime example is the changing paradigm of thought on retinopathy of prematurity and oxygen. After oxygen exposure was shown to have a causal role in the development of retinopathy of prematurity, restricted oxygen therapy was universally implemented. Several randomized, controlled trials subsequently demonstrated that oxygen restriction may result in a lower incidence of retinopathy of prematurity, but may increase mortality.[15,16] The appropriate oxygen targets in prematurity are still debated and this example demonstrates that it can be difficult to adopt an intervention when data on possible consequences are limited or unclear. In some circumstances, however, the delay in dissemination and uptake of evidence-based protocols can cause undue harm. For example, a consensus statement on the beneficial effects of antenatal steroids on perinatal outcomes was released by the National Institute of Health in 1994; however, there was significant delay in the uptake of this intervention across hospitals nationwide, and there continues to be variation in implementation.[7,17]

The recognition of which new therapies are evidence based enough to adopt can be especially challenging in the current era of the ever-increasing availability of information and medical literature. Clinicians, therefore, rely on multiple stakeholders to learn about the appropriate evidence base for their practice. Clinicians who lack a community for clinical practice discussion may find it particularly challenging to discern what new therapies are appropriate to adopt. Payers and regulatory agencies may not be fully aware of the latest evidence-based practices. In these instances, a larger network of health care providers could inform incentive structures for changing practice (**Fig. 1**).

Even when the best evidence is recognized, it can be challenging to translate into practice, owing to the complex circumstances that are typical of perinatal health

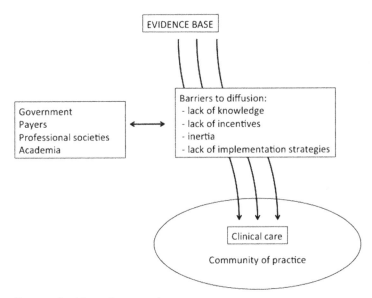

Fig. 1. Diffusion of evidence into practice.

care. Antenatal corticosteroids as a beneficial treatment before preterm delivery could be considered an 'easy' practice to adopt. Nevertheless, wide variation in administration continues to exist. Notably, hospitals that are actively performing quality improvement achieve higher rates of administration.[12,17] Many other evidence-based practices are complex in their implementation, requiring a combination of technical and behavioral adaptations. For example, novel evidence regarding the use of therapeutic hypothermia for asphyxia, better thermoregulation in the delivery room, or early noninvasive respiratory support for preterm infants may be easier concepts to understand than to actually implement in the clinical setting.

In this context, state collaboratives can play an important role in more effective and efficient dissemination and implementation of evidence-based protocols to its participant members. These networks draw on a local community of hospitals, clinicians, and sometimes partner stakeholders, such as public health professionals and family advocates, working together to improve perinatal outcomes.[18] They play a vital role in effectively providing a learning laboratory and a platform for continuous quality improvement.

In addition to gathering data and curating evidence, regional collaboratives harness local community wisdom and create a standardized workflow that can be applied to specific settings. Ideally, collaboratives should be used to disseminate "best practices" for a given benchmarking effort; however, in many cases, the extensive research, controlled trials, and verification may not exist to have a "best practice." In these situations, collaboratives can play a vital role in disseminating and testing "potentially better practices," a term coined by Paul Plsek that is now widely used to describe health care benchmarking efforts.[19] This terminology implies that we are always looking for practices that might lead to improvement, but we may not truly know whether certain practices are better until they are implemented and the consequences are measured to determine whether there is an actual improvement in a local context. If there is improvement, these "potentially better practices" can then be revised and generalized to apply to other settings.[19] Most neonatal intensive care units (NICUs) hope to improve the care they provide to patients and families through individual quality improvement projects; however, state-based quality collaboratives allow coordinated improvement efforts at a regional scale. Statewide collaborative improvement initiatives do not replace, but instead are meant to spur on, support, and build on each hospital's individual quality improvement efforts.

FRAMEWORK FOR COLLABORATIVE QUALITY IMPROVEMENT

The Vermont Oxford Network (VON) provided the framework for the development of regional perinatal quality care collaboratives. The VON is a voluntary collaboration of health care professionals from NICUs around the world, with a mission to improve health care for newborns through coordinated research, education, and quality improvement projects. The VON maintains one of the largest databases on high-risk infants from more than 1000 centers. The database is used for quality improvement projects, clinical trials, and as a way to provide confidential feedback and center-specific reports.[20] The VON has also established both in-person and Internet-based quality improvement collaboratives that have demonstrated significant improvement in various aspects of newborn care, including reducing infection rates, reducing the incidence of chronic lung disease, and promoting evidence-based surfactant use.[21,22] Although participation in national collaborative initiatives can have a wide reach in facilitating broad quality improvement projects, regional collaboratives may have characteristics that allow different advantages. State or regional collaboratives can provide contextual understanding for hospitals sharing similar regulatory patterns or patient populations. Individual regions may have specific characteristics or needs that may not be as well-addressed by a broader national collaborative. By taking a region's economic, geographic, and sociodemographic characteristics into account, and by relying on local and trusted expertise, regional collaboratives are able to design and implement initiatives that are best suited to the needs of their individual members.[23]

EXAMPLES OF STATE COLLABORATIVES AND THEIR SUCCESSES

The VON, the Centers for Disease Control and Prevention (CDC), and state health departments have partnered with statewide quality collaboratives and have established successful initiatives to improve treatment practices and outcomes.[18] From information available through the CDC and other sources, we identified at least 31 states with established or emerging perinatal quality collaboratives. We highlight several examples of their significant progress in addressing quality and safety gaps (**Table 1**).[24] Further descriptions of successes in statewide quality improvement are well-described elsewhere.[25]

The California Perinatal Quality Care Collaborative (CPQCC) was founded in 1997 as the first statewide perinatal collaborative organization. It is one of the most comprehensive statewide collaboratives in that it has near population-based membership, including more than 90% of all neonates in approximately 140 NICUs. It also involves branches in maternal, neonatal, and high-risk infant follow-up, and maintains linked data registries, combining clinical with regulatory data (such as vital statistics and reimbursement figures).[23] CPQCC activities include audit and feedback, applied quality improvement activities with its members, and research. Its members have published widely in the areas of quality improvement,[26–28] quality measurement science,[29–32] and epidemiologic trends and associations.[33–36] These activities are interconnected and have informed each other. One of the goals of the CPQCC has

Table 1
Examples of quality improvement initiatives by state collaboratives

	CA	CO	FL	GA	IL	MA	MI	MS	NE	NH/ ME/VT	NY	NC	OH	OK	TN	TX	UT	WV	WI
Antenatal steroids	✓	—	✓	—	—	—	—	—	—	—	✓	—	✓	—	✓	—	—	—	—
Antimicrobial stewardship	✓	✓	—	—	—	—	—	—	—	—	—	✓	—	✓	✓	—	—	—	—
Vital statistics and birth certificate accuracy	—	—	✓	—	✓	—	—	—	—	✓	—	—	✓	—	—	—	—	—	—
Nosocomial and central-line associated bloodstream infections	✓	—	—	—	—	—	✓	—	—	—	✓	✓	✓	—	✓	—	—	—	—
Congenital heart disease screening	—	—	✓	✓	—	—	—	—	—	—	✓	✓	—	✓	✓	—	—	—	—
Delivery room management	✓	—	—	—	—	—	—	✓	—	—	—	—	—	—	✓	—	—	—	—
Reducing early- elective deliveries/ primary C-sections	✓	—	✓	—	✓	✓	—	—	✓	—	✓	✓	✓	—	✓	✓	—	✓	—
Hospital duration of stay	✓	—	—	—	—	—	—	—	—	—	—	—	—	—	—	—	—	—	—
Human milk/ breastfeeding promotion/ nutrition	✓	—	✓	—	—	✓	—	✓	✓	—	✓	✓	✓	✓	✓	✓	—	✓	✓
Neonatal abstinence syndrome	—	—	✓	—	—	✓	✓	—	—	✓	—	✓	✓	—	—	—	✓	—	—

Not a comprehensive list of all statewide activities.

Data from the Centers for Disease Control and Prevention (CDC). State Perinatal Quality Collaboratives. 2017. Available at: https://www.cdc.gov/reproductivehealth/maternalinfanthealth/pqc-states.html. Accessed June 17, 2017.

been to construct a single database that can be used to inform process and outcomes improvement at both the hospital and community levels on the continuum from maternal to neonatal care.[23] Through linkage of this database to other population-based datasets within California, such as vital statistics and hospital discharge data, the CPQCC has been able to describe epidemiologic trends and resource use across the state, and to identify quality gaps that lead to improvement initiatives. CPQCC quality improvement projects have resulted in improved respiratory outcomes (with promotion of antenatal steroid use), fewer nosocomial infections, more human milk feedings, safer delivery room care, shorter durations of stay, and better antimicrobial stewardship.[37]

The New York State Perinatal Quality Collaborative has partnered with the CDC and the New York State Department of Health to promote initiatives to provide the safest care for women and infants through evidence-based interventions. This collaborative has been successful in achieving a 75% reduction in scheduled deliveries without a medical indication before $38^{6/7}$ weeks gestation among 78 hospitals.[18] Through the implementation of central line care bundles and central line maintenance checklists, their work has led to a 67% decrease in rates of central line–associated bloodstream infections in 18 regional referral NICUs. Conference calls, statewide workshops, and periodic surveys were used to promote implementation of these interventions.[38]

The Perinatal Quality Collaborative of North Carolina is another voluntary, statewide organization that has focused on providing high-value perinatal care through partnerships with the North Carolina Division of Medical Assistance, the March of Dimes, and the University of North Carolina School of Medicine. This organization has created several initiatives that include establishing an immunization registry, reducing catheter-associated bloodstream infections, eliminating elective deliveries before 39 weeks of gestation, improving care of neonatal abstinence syndrome, and promoting the use of human milk and breastfeeding in preterm and term infants. Their initiative to reduce early term elective births involved 33 hospital teams that participated in in-person learning sessions, regional meetings, webinars, and a website to disseminate data and exchange information among participating teams. Each team developed their own action plan for reducing elective deliveries that was based on their individual practices and needs. Over a 9-month period, the participating hospitals collectively decreased the early term elective deliveries by 45%.[39]

Tennessee is another state that has established an effective perinatal quality collaborative organization. The Tennessee Initiative for Perinatal Quality Care began as a data-sharing opportunity among NICUs in 2008 that has grown into an active statewide quality improvement organization. Their projects have included establishing evidence-based approaches to antenatal steroid implementation, congenital heart disease screening, neonatal abstinence syndrome, breastfeeding promotion, and neonatal resuscitation. One example of their initiatives was the creation of the Undetected Critical Congenital Heart Disease Registry, in partnership with pediatric cardiologists and the Tennessee Department of Health, to identify newborns discharged from the hospital with undiagnosed critical congenital heart disease. A review of the registry revealed an undetected critical congenital heart disease incidence of 15 per 100,000 live births in 2011.[40] To address these missed diagnoses, Tennessee implemented a statewide pulse oximetry screening program for critical congenital heart disease in 2013. The established statewide registry through the Tennessee Initiative for Perinatal Quality Care is being used to monitor the impact of the screening program.[41]

The Ohio Perinatal Quality Collaborative (OPQC), founded in 2007, has focused on improving birth data and prematurity outcomes. Through online training modules, webinars, and site visits, the OPQC has improved the quality of data in their state's birth registry, the Integrated Perinatal Health Information system, which has now become an extensive population-based dataset. As a result of this project, antenatal corticosteroid administration rates are more accurately reflected in Ohio's birth registry and the information available through this dataset can be used for quality improvement activities across the state.[18]

There are several examples of how statewide organizations are able to learn from each other and replicate successful initiatives. Similar to the CPQCC, the OPQC has developed online toolkits on optimizing antenatal steroid use with the hope of improving administration rates across the state. The Illinois Perinatal Quality Collaborative established a Birth Certificate Accuracy Initiative in 2014 to improve data collection and quality, modeling their initiative after the OPQC project.[42]

STRATEGIES USED BY STATEWIDE COLLABORATIVES

Statewide collaboratives use the strengths of larger communities of practice to facilitate various strategies for implementation and dissemination of evidence-based practice. The Institute for Healthcare Improvement (IHI) has provided a framework for improvement work through the use of the Model for Improvement in addition to the Breakthrough Series model. The Model for Improvement involves addressing 3 fundamental questions and implementing Plan–Do–Study–Act cycles. The 3 key questions are: What are we trying to accomplish? How will we know that a change is an improvement? What change can we make that will result in improvement? This model has been used successfully by several health care organizations to test change and improve health care outcomes.[43] The IHI Breakthrough Series model is the most extensively evaluated and used model for collaborative initiatives and was designed to help health care organizations make improvements in quality while reducing costs. In this model, a topic is first identified for which there is a large gap between what is known based on existing evidence and what is actually done in clinical practice. A team of expert faculty is then assembled to develop specific content and evidence-based guidelines. Organizations are subsequently invited to join the collaborative and multidisciplinary teams composed of individuals from participating organizations are created to participate in the collaborative process. The teams engage in Learning Sessions, which are in-person meetings where they learn improvement techniques from experts and share their experiences with implementing new practices. In between these sessions, the teams are implementing the changes at their individual institutions and submitting monthly progress reports for the entire collaborative to review. Teams continue to learn from one another through monthly conference calls, exchange of reports, and posting of performance data. At the end of the collaborative, the teams summarize their results and lessons learned and present to nonparticipating organizations at conferences.[44] This model has been used by several regional collaboratives to disseminate evidence-based guidelines and translate these guidelines into action. An example of an application of this model is seen in **Fig. 2**, illustrating a recent collaborative effort in antibiotic stewardship.

As noted, the CPQCC has used the principles established by IHI for quality improvement initiatives.[27,45] The success of CPQCC's collaborations have largely stemmed from the Perinatal Quality Improvement Panel (PQIP), which is the quality action arm of CPQCC. PQIP uses CPQCC data and relevant literature to recommend quality improvement initiatives, develop toolkits and workshops, and establish benchmarks for improvement. PQIP members represent experts in quality improvement and clinical care, physicians, and nurses from a wide variety of hospital settings including community, academic, private, and public institution, and from across regions. The PQIP membership also includes officials from public health departments and other statewide stakeholders. The work of the committee is divided into 4 subcommittees that focus on research, data, education, and infrastructure (**Box 1**).

With oversight of the general committee, the Data Interface and Opportunities Committee establishes clinically relevant targets that have the potential for improvement. This committee also aims to improve the web-based reporting platform that is available to members to identify quality gaps, trends over time, and tools for performing quality improvement, such as run charts (**Fig. 3**).

Recommendations are made by the Data Interface and Opportunities Committee and the general PQIP committee based on existing evidence and are compiled into toolkits. The infrastructure subcommittee leads the development of these toolkits by partnering with subject matter experts across the state. The toolkits contain several

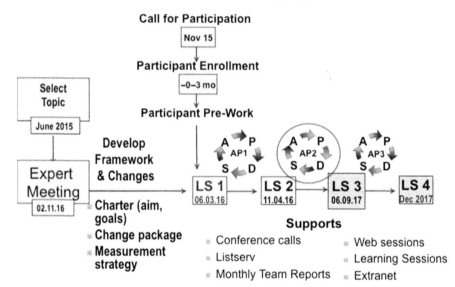

Fig. 2. An application of the Model for Improvement from the Institute for Healthcare Improvement. AP, action plan; LS, learning session; PDSA, plan–do–study–act; QI, quality improvement. (*From* Langley GJ, Nolan KM, Norman CL, et al. The improvement guide: a practical approach to enhancing organizational performance (2nd edition). San Francisco: Jossey-Bass Publishers; 2009; and Institute for healthcare improvement. The breakthrough series: IHI's collaborative model for achieving breakthrough improvement. Boston: Institute for Healthcare Improvement; 2003.)

components: a summary of the relevant literature, examples of specific policies and procedures, quality improvement strategies, data collection tools, and benchmarks and strategies to achieve the established goals.[37] The CPQCC and PQIP have created toolkits that target a number of important interventions regarding newborn care, including antenatal corticosteroid therapy, postnatal steroid use, nutritional support for very low birthweight infants, delivery room management, and prevention of neonatal hospital-acquired infections.

In conjunction with the toolkits, the PQIP has led in-person quality improvement workshops. These workshops enable multidisciplinary teams from units across the state to gather and address problems and strategies for specific improvement projects. Teams complete preworkshop exercises that introduce them to the toolkit elements, attend didactic presentations by regional experts in the topic, and participate in small group sessions to discuss barriers to implementation of the toolkit recommendations and strategies for overcoming any challenges at their institution. These workshops also provide an opportunity for collaboration among groups. This strategy of data collection and analysis, toolkit development, and workshop facilitation has been used successfully by the CPQCC for initiatives such as central line infection reduction.[37,46]

Workshops and other quality improvement education sessions are led by the PQIP Education Subcommittee. In addition to regular email distribution and regional training programs, a key dissemination point has been the annual meeting of the

---

Box 1
Structure of the California Perinatal Quality Care Collaborative Perinatal Quality Improvement Panel committees

Research

1. Evaluate quality improvement projects.

2. Publish toolkits.

3. Advance quality improvement science.

Data interface and opportunities

1. Explore California Perinatal Quality Care Collaborative databases.

2. Improve user interface of web reporting tools.

Education

1. Market and disseminate toolkits.

2. Plan annual meeting for statewide quality improvement education.

Infrastructure

1. Plan and implement collaborative quality improvement activities.

2. Innovate new approaches to quality improvement.

3. Update toolkits.

California Association of Neonatologists, with the 23rd such meeting having taken place in March 2017. Before that meeting, there is a full day dedicated to education and collaborative sharing in quality improvement work and strategies, currently capped off by an evening poster session of presenting local and regional quality improvement work.

The PQIP Research Subcommittee is tasked with evaluating CPQCC quality improvement activities and advancing the science of quality improvement, which can then inform future statewide work. Recent projects have included comparing the results of a group of NICUs using the IHI model collaboratively versus NICUs working individually on a specific quality improvement project. These studies demonstrated greater improvements in targeted outcomes by hospitals that participated in a collaborative quality improvement group as compared with hospitals that pursued individual efforts.[45,47]

In addition to the specific work by the committees noted, the involvement of volunteers from across the state and from a variety of settings has opened up a community of practice in which members can reach out to other members to get advice or demonstrate and recommend best practices. Through the structure provided in the statewide collaborative, hospitals and providers who may not have had experience with quality improvement or with newer clinical strategies have the opportunity to learn about quality measures and quality improvement concepts and techniques, and can also collaborate more easily with experts in the field. When initiatives are instituted, organizations can share their approaches on what has worked well or not, and can learn from each other.

The opportunity to collect and share data and measure specific outcomes also allows individual units to compare their performance to other hospitals in the network. Traditionally, the goal in perinatal statewide collaboratives has not been singling out hospitals that are performing below expectations, but instead to set a standard of care that all hospitals should strive to achieve.[23] The collaborative environment,

A

NICU Operations

Live Births	Inborn Admission Percent	NICU Admissions	CPQCC Small Babies	CPQCC Big Babies
3,056	11.42%	476	68	149

Acute Transports-Out	TRIPS @ Destination NICU Admit	TRIPS Change Eval to NICU Admit	Out-the-Door Time to Destination	With at least 1 Major Surgery
28	6.68	−1.84	7.25	1

VON Small Babies

Baby Monitor	Survival w/out Major Morbidity	Growth Velocity	Median PMA at Home Discharge
Under Development	55.41%	12.05	39 / 3

ANS (JC) Treatment	ROP Exam at Appropriate PMA	Chronic Lung Disease	NEC at this NICU	Home on Human Milk Nutrition
95.24%	100	37.58%	0.00	53.66%

Big Babies

Early Sepsis	Moderate/Severe HIE	Active Cooling Volume	High Acuity
0.66%	0.00	0	31.54%

Infection Control   **HRIF**

Late Infection at this NICU	CLABSI	ABX Use	HRIF Referral	Core Visit 1 at Recommended Age
14.16%	1.07 % Line Days	28.45%	100	41.03%

Fig. 3. Examples of California Perinatal Quality Care Collaborative (CPQCC) web-based reports. (*A*) Displays a general "dashboard" for quickly viewing a summary of key measures. (*B*) A "quick look" feature can delve further at trends at the individual neonatal intensive care unit (NICU) on measures such as chronic lung disease. (*C*) A control/run chart feature can help with active quality improvement tracking. (*D*) A detailed table option can allow for further evaluation of subsets of infants. ABX, antibiotics; ANS, antenatal steroids; CLABSI, central line-associated bloodstream infection; HIE, hypoxic ischemic encephalopathy; NEC, necrotizing enterocolitis; PMA, postmenstrual age; ROP, retinopathy of prematurity; VON, Vermont Oxford Network.

B

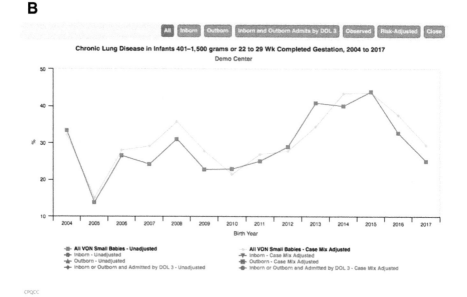

Fig. 3. (*continued*).

C

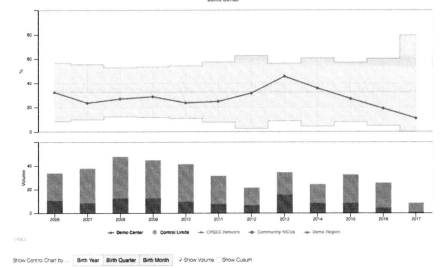

Fig. 3. (continued).

D

Chronic Lung Disease (CLD)

All CPQCC NICU Admissions of Infants 401 to 1,500 grams or 22 to 29 wk of Gestation born in 2004 to 2017

This report is final for years 2016 and earlier. The report is preliminary for 2017 as the data collection is on-going.

California Perinatal Quality Care Collaborative (CPQCC)

DEMO CENTER

	Center			CPQCC Network		
	N	Total	%	N	Total	%
2004 through 2016						
≤24 6/7 wk	6	11	54.5	2,961	4,511	65.6
25 0/7 – 25 6/7 wk	8	14	57.1	2,465	4,410	55.9
26 0/7 – 26 6/7 wk	17	24	70.8	2,414	5,511	43.8
27 0/7 – 27 6/7 wk	6	21	28.6	2,197	6,734	32.6
28 0/7 – 28 6/7 wk	4	27	14.8	1,803	8,234	21.9
29 0/7 – 29 6/7 wk	5	38	13.2	1,382	9,888	14.0
≥30 0/7 wk	12	100	12.0	2,002	22,775	8.8
Total	58	235	24.7	15,224	62,063	24.5
2017						
≤24 6/7 wk	1	1	100	81	134	60.4
25 0/7 – 25 6/7 wk	0	1	0.0	59	103	57.3
26 0/7 – 26 6/7 wk	NA	0	NA	57	146	39.0
27 0/7 – 27 6/7 wk	1	3	33.3	44	174	25.3
28 0/7 – 28 6/7 wk	0	3	0.0	59	271	21.8
29 0/7 – 29 6/7 wk	0	1	0.0	44	302	14.6
≥30 0/7 wk	0	1	0.0	63	880	7.2
Total	2	10	20.0	407	2,010	20.2
2016						
≤24 6/7 wk	1	1	100	234	341	68.6
25 0/7 – 25 6/7 wk	1	1	100	175	307	57.0
26 0/7 – 26 6/7 wk	NA	0	NA	180	460	39.1
27 0/7 – 27 6/7 wk	0	2	0.0	143	463	30.9
28 0/7 – 28 6/7 wk	0	2	0.0	130	652	19.9
29 0/7 – 29 6/7 wk	0	1	0.0	92	704	13.1
≥30 0/7 wk	1	7	14.3	134	1,769	7.6
Total	3	14	21.4	1,088	4,696	23.2
2015						

Fig. 3. (continued).

synergistic learning network, and positive peer pressure can generate and sustain quality gains.

OTHER ADVANTAGES TO STATEWIDE COLLABORATIVE STRUCTURES

By joining together as a group across a state, neonatologists and NICU leaders can become an important resource for health care policymakers to help guide policies and regulations that focus on providing optimal care for mothers and children. Each state government has its own structure of financing health care, regulatory environment, and other potential stakeholders that may function at the state level. By working together for common purposes, the group may be better able to change policies that will allow for the implementation of the most up-to-date evidence-based practice. A recent fruitful collaboration between the state and the CPQCC is evidenced in efforts to promote antibiotic stewardship. A collaborative effort to reduce the unnecessary use of antibiotics emerged from a scientific collaboration, highlighting the enormous variation in antibiotic use rates across CPQCC NICUs.[48] This situation is also an example of how state collaborative work can spearhead national efforts; this topic has been picked up and targeted for improvement by the VON and the CDC.

CHALLENGES

Despite the examples of successful state initiatives and the advantages that have been discussed, a number of barriers to the initiation and sustainment of quality improvement collaboratives exist at the level of the statewide organization and at the level of the individual participating hospital or unit.

Initiating a quality care collaborative and obtaining funding to sustain the organization can be challenging. For many established quality care collaboratives, partnerships with the CDC, VON, state health departments, university medical centers, or private organizations like the March of Dimes have been vital to the maintenance of these organizations. Even with these partnerships, many collaboratives still rely on additional independent grants from public and private organizations. Quality collaboratives need to leverage the resources of critical stakeholders, and must also keep these stakeholders engaged to sustain funding.[49] The stakeholders, such as physician groups, consumer organizations, hospital administrators, or parent groups, may all have different priorities and varying opinions on what quality issues are most important. Discussions must be held to ensure that all involved parties agree to address a common goal, and the organization must be structured to achieve value with minimal risk for each group.[23]

There are also significant challenges in large-scale data collection and dissemination. The primary goal of a quality care collaborative is to collect high-quality and reliable data, translate those data into practical information and guidelines, and transform that information into action to improve care and outcomes. This task is not easy. Self-reported data by individual institutions can be subject to reporting bias through inaccurate reporting and possible underreporting of poor outcomes. Education of those who are performing data entry is required, as well as regular audits of data accuracy, for the data collected to be able to be used appropriately and effectively.[50]

At an individual unit level, additional obstacles arise from participating in a collaborative quality improvement effort. Many NICUs are already involved in their own quality improvement initiatives and may have priorities established by their own unit or hospital. They may also be participating in national organizations like the VON or other large provider groups. Units and providers may face the competing demands of having to meet quality expectations established by the hospital, the regional collaborative, and the national collaborative. The pressure of full participation in all of these initiatives can be quite taxing and there may be an overwhelming amount of material and ideas.[49,50] Furthermore, after the initial investment in participating in a project, we are still learning about the factors that promote sustainment of gains made during that increased period of effort.[51]

A unit may also not have the staff, financial resources, or quality expertise to test and implement an initiative effectively. Individual units should set realistic targets and priorities for what they are capable of achieving. Even if it is difficult to be involved in a statewide quality improvement initiative, the unit may still benefit from other aspects of the collaborative, including the dissemination of resources and information, the ability to network with experts, and involvement in a community that can facilitate other quality work.

Another challenge is that it can be difficult to motivate and share information with staff and stakeholders who are not able to attend the collaborative sessions and who may not feel fully committed to an initiative. Structural interventions that promote the spread of quality improvement thinking and methodology to all frontline workers may prove useful in this regard, but require further testing.[52]

Although statewide collaboratives can better address specific regional characteristics, significant differences exist between hospitals and patient populations within a state, and the local context may prove a barrier to implementation for hospitals with dissimilar capacities and characteristics.[50] Some of these challenges can be addressed by discussions held at the collaborative learning sessions, where units review their experiences and progress, and groups discuss how initiatives can be tailored to an individual unit's needs. As difficult as it is to ensure participating hospitals and units remain involved, it can be even more difficult to attract and engage units that are not involved in the collaborative. Many units remain unengaged in regional collaboratives because of the numerous practical challenges highlighted herein. Without majority participation in a region, the reach of a quality care collaborative may be limited, especially in larger states. Although larger states may struggle with member engagement, smaller state collaboratives may face their own unique challenges. Smaller states have fewer economies of scale for data center, evaluation, and improvement tasks. It may also be difficult to find local trusted expertise and leadership for clinical topics and engagement by members for necessary quality improvement work. In addition, smaller state collaboratives may find it challenging to establish quality improvement initiatives that reach statistical significance owing to a limited sample size of NICUs and patients. One solution is for these states to form a multistate collaborative, such as the Northern New England Perinatal Quality Improvement Network, which includes NICUs in New Hampshire, Maine, and Vermont.

With continued innovation and collaboration, additional opportunities for optimizing quality improvement approaches to the context of individual NICUs exist within state collaboratives. For example, we have found regional differences across networks within California, which may relate to organizational features of health systems that drive quality.[17] However, the ability of higher performing units or networks to serve as mentors remains largely untapped. The promotion of these regional "network quality improvement" projects may be an extension of the larger statewide collaborative structure. In many respects, the potential for statewide collaboratives to advance health care is still in its early stages.

FUTURE WORK

Since the start of the CPQCC in 1997, and the subsequent formation of other perinatal state collaboratives, we have seen many innovative strategies to disseminate and implement evidence-based practices in the NICU. Although we have described some of the successful strategies that have resulted in the improvement of care and outcomes for thousands of infants through these efforts, many opportunities for further advancement in quality improvement strategies remain. State collaboratives have and can continue to function as experimentation and innovation "laboratories" for this purpose. Examples include improvement efforts at the micronetwork level, fostered by our emerging ability to display empirical provider networks[32]; mentored minicollaboratives that bring together high and low performing units; push reporting of quality outlier status to alert NICUs of opportunities for improvement; engagement of family members in improvement work or family-guided collaborative efforts; and transdisciplinary collaboratives that allow the NICU community to interface with obstetric and pediatric providers, as well as community liaisons.

All politics is local, and so is care delivery. State collaboratives are ideally positioned to leverage the social connectivity and provider professionalism in their environments to promote ongoing improvements in care.

REFERENCES

1. Institute of Medicine (IOM). To err is human. Washington, DC: National Academy Press; 1999.
2. Institute of Medicine Committee on Quality of Health Care in America. Crossing the quality chasm: a new health system for the 21st century. Washington, DC: National Academy Press; 2001.
3. Cutler DM, Rosen AB, Vijan S. The value of medical spending in the United States, 1960-2000. N Engl J Med 2006;355(9):920–7.
4. Squires DA. Explaining high health care spending in the United States: an international comparison of supply, utilization, prices, and quality. Issue Brief (Commonw Fund) 2012;10:1–14.
5. Nolte E, McKee M. Variations in amenable mortality–trends in 16 high-income nations. Health Policy 2011;103(1):47–52.
6. Morris ZS, Wooding S, Grant J. The answer is 17 years, what is the question: understanding time lags in translational research. J R Soc Med 2011;104(12): 510–20.
7. Hanney S, Mugford M, Grant J, et al. Assessing the benefits of health research: lessons from research into the use of antenatal corticosteroids for the prevention of neonatal respiratory distress syndrome. Soc Sci Med 2005;60(5):937–47.
8. Lapcharoensap W, Gage SC, Kan P, et al. Hospital variation and risk factors for bronchopulmonary dysplasia in a population-based cohort. JAMA Pediatr 2015;169(2):e143676.
9. Lee HC, Bennett MV, Schulman J, et al. Accounting for variation in length of NICU stay for extremely low birth weight infants. J Perinatol 2013;33(11):872–6.
10. Lee HC, Durand DJ, Danielsen B, et al. Hospital variation in medical and surgical treatment of patent ductus arteriosus. Am J Perinatol 2015;32(4):379–86.
11. Lee HC, Gould JB. Factors influencing breast milk versus formula feeding at discharge for very low birth weight infants in California. J Pediatr 2009;155(5): 657–62.e1-2.
12. Lee HC, Lyndon A, Blumenfeld YJ, et al. Antenatal steroid administration for premature neonates in California. Obstet Gynecol 2011;117(3):603–9.
13. To err is human: building a safer health system. Washington, DC: National Academy Press, Institute of Medicine; 2000.

14. Lenfant C. Shattuck lecture–clinical research to clinical practice–lost in translation? N Engl J Med 2003;349(9):868–74.

15. Sola A, Chow L, Rogido M. Retinopathy of prematurity and oxygen therapy: a changing relationship. An Pediatr (Barc) 2005;62(1):48–63 [in Spanish].

16. Fleck BW, Stenson BJ. Retinopathy of prematurity and the oxygen conundrum: lessons learned from recent randomized trials. Clin Perinatol 2013;40(2):229–40.

17. Profit J, Goldstein BA, Tamaresis J, et al. Regional variation in antenatal corticosteroid use: a network-level quality improvement study. Pediatrics 2015;135(2): e397–404.

18. Henderson ZT, Suchdev DB, Abe K, et al. Perinatal quality collaboratives: improving care for mothers and infants. J Womens Health (Larchmt) 2014; 23(5):368–72.

19. Plsek PE. Quality improvement methods in clinical medicine. Pediatrics 1999; 103(1 Suppl E):203–14.

20. Horbar JD, Soll RF, Edwards WH. The Vermont Oxford Network: a community of practice. Clin Perinatol 2010;37(1):29–47.

21. Horbar JD, Carpenter JH, Buzas J, et al. Collaborative quality improvement to promote evidence based surfactant for preterm infants: a cluster randomised trial. BMJ 2004;329(7473):1004.

22. Horbar JD, Rogowski J, Plsek PE, et al. Collaborative quality improvement for neonatal intensive care. NIC/Q Project Investigators of the Vermont Oxford Network. Pediatrics 2001;107(1):14–22.

23. Gould JB. The role of regional collaboratives: the California Perinatal Quality Care Collaborative model. Clin Perinatol 2010;37(1):71–86.

24. Centers for Disease Control and Prevention (CDC). State Perinatal Quality Collaboratives. 2017. Available at: https://www.cdc.gov/reproductivehealth/ maternalinfanthealth/pqc-states.html. Accessed June 17, 2017.

25. Gupta M, Donovan EF, Henderson Z. State-based perinatal quality collaboratives: pursuing improvements in perinatal health outcomes for all mothers and newborns. Semin Perinatol 2017;41(3):195–203.

26. Wirtschafter DD, Powers RJ, Pettit JS, et al. Nosocomial infection reduction in VLBW infants with a statewide quality-improvement model. Pediatrics 2011; 127(3):419–26.

27. Lee HC, Kurtin PS, Wight NE, et al. A quality improvement project to increase breast milk use in very low birth weight infants. Pediatrics 2012;130(6):e1679–87.

28. Wahid N, Bennett MV, Gould JB, et al. Variation in quality report viewing by providers and correlation with NICU quality metrics. J Perinatol 2017;37(7):893–8.

29. Profit J, Gould JB, Draper D, et al. Variations in definitions of mortality have little influence on neonatal intensive care unit performance ratings. J Pediatr 2013; 162(1):50–5.e2.

30. Profit J, Kowalkowski MA, Zupancic JA, et al. Baby-MONITOR: a composite indicator of NICU quality. Pediatrics 2014;134(1):74–82.

31. Lee HC, Bennett MV, Schulman J, et al. Estimating length of stay by patient type in the neonatal intensive care unit. Am J Perinatol 2016;33(8):751–7.

32. Kunz SN, Zupancic JA, Rigdon J, et al. Network analysis: a novel method for mapping neonatal acute transport patterns in California. J Perinatol 2017;37(6): 702–8.

33. Griffin IJ, Lee HC, Profit J, et al. The smallest of the small: short-term outcomes of profoundly growth restricted and profoundly low birth weight preterm infants. J Perinatol 2015;35(7):503–10.

34. Kastenberg ZJ, Lee HC, Profit J, et al. Effect of deregionalized care on mortality in very low-birth-weight infants with necrotizing enterocolitis. JAMA Pediatr 2015; 169(1):26–32.

35. Ngo S, Profit J, Gould JB, et al. Trends in patent ductus arteriosus diagnosis and management for very low birth weight infants. Pediatrics 2017;139(4) [pii: e20162390].

36. Profit J, Gould JB, Bennett M, et al. Racial/ethnic disparity in NICU quality of care delivery. Pediatrics 2017;140(3) [pii:e20170918].

37. Wirtschafter DD, Powers RJ. Organizing regional perinatal quality improvement: global considerations and local implementation. Neoreviews 2004;5:50–9.

38. Schulman J, Stricof R, Stevens TP, et al. Statewide NICU central-line-associated bloodstream infection rates decline after bundles and checklists. Pediatrics 2011; 127(3):436–44.

39. Berrien K, Devente J, French A, et al. The perinatal quality collaborative of North Carolina's 39 weeks project: a quality improvement program to decrease elective deliveries before 39 weeks of gestation. N C Med J 2014;75(3):169–76.

40. Mouledoux JH, Walsh WF. Evaluating the diagnostic gap: statewide incidence of undiagnosed critical congenital heart disease before newborn screening with pulse oximetry. Pediatr Cardiol 2013;34(7):1680–6.

41. Tennessee Initiative for Perinatal Quality Care. Available at: https://tipqc.org/. Accessed July 2, 2017.

42. Illinois Perinatal Quality Collaborative - Birth Certificate Accuracy Initiative. Available at: http://ilpqc.org/Birth-Certificate-Accuracy-Initiative. Accessed June 29, 2017.

43. Langley GJ, Nolan KM, Norman CL, et al. The improvement guide: a practical approach to enhancing organizational performance. 2nd edition. San Francisco (CA): Jossey-Bass Publishers; 2009.

44. Institute for Healthcare Improvement. The breakthrough series: IHI's collaborative model for achieving breakthrough improvement. Boston: Institute for Healthcare Improvement; 2003.

45. Lee HC, Powers RJ, Bennett MV, et al. Implementation methods for delivery room management: a quality improvement comparison study. Pediatrics 2014;134(5): e1378–86.

46. Powers RJ, Wirtschafter D, Perinatal Quality Improvement Panel of the California Perinatal Quality Care Collaborative. Prevention of Group B streptococcus early-onset disease: a toolkit by the California Perinatal Quality Care Collaborative. J Perinatol 2010;30(2):77–87.

47. Lapcharoensap W, Bennett MV, Powers RJ, et al. Effects of delivery room quality improvement on premature infant outcomes. J Perinatol 2017;37(4):349–54.

48. Schulman J, Dimand RJ, Lee HC, et al. Neonatal intensive care unit antibiotic use. Pediatrics 2015;135(5):826–33.

49. Louis JM. Promise and challenges of maternal health collaboratives. Clin Obstet Gynecol 2015;58(2):362–9.

50. Devers KJ, Foster L, Brach C. Nine states' use of collaboratives to improve children's health care quality in Medicaid and CHIP. Acad Pediatr 2013;13(6 Suppl): S95–102.

51. Stone S, Lee HC, Sharek PJ. Perceived factors associated with sustained improvement following participation in a Multicenter Quality Improvement Collaborative. Jt Comm J Qual Patient Saf 2016;42(7):309–15.

52. James B, Ward A. Introduction to 100% participation. 2016. Available at: https://www.youtube.com/watch?v=-JmqvzXpGDU. Accessed September 7, 2017.

Antenatal Corticosteroids
Who Should We Be Treating?

Whitney A. Booker, MD*, Cynthia Gyamfi-Bannerman, MD, MSc

KEYWORDS

- Antenatal corticosteroids • Prematurity • Preterm birth • Preterm labor
- Respiratory distress syndrome

KEY POINTS

- Antenatal corticosteroids are a crucial treatment in improving neonatal outcomes for those patients at risk for preterm birth.
- Reduction in neonatal morbidities include respiratory distress syndrome, intraventricular hemorrhage, and necrotizing enterocolitis.
- Therapeutic benefits have been demonstrated as early as 23 weeks' gestation, and recent data have supported neonatal benefit through the late preterm period.

INTRODUCTION

One of the most important antenatal therapies to improve outcomes for patients at risk for preterm birth is antenatal corticosteroids.[1,2] As early as 1969, Liggins[2] noted that lambs who received glucocorticoids and then delivered prematurely had lungs that remained partially expanded. This preliminary evidence led to a randomized, controlled trial of betamethasone therapy on 282 mothers who were at risk for preterm delivery, to assess the effect of steroids on neonatal morbidity and mortality. They found that in pregnancies at risk for premature delivery, when treated with corticosteroids, infants demonstrated a decreased risk of respiratory distress syndrome (RDS) compared with those not treated with steroids.[3] Additionally, they found that early neonatal mortality was 3.2% in the antenatal corticosteroid treated group and 15.0% in the controls ($P = .01$). From these early studies, Liggins[3] hypothesized that glucocorticoids caused premature liberation of surfactant into the alveoli, by induction of an enzyme related to the biosynthesis of surfactant.

The authors of this article have no commercial or financial conflicts of interests, and no funding sources were used in the composition of this article.
Division of Maternal-Fetal Medicine, Department of Obstetrics and Gynecology, College of Physicians and Surgeons, Columbia University Medical Center, 622 West 168th Street, PH 16-66, New York, NY 10032, USA
* Corresponding author.
E-mail address: wb2322@cumc.columbia.edu

Clin Perinatol 45 (2018) 181–198
https://doi.org/10.1016/j.clp.2018.01.002
0095-5108/18/© 2018 Elsevier Inc. All rights reserved.

Mechanism of Action

Antenatal corticosteroids affect the fetal lungs through multiple processes (**Box 1**). They stimulate development of both type I and type II pneumocytes, which are surface epithelial cells of the lung alveoli. Type II pneumocytes contain phospholipid multilamellar bodies, the precursors to pulmonary surfactant.[4] The saccular stage of lung development begins at 24 to 28 weeks' gestation and is when type II pneumocytes first appear. It is at this phase that steroid administration has the clear capability to induce type II pneumocytes to increase surfactant production.[5] Additionally, glucocorticoids act to increase lung compliance and maximal lung volume, as well as to reduce protein extravasation from the pulmonary vasculature to the airspace, thereby helping to clear lung fluid before delivery. These biochemical and structural effects on the lung are the basis for improved clinical outcomes after glucocorticoid treatment.[4]

Clinical Efficacy

RDS is a syndrome most commonly diagnosed in premature neonates, clinically characterized by tachypnea, tachycardia, chest wall retractions, expiratory grunting, and nasal flaring. It likely occurs owing to insufficient production of pulmonary surfactant and structural immaturity of the lungs. The incidence of RDS increases with earlier gestational ages, and is highest in infants before 28 weeks' gestation.[6] Approximately 1% of newborn infants are affected by RDS and it is the leading cause of death in babies who are born prematurely.[6,7] The introduction of antenatal steroids for the acceleration of fetal lung maturity and the development of exogenous surfactant has demonstrated reduced rates of RDS in randomized trials worldwide.[8] A recent 2017 Cochrane review of all randomized trials comparing treatment with antenatal corticosteroids versus placebo in patients at risk for preterm birth demonstrated a significant

---

Box 1
Effects of antenatal corticosteroids on fetal lungs

Anatomy and biochemistry
  Thinning of the mesenchyme of the alveolar-capillary structure
  Increased saccular and alveolar gas volumes
  Decreased alveolar septation
  Increased antioxidant volumes
  Increased surfactant

Physiology
  Increase compliance
  Improved gas exchange
  Decreases epithelial permeability
  Protection of the preterm lung from injury during resuscitation

Interactions with exogenous surfactant
  Improved surfactant treatment responses
  Improved surfactant dosage–response curve
  Decreases inactivation of surfactant

Clinical
  Decreases incidence of respiratory distress syndrome
  No effect on the incidence on bronchopulmonary dysplasia
  Decreased mortality

(*From* Jobe AH, Kamath-Rayne BD. Fetal lung development and surfactant. In: Creasy RK, Resnik R, Greene MF, et al, editors. Creasy and Resnik's maternal-fetal medicine: principles and practice. Philadelphia: Elsevier/Saunders; 2014. p. 184; with permission.)

reduction in overall RDS (relative risk [RR], 0.66; 95% confidence interval [CI], 0.56–0.77) as well as moderate to severe RDS (RR, 0.59; 95% CI, 0.38–0.91). Additionally, neonates exposed to antenatal corticosteroids had a reduced need for mechanical ventilation (RR, 0.68; 95% CI, 0.56–0.84).[8]

Additional common complications of prematurity include intraventricular hemorrhage (IVH) and necrotizing enterocolitis. In preterm infants born before 26 weeks' gestation, the frequency of IVH is between 20% and 30%.[9] Bleeding into the central nervous system owing to impaired cerebral blood flood and immature delicate fetal blood vessels in the germinal matrix tissue results in hemorrhage into the ventricular system.[10] Antenatal corticosteroids promote circulatory stability in the vulnerable vascular germinal matrix. The clinical benefit of therapy was demonstrated in a 2017 systematic review with a reduction of neonatal IVH (RR, 0.55; 95% CI, 0.40–0.76).[8] However, the precise molecular mechanism of action of how antenatal corticosteroids reduce IVH is unclear.[11] Vascular endothelial growth factor promotes angiogenesis in the germinal matrix, which in rabbit models has been thought to contribute to increased vascular fragility and hemorrhage.[12] In vitro, the downregulation of vascular endothelial growth factor is accomplished by glucocorticoids, resulting in the suppression of angiogenesis in various disease models.[13,14] Additional growth factors, as upregulated by glucocorticoids, have been found to play a key role in maturation of the vasculature in immature blood vessels.[15] Necrotizing enterocolitis affects almost 10% of preterm infants and carries a mortality rate of up to 35%.[6] The beneficial effects of corticosteroid administration have been demonstrated in both animal[16] and human models,[17,18] and have been shown to accelerate maturation of the intestinal mucosal barrier. A 2017 Cochrane review similarly found necrotizing enterocolitis to be significantly reduced with antenatal steroid therapy (RR, 0.50; 95% CI, 0.32–0.78).[8] Additionally, antenatal corticosteroids have been shown to decrease neonatal mortality (RR, 0.69; 95% CI, 0.59–0.81) and decrease rates of systemic infection in the first 48 hours of life (RR, 0.60; 95% CI, 0.41–0.88; **Table 1**).[8]

GESTATIONAL AGE CONSIDERATIONS TO ANTENATAL CORTICOSTEROID ADMINISTRATION

The recommended gestational age for the administration of antenatal corticosteroids is based on studies that have demonstrated that therapy can result in improved neonatal morbidity and mortality. The American College of Obstetricians and Gynecologists recommends a single course of corticosteroids for women between 24 0/7 weeks' and 33 6/7 weeks' gestation, and recently extended this recommendation to include late preterm pregnancies (34 0/7–36 5/7 weeks' gestation). Antenatal steroids may also be considered for pregnant women as early as 23 0/7 weeks' gestation, who are at risk of preterm delivery within 7 days.[19]

Periviable

The prevalence of periviable birth ranges from 0.03% to 1.9%.[20] These early deliveries account for more than 40% of neonatal deaths.[21] Neonatal morbidity and mortality is affected by many factors, including gestational age and birth weight, as well as a variety of antecedent maternal and fetal medical problems. The *Eunice Kennedy Shriver* National Institute of Child and Human Development (NICHD) Neonatal Research Network developed an easily accessible online calculator to estimate the overall and intact survival for extremely low birth weight neonates.[22] The risk of common neonatal outcomes near the limit of viability are numerous, including moderate or profound neurodevelopmental impairment or death. The group assessed 5 clinical

Table 1
Neonatal clinical outcomes with administration of antenatal corticosteroids: treatment versus no treatment

Outcomes	Anticipated Absolute Effects (95% CI)		Relative Effect (95% CI)	Number of Participants (Studies)
	Risk with Placebo/ No Treatment	Risk with Corticosteroids		
Chorioamniotis	Study population 48 per 1000	40 per 1000 (32–51)	RR 0.83 (0.66–1.06)	5546 (15 RCTs)
Perinatal deaths	Study population 102 per 1000	73 per 1000 (59–91)	Average RR 0.72 (0.58–0.89)	6729 (15 RCTs)
Respiratory distress syndrome	Study population 176 per 1000	116 per 1000 (98–135)	Average RR 0.66 (0.56–0.77)	7764 (28 RCTs)
Intraventricular hemorrhage	Study population 51 per 1000	28 per 1000 (20–39)	Average RR 0.55 (0.40–0.76)	6093 (16 RCTs)
Mean birthweight (g)	Absolute risks not calculated		Mean birthweight was 18.47 g less (40.83 g less to 3.90 g more)	6182 (16 RCTs)

Abbreviations: CI, confidence interval; RCT, randomized, controlled trial; RR, relative risk.
Adapted from Roberts D, Dalziel S. Antenatal corticosteroids for accelerating fetal lung maturation for women at risk of preterm birth. Cochrane Database Syst Rev 2006. (3):CD00445; with permission.

factors: gestational age between 22 and 25 weeks, birthweight (401–1000 g), plurality, neonatal gender, and if antenatal corticosteroids were administered within 7 days of delivery.[23,24]

The biologic plausibility that corticosteroids will be efficacious in the periviable period is based on data related to perinatal mortality. However, sequential phases of fetal lung development also suggest a role for pulmonary benefit. Alveolar development is detected as early as 22 weeks' gestation.[25] Research studies in both the laboratory setting[5] as well as in clinical observational studies[26,27] support the use of corticosteroid administration in the periviable period. The *Eunice Kennedy Shriver* NICHD Neonatal Research Network published observational data that demonstrated a significant reduction in death or neurodevelopmental impairment at 18 to 22 months for neonates who had been exposed to antenatal corticosteroids and born at 23 weeks' gestation (83.4% steroids vs 90.5% without steroids; adjusted odd ratio [AOR], 0.58; 95% CI, 0.42–0.80), 24 weeks' gestation (68.4% steroids vs 80.3% without steroids; AOR, 0.62; 95% CI, 0.49–0.78), and 25 weeks' gestation (52.7% steroids vs 67.9% without steroids; AOR, 0.61; 95% CI, 0.50–0.74). Of note, at 22 weeks' gestation there was no significant difference in these outcomes (90.2% steroids vs 93.1% without steroids; AOR, 0.81; 95% CI, 0.29–2.21). In infants that were born at 22 weeks' gestation receiving steroids, the only outcome that was significantly less was death or necrotizing enterocolitis (73.5% with steroids vs 84.5% without steroids; AOR, 0.54; 95% CI, 0.30–0.97). They also demonstrated that exposure to antenatal corticosteroids in infants born between 23 and 25 weeks' gestation decreased the incidence of death, IVH, periventricular leukomalacia, and necrotizing enterocolitis.[28]

Additional prospective cohort studies have demonstrated that, among infants born from 23 to 34 weeks' gestation, antenatal exposure to corticosteroids compared with no exposure was associated with lower mortality and morbidity at most gestations.[29] However, despite these improved outcomes in the periviable period, significant neonatal morbidity and mortality still exist. When delivery is anticipated in this gestational age window, health care providers must provide both medical information in parallel with emotional support for families faced with these complex and ethically challenging decisions. The NICHD Neonatal Research Network has compiled outcome data on extremely preterm infants and created an online tool to help providers provide estimated rates of neonatal morbidity and mortality based on delivery characteristics (**Fig. 1**). Each patient and their family must receive informed consent and be provided with options in both declining and accepting interventions based on their values and personal circumstances.

24 0/7 to 33 6/7 Weeks

In 1994, the National Institutes of Health held a consensus conference on the use of antenatal corticosteroids for fetal maturation in all fetuses between 24 and 34 weeks' gestation owing to underuse in the 1980s and early 1990s.[30] Administration in this gestational age window is recommended by the American College of Obstetricians and Gynecologists. Additionally, a recent 2017 Cochrane metaanalysis reinforces the beneficial effects and supports the continued used of antenatal corticosteroids to be considered part of routine therapy for patients at risk for preterm delivery between 24 and 34 weeks' gestation. Steroid treatment at this gestational age was associated with a reduction in perinatal death, neonatal death, RDS, moderate to severe RDS, IVH, necrotizing enterocolitis, need for mechanical ventilation, and systemic infections in the first 48 hours of life.[8] Based on these data, it seems that between 24 and 34 weeks' gestation there is an optimal therapeutic window for steroid-induced reprograming of lung development.

Late Preterm Pregnancies

In women between 34 0/7 weeks and 36 6/7 weeks' gestation at risk of preterm birth within 7 days, and who have not received a previous dose of antenatal corticosteroids, the American College of Obstetricians and Gynecologists recommend a single course of betamethasone.[19] The implementation of steroids in this late preterm birth period is also supported by the Society for Maternal Fetal Medicine.[31] This cohort of patients is particularly important to capture, because 70% of all preterm births occur in the late preterm period.[32] The data to support late preterm steroid administration stem from the Antenatal Late Preterm Steroids trial, which was conducted by the *Eunice Kennedy Shriver* NICHD, Maternal-Fetal Medicine Units (MFMU) Network.[33] This was a double-blinded, placebo-controlled, randomized, controlled trial assessing women with a singleton gestation, who were at high risk for preterm birth between 34 0/7 and 36 6/5 weeks' gestation between 2010 and 2015. To be eligible, women had to present with either preterm labor with a cervix that was at least 3 cm dilated or 75% effaced, preterm premature rupture of membranes, or with an indication for a planned late preterm delivery between 24 hours and 7 days of assessment. In 2831 subjects, the study demonstrated a significant decrease in the primary outcome, the need for respiratory support within the first 72 hours of life (14.4% vs 11.6%; RR, 0.80; 95% CI, 0.66–0.97). Additionally, they demonstrated significant decreases in the rates of severe respiratory morbidity, bronchopulmonary dysplasia, transient tachypnea of the newborn, the need for resuscitation at birth, and the need for postnatal surfactant. Compared with placebo, patients treated with steroids had no

Enter the characteristics below	
Gestational Age *(Best Obstetric Estimate in Completed* *Weeks)*	*Select Age* ⬇
Birth Weight *(401 to 1000 grams)*	*grams*
Sex	*Female/Male*
Singleton Birth	*Yes/No*
Antenatal Corticosteroids *(Within Seven Days Before Delivery)*	*Yes/No*

Estimated outcomes for infants in the NRN sample are as follows:

Outcomes	Outcomes for All Infants	Outcomes for Mechanically Ventilated Infants
Survival	____ %	____ %
Survival Without Profound Neurodevelopmental Impairment	____ %	____ %
Survival Without Moderate to Severe Neurodevelopmental Impairment	____ %	____ %
Death	____ %	____ %
Death or Profound Neurodevelopmental Impairment	____ %	____ %
Death or Moderate to Severe Neurodevelopmental Impairment	____ %	____ %

Fig. 1. Rates of neonatal morbidity and mortality based on delivery characteristics.

increased risk of clinical chorioamniotis, endometritis, or cesarean delivery. Neonates treated with betamethasone did have an increased risk of hypoglycemia (24% vs 14.9%; RR, 1.61; 95% CI, 1.38–1.88), but these rates were similar to those expected in late preterm neonates.[34] This Advanced Paediatric Life Support multicenter study is the largest randomized clinical trial to date assessing the benefits of antenatal corticosteroids in the late preterm period, and their findings are consistent with several other randomized, controlled trials on the benefits of antenatal corticosteroids before 34 weeks' gestation.[8,35] As summarized in a large metaanalysis, including 6 trials, infants of mothers who received antenatal corticosteroids at 34 0/7 to 36 6/7 weeks had a significantly lower incidence of transient tachypnea of the newborn (RR, 0.72; 95% CI, 0.56–0.92), severe RDS (RR, 0.60; 95% CI, 0.33–0.94), and use of surfactant (RR, 0.61; 95% CI, 0.38–0.99).[35]

Early Term

Neonates delivered in the early term period (between 37 0/7 and 38 6/7) are at increased risk for adverse outcomes compared with neonates delivered at and after 39 weeks' gestation.[36] Infants born at 37 0/7 weeks to 37 6/7 weeks are at 1.7 times increased risk for respiratory complications than those born between 38 0/7 and 38 6/7 weeks' gestation; and these neonates are at 2.4 times increased risk than those born between 39 0/7 and 39 6/7 weeks' gestation.[37] Additionally, it is known that infants born by cesarean section are at increased risk for the most significant neonatal morbidity in the early term period, namely, RDS and transient tachypnea of the newborn.[35,38] The administration of antenatal corticosteroids after 37 weeks in this early term cohort has shown to be beneficial in select populations. The Antenatal Steroids for Term Caesarean Section (ASTECS) randomized trial tested whether steroids reduce respiratory distress in neonates born by elective cesarean section at term. The treatment group received betamethasone 48 hours before delivery. They found significantly decreased rates in their primary outcome of RDS requiring admission to the neonatal intensive care unit (0.051 in the control group vs 0.024 in the treatment group; RR, 0.46; 95% CI, 0.23–0.93). These findings imply that babies born by elective cesarean section after 37 weeks' gestation can benefit from antenatal corticosteroids.[39]

Additionally, in a 2016 metaanalysis of 3 randomized trials of antenatal corticosteroids administered 48 hours before a scheduled cesarean section after 37 0/7 weeks, there was an appreciable reduction of transient tachypnea of the newborn (3% vs 7%; RR, 0.38; 95% CI, 0.25–0.57), respiratory distress system (2.7% vs 6.7%; RR, 0.40; 95% CI, 0.27–0.59), and the use of mechanical ventilation (0.7% vs 3.6%; RR, 0.19; 95% CI, 0.08–0.43). Additionally seen were higher APGAR scores at 1 and 5 minutes, reductions in time on oxygen, maximum inspired oxygen, and the duration of stay in the neonatal intensive care unit.[35]

IT IS ALL ABOUT TIMING

The administration of antenatal corticosteroids should include a thoughtful review of timing. The optimal time to administer steroids before delivery cannot be predicted in most cases.[40,41] The ideal therapeutic window after administration is when delivery occurs 24 hours to 7 days after a complete course of treatment.[42–44] The minimal amount of time required between receiving steroids and delivery to define an improved neonatal outcome has not been predicted precisely. Therefore, there are very few cases when delivery is considered imminent where therapy should be withheld. In a 2017 multicenter, population-based prospective cohort study gathering data from 11 European countries, outcomes demonstrated that the administration of steroids was associated with a decrease in mortality, reaching a plateau with more than 50% risk reduction after an administration-to-birth interval of 18 to 36 hours. A simulation of steroids administered 3 hours before delivery compared with those who did not receive steroids showed an estimated decrease in neonatal mortality would be 26%.[45] Similar benefits were seen in observational studies with a decrease in the need for vasopressors as well as a decreased risk of IVH and neonatal death, even with incomplete courses of steroids.[46]

At the other end of the spectrum, there have been some studies to show a decreasing therapeutic benefit if steroids are administered more than 7 days before delivery.[44,47] The frequency of RDS has been found to be higher in infants delivering more than 1 week after steroid exposure.[43] And in infants delivering more than 14 days after steroid exposure, there is an associated increased risk for ventilator support and surfactant use.[48,49]

In terms of incomplete doses, clinical results are variable. In extreme prematurity, even the receipt of a partial course of antenatal corticosteroids has been shown to have improved neonatal outcomes.[50] However, other studies looking at the time interval from steroid exposure to delivery in very low birth weight infants have demonstrated no statistically significant improvement with respect to RDS treated with surfactant, IVH, necrotizing enterocolitis, or death.[51]

The Choice of Antenatal Corticosteroid

Historically, betamethasone and dexamethasone have both been acceptable options for corticosteroid therapy for effectively accelerating fetal lung maturity, because they differ by only 1 methyl group.[52] In a 2013 Cochrane review, 12 randomized trials were included to assess the superiority of 1 corticosteroid over the other. They found that dexamethasone was associated with a reduced risk of a reduced risk of IVH compared with betamethasone (RR, 0.44; 95% CI, 0.21–0.92). However, no statistically significant differences were noted for the other primary outcomes, including RDS (RR, 1.06; 95% CI, 0.88–1.27) and perinatal death (RR 1.41; 95% CI, 0.54–3.67). Additionally, those infants exposed to dexamethasone had a significantly shorter stay in the neonatal intensive care unit (mean difference, −0.91; 95% CI, −1.71 to −0.05).[53] In comparison, Lee and colleagues[54] found that prenatal betamethasone exposure was associated with a decreased likelihood of impaired neurodevelopmental status and reduced risk of hearing impairment when compared with dexamethasone. In a 2000 Consensus Panel convened by the NICHD, no significant scientific evidence supported the preferential benefit of betamethasone over dexamethasone. The American College of Obstetricians and Gynecologists notes the inconsistency of these data, and that no sufficient evidence supports the recommendation of one corticosteroid regimen over the other.[19]

The standard treatment dose should consist of either (i) two 12-mg doses of betamethasone given intramuscularly 24 hours apart or (ii) four 6-mg doses of dexamethasone administered intramuscularly every 12 hours.[55] Compared with intramuscular dexamethasone, neonates given oral dexamethasone had a significantly increased incidence of neonatal sepsis (RR, 8.48; 95% CI, 1.11–64.93); no statistical differences were seen for other outcomes.[53]

When to Rescue

The American College of Obstetricians and Gynecologists recommend a single repeat course of antenatal corticosteroids should be considered if (i) the patients is less than 34 0/7 weeks' gestation, (ii) she is at imminent risk of delivery within the next 7 days, and (iii) her prior course of antenatal corticosteroids was administered more than

14 days ago.[19] These recommendations are evidenced from a 2015 systematic review of 10 randomized trials, who had already received a single course of corticosteroids 7 or more days previously, and were considered to be still at risk for preterm birth. The authors concluded that, compared with no repeat corticosteroid treatment, repeat administration reduced the risk of primary outcomes, including RDS (RR, 0.83; 95% CI, 0.75–0.91), and composite serious infant outcome (RR, 0.84; 95% CI, 0.75–0.94). When evaluating long-term childhood outcomes, no significant harm or benefit was observed.[56] Given these results, depending on the clinical scenario, rescue corticosteroids could be considered as early as 7 days from the prior dose if the second course will be completed at less than 34 weeks' gestation.

SAFETY SURROUNDING THE USE OF ANTENATAL CORTICOSTEROIDS
Maternal Safety

Maternal therapy is overall well-tolerated and systematic reviews have confirmed no increased risk of maternal death, chorioamnionitis, or endometritis.[8] Betamethasone has low mineralocorticoid activity in comparison with other corticosteroids, so even in patients with severe preeclampsia, no worsening maternal outcomes have been demonstrated, and hypertension is not a contraindication to therapy. A small increased risk of gestational diabetes has been reported.[57] Studies have demonstrated a transient leukocytosis within 7 days of administration.[58] The steroid effect can occur within hours after the first dose and may last up to 1 week. Additionally, a resultant leukocytosis has been observed, with a return to baseline within approximately 3 days.[59,60]

Fetal Safety

Fetal outcomes have been studied to assess for safety profile. Observational studies have noted associated transient decreases in variability on external fetal heart rate monitoring[61,62] and occasionally reduced scores on the biophysical profile for fetal breathing and body movements.[63,64] A prospective study examining betamethasone administration in fetuses between 26 and 32 weeks' gestation observed that body movements were reduced on day 2 by 50% ($P<.01$), and breathing movements were largely absent on day 2 ($P<.01$); all values returned to baseline on day 4.[65] Additionally observed was a transient improvement in umbilical artery end-diastolic flow, lasting up to 3 days.[66,67] Additionally, the NICHD MFMU demonstrated that repeated doses was associated with a decrease in placental growth in a dose-dependent fashion.[68]

Neonatal Safety

The clinical effects on perinatal outcomes have mostly been related to the numbers of courses, and have been predominately studied before 34 weeks' gestation. In terms of single course, a large 2017 Cochrane review demonstrated no increased risk of either neonatal infection or small-for-gestational age infants.[8] However, this neonatal safety profile was not supported with multidose regimens.

Initially in 2006, the Australasian Collaborative Trial of Repeated Doses of Steroids demonstrated a neonatal benefit of weekly courses of antenatal corticosteroids,[69] and these results were supported in a Cochrane systematic review.[70] This dose–response relationship was further explored in 2008 in the Multiple Courses of Antenatal Corticosteroids for Preterm Birth (MACS) randomized, controlled trial. Infants exposed to multiple courses of steroids weighed less at birth than those exposed to placebo (2216 g vs 2330 g; $P = .0026$), were shorter (44.5 vs 45.4 cm; $P<.001$) and had a smaller head circumference (31.1 cm vs 31.7 cm; $P<.001$).[71] Additionally, in a 2006 study by the NICHD MFMU Network, repeated courses of corticosteroids demonstrated a reduction in multiples of the birth weight median by gestational age (0.88 vs 0.91; $P = .01$), and more neonates weighing less than the 10th percentile (23.7 vs 15.3%; $P = .02$). Significant weight reductions occurred for the group receiving 4 or more courses. From this study, these investigators were able to demonstrate that repeated courses of antenatal corticosteroids do not improve the composite neonatal outcomes, and is also accompanied by a decrease in birth weight and an increase in the number of small-for-gestational age infants.[72] In addition to reduction in birth weight, the administration of multiple courses of steroids in patients with preterm labor before 34 weeks' gestation has been associated with an increased risk of perinatal infection and sepsis-related neonatal death.[73] Long-term follow-up data on multidose regimens are inconclusive. A 2007 study by the NICHD MFMU demonstrated that children who had been exposed to multiple versus single courses did not differ significantly in childhood Bayley scores or anthropometric measurements. However, although not significantly different, they did find a higher rate of cerebral palsy among children who had been exposed to 4 or more doses.[74] Nevertheless, the 2- and 5-year follow-up data on multiple course regimens have not shown to affect pediatric mortality or disability.[75,76] From these studies and concerns for neonatal harm, as well as the balance of risks and benefits, the American College of Obstetricians and Gynecologists do not recommend multiple courses of steroids.[19]

Neonatal outcomes are less well-studied in patients receiving steroids in the late term period. One of the greatest concerns is an increased incidence of neonatal hypoglycemia that, if prolonged or persistent, can be associated with developmental delay and physical growth defects.[77] The ALPS trial did find that in patients receiving treatment between 34 0/7 weeks and 36 5/7 weeks, neonatal hypoglycemia occurred more frequently (24% vs 15%; RR, 1.60; 95% CI, 1.37–1.89); however, this event did not result adverse events related to the hypoglycemia.[33] Additionally, adverse events related to hypoglycemia were similar to those reported in the general population of late preterm infants.[33] In a systematic review and metaanalysis, steroids given after 34 weeks' gestation did not result in any long-term neurologic or cognitive outcomes at ages 8 to 15 years[39]; however, the long-term safety of antenatal corticosteroid administration at term is still not well-studied and not currently recommended in the United States. Further studies are needed to assess the long-term neurodevelopmental outcomes of children exposed to corticosteroids at this gestational age.

CONSIDERATIONS FOR SPECIAL POPULATIONS
Multiple Gestations and Obesity

Previous theoretic concerns that the added maternal plasma volume in multiple gestations could decrease the neonatal benefits of the traditional dosing of antenatal corticosteroids have not been validated.[78] Compared with singletons, maternal and umbilical cord serum betamethasone concentrations have not been shown to be significantly different.[79] Similarly, obesity can affect the volume of distribution. And even though the blood flow per gram of fat in a normal weight individual is more than that of a morbidly obese patient,[80] no differences in betamethasone concentrations were seen in obese versus nonobese women.[79] After preterm steroid prophylaxis, infants of obese women have not been shown to receive more pulmonary surfactant than preterm infants of nonobese women (odds ratio, 0.67; 95% CI, 0.13–1.40).[81] Additionally, maternal body mass index has not been shown to affect neonatal morbidities in those receiving steroids.[82]

The clinical outcomes studies to support the therapeutic benefit of antenatal corticosteroids in twin pregnancy are contradictory. In a secondary analysis of twins delivered between 24 0/7 and 36 6/7 weeks, the primary outcome of RDS was not reduced in those twins receiving steroids.[83] However, other studies have shown that as early as 22 weeks, steroid exposure has proven to be beneficial in multiple gestations. In comparing exposure with nonexposure, twins born between 22 and 28 weeks receiving steroids have been associated with a lower risk of in-hospital mortality (adjusted RR, 0.87; 95% CI, 0.78–0.96).[84] This therapeutic benefit in twins was demonstrated in a recent retrospective cohort study using data on twins born between 24 0/7 and 33 6/7 weeks. Neonatal outcomes were compared in those who received a completed course of antenatal corticosteroids 1 to 7 days before birth and those who did not, and found a clinically significant decrease in neonatal mortality, short-term respiratory morbidity, and severe neurologic injury that is similar in magnitude to that observed among singletons.[85] Additional studies in twins have supported a significant reduction in RDS when the steroid to delivery interval was between 2 and 7 days (aOR, 0.419; 95% CI, 0.181–0.968; $P = .42$).[86] As seen in singletons, optimal therapeutic neonatal benefit is not demonstrated exceeding an interval of 7 days to delivery.[87] Also of note, exposure to rescue steroids has been associated with improved neonatal outcomes.[88]

To date, there has not been a large enough sample size or a randomized, controlled trial to confirm a therapeutic benefit of steroid administration in twin pregnancy. However, the American College of Obstetricians and Gynecologists recommend that twin gestations at risk for preterm birth received the same standard regimen as that recommended for a singleton pregnancy.[19]

Maternal Glycemia Associated with Steroid Administration

Although antenatal corticosteroid therapy has been found to cause a transient hyperglycemia, administration to women with diabetes in pregnancy is still recommended. Because direct evidence on the effectiveness and safety of steroids is lacking for this cohort of patients,[89] close observation is warranted. The glycemic effect of steroids begins about 12 hours after administration of the first dose, and lasts up to 5 days after the second dose.[90] Glucose levels increase in both patients with and without diabetes, although the mean maximum glucose levels have been seen to be higher for those with diabetes than without (205 mg/dL vs 173 mg/dL; $P<.01$).[91] Additionally, studies have supported these findings, seeing glucose levels increase by 33% to 48% in diabetic patients and by 16% to 33% in those without diabetes.[92]

A standardized protocol for preventing hyperglycemia during the treatment of diabetic patients receiving antenatal corticosteroids has not yet been established. Retrospective data have demonstrated that the requirement for insulin is greatest 9 to 10 hours after each dose of betamethasone.[93] Glycemic control and monitoring was dependent on the underlying nature of the diabetes, and how well the patient was controlled at baseline. The National Institute for Health and Clinical Excellence guidelines on the management of diabetes in pregnancy recommend that diabetic women receiving steroids should have additional insulin, although a specific protocol has not been designed. Based on studied patients in the United Kingdom, Kaushal and colleagues[94] have established a protocol. Subcutaneous insulin and diet are continued from the first dose of corticosteroids until 12 hours after the second, and then supplementary intravenous insulin is infused according to hourly blood glucose measurements. Their protocol includes 4 graded sliding scales. The initial scale is selected based on the patient's current subcutaneous insulin dose, and it is advanced if the blood glucose is 10.1 mmol/L or more for 2 consecutive hours. Some protocols have demonstrated a need for increasing the insulin dose from 20%[95] to 40% shortly after steroid treatment is needed to prevent severe dysregulation of metabolic control.[96] This management decision should individualized to the patient, and a proactive approach is needed to ensure optimal outcomes.

Infection and Preterm Premature Rupture of Membranes

The American College of Obstetricians and Gynecologists recommend that antenatal corticosteroids be administered to patients with preterm premature rupture of membranes, because it has been shown to decrease neonatal mortality, RDS, IVH, and necrotizing enterocolitis.[8,97,98] However, the neonatal benefit of patients with preterm premature rupture of membranes at less than 28 weeks' gestation is less clear.[99] Additionally, owing to insufficient evidence, the American College of Obstetricians and Gynecologists does not recommend for or against a rescue course of corticosteroids at any gestational age.[100]

The use of betamethasone has been found to cause a leukocytosis.[101] In patients with preterm premature rupture of membranes who are treated with steroids, there is no difference in chorioamnionitis or RDS.[102] And even in patients with confirmed histologic chorioamniotis, antenatal steroids have been found to be associated with less neonatal mortality and morbidity.[103,104] Additionally, a second maternal antenatal corticosteroid course has not been associated with an increased rate of chorioamnionitis[105] or neonatal sepsis.[106]

SUMMARY

Antenatal corticosteroids remain one of the most powerful tools in our armamentarium to fight the neonatal complications of prematurity. The rate of preterm birth continues to increase, and we must stay equipped to battle the morbidity and mortality that it brings. Over 40 years ago, Liggins and Howie introduced the beneficial effects on newborn lungs leading to less respiratory disease. Since that time, numerous additional therapeutic benefits have been described, including the reduction of neonatal death, IVH, and necrotizing enterocolitis. With advancing technologies and knowledge, the cusp of viability continues to broaden, and with this comes great responsibility to use our knowledge and tools to improve outcomes for patients. Concurrently, we must commit ourselves to providing patients with a thorough understanding, not only of the benefit, but also the limitations of these interventions in the management of preterm birth.

REFERENCES

1. Roberts D, Dalziel S. Antenatal corticosteroids for accelerating fetal lung maturation for women at risk of preterm birth. Cochrane Database Syst Rev 2006;(3):CD004454.
2. Liggins GC. Premature delivery of foetal lambs infused with glucocorticosteroids. J Endocrinol 1969;45:515–23.
3. Liggins GC, Howie RN. A controlled trial of antepartum glucocorticoid treatment for prevention of the respiratory distress syndrome in premature infants. Pediatrics 1972;50(4):515–25.
4. Ballard PL, Ballard RA. Scientific basis and therapeutic regimens for use of antenatal glucocorticoids. Am J Obstet Gynecol 1995;173(1):254–62.
5. Gonzales LW, Ballard PL, Ertsey R, et al. Glucocorticoids and thyroid hormones stimulate biochemical and morphological differentiation of human fetal lung in organ culture. J Clin Endocrinol Metab 1986;62(4):678–91.

6. Stoll BJ, Hansen NI, Bell EF, et al. Neonatal outcomes of extremely preterm infants from the NICHD Neonatal Research Network. Pediatrics 2010;126(3): 443–56.

7. Rodriguez RJ, Martin RJ, Fanaroff AA. Fanaroff and Martin's neonatal-perinatal medicine: diseases of the fetus and infant. 7th edition. St Louis (MO): Elsevier Mosby; 2002. p. 1001–11.

8. Roberts D, Brown J, Medley N, et al. Antenatal corticosteroids for accelerating fetal lung maturation for women at risk of preterm birth. Cochrane Database Syst Rev 2017;(3):CD004454.

9. Allen KA. Treatment of intraventricular hemorrhages in premature infants: where is the evidence? Adv Neonatal Care 2013;13(2):127–30.

10. Bassan H. Intracranial hemorrhage in the preterm infant: understanding it, preventing it. Clin Perinatol 2009;36(4):737–62, v.

11. Vinukonda G, Dummula K, Malik S, et al. Effect of prenatal glucocorticoids on cerebral vasculature of the developing brain. Stroke 2010;41(8):1766–73.

12. Ballabh P, Xu H, Hu F, et al. Angiogenic inhibition reduces germinal matrix hemorrhage. Nat Med 2007;13(4):477–85.

13. Yano A, Fujii Y, Iwai A, et al. Glucocorticoids suppress tumor angiogenesis and in vivo growth of prostate cancer cells. Clin Cancer Res 2006;12(10):3003–9.

14. Kasselman LJ, Kintner J, Sideris A, et al. Dexamethasone treatment and ICAM-1 deficiency impair VEGF-induced angiogenesis in adult brain. J Vasc Res 2007; 44(4):283–91.

15. Armulik A, Abramsson A, Betsholtz C. Endothelial/pericyte interactions. Circ Res 2005;97(6):512–23.

16. Israel EJ, Schiffrin EJ, Carter EA, et al. Prevention of necrotizing enterocolitis in the rat with prenatal cortisone. Gastroenterology 1990;99(5):1333–8.

17. Bauer CR, Morrison JC, Poole WK, et al. A decreased incidence of necrotizing enterocolitis after prenatal glucocorticoid therapy. Pediatrics 1984; 73(5):682–8.

18. Halac E, Halac J, Begue EF, et al. Prenatal and postnatal corticosteroid therapy to prevent neonatal necrotizing enterocolitis: a controlled trial. J Pediatr 1990; 117(1 Pt 1):132–8.

19. American College of Obstetricians and Gynecologists' Committee on Obstetric Practice, Society for Maternal– Fetal Medicine. Committee opinion no.677: antenatal corticosteroid therapy for fetal maturation. Obstet Gynecol 2016;128(4): e187–194.

20. Chauhan SP, Ananth CV. Periviable births: epidemiology and obstetrical antecedents. Semin Perinatol 2013;37(6):382–8.

21. American College of Obstetricians and Gynecologists and the Society for Maternal–Fetal Medicine, Ecker JL, Kaimal A, Mercer BM, et al. Periviable birth: interim update. Am J Obstet Gynecol 2016;215(2):B2–12.e1.

22. NICHD Neonatal Research Network (NRN) Online Calculator. Available at: https://www1.nichd.nih.gov/epbo-calculator/Pages/epbo_case.aspx. Accessed February 12, 2018.

23. Tyson JE, Parikh NA, Langer J, et al. Intensive care for extreme prematurity–moving beyond gestational age. N Engl J Med 2008;358(16):1672–81.

24. Stoll BJ, Hansen NI, Bell EF, et al. Trends in care practices, morbidity, and mortality of extremely preterm neonates, 1993-2012. JAMA 2015;314(10):1039–51.

25. Chetty A, Andersson S, Lassus P, et al. Insulin-like growth factor-1 (IGF-1) and IGF-1 receptor (IGF-1R) expression in human lung in RDS and BPD. Pediatr Pulmonol 2004;37(2):128–36.

26. Abbasi S, Oxford C, Gerdes J, et al. Antenatal corticosteroids prior to 24 weeks' gestation and neonatal outcome of extremely low birth weight infants. Am J Perinatol 2010;27(1):61–6.

27. Park CK, Isayama T, McDonald SD. Antenatal corticosteroid therapy before 24 weeks of gestation: a systematic review and meta-analysis. Obstet Gynecol 2016;127(4):715–25.

28. Carlo WA, McDonald SA, Fanaroff AA, et al. Association of antenatal corticosteroids with mortality and neurodevelopmental outcomes among infants born at 22 to 25 weeks' gestation. JAMA 2011;306(21):2348–58.

29. Travers CP, Clark RH, Spitzer AR, et al. Exposure to any antenatal corticosteroids and outcomes in preterm infants by gestational age: prospective cohort study. BMJ 2017;356:j1039.

30. Effect of corticosteroids for fetal maturation on perinatal outcomes. NIH consensus development panel on the effect of corticosteroids for fetal maturation on perinatal outcomes. JAMA 1995;273(5):413–8.

31. Implementation of the use of antenatal corticosteroids in the late preterm birth period in women at risk for preterm delivery. Am J Obstet Gynecol 2016; 215(2):B13–5.

32. Hamilton BE, Martin JA, Osterman MJ, et al. Births: final data for 2014. Natl Vital Stat Rep 2015;64(12):1–64.

33. Gyamfi-Bannerman C, Thom EA, Blackwell SC, et al. Antenatal betamethasone for women at risk for late preterm delivery. N Engl J Med 2016;374(14):1311–20.

34. Harris DL, Weston PJ, Harding JE. Incidence of neonatal hypoglycemia in babies identified as at risk. J Pediatr 2012;161(5):787–91.

35. Saccone G, Berghella V. Antenatal corticosteroids for maturity of term or near term fetuses: systematic review and meta-analysis of randomized controlled trials. BMJ 2016;355:i5044.

36. American College of Obstetricians and Gynecologists. ACOG committee opinion no. 561: nonmedically indicated early-term deliveries. Obstet Gynecol 2013;121(4):911–5.

37. Prefumo F, Ferrazzi E, Di Tommaso M, et al. Neonatal morbidity after cesarean section before labor at 34(+0) to 38(+6) weeks: a cohort study. J Matern Fetal Neonatal Med 2016;29(8):1334–8.

38. Zanardo V, Simbi AK, Franzoi M, et al. Neonatal respiratory morbidity risk and mode of delivery at term: influence of timing of elective caesarean delivery. Acta Paediatr 2004;93(5):643–7.

39. Stutchfield PR, Whitaker R, Gliddon AE, et al. Behavioural, educational and respiratory outcomes of antenatal betamethasone for term caesarean section (ASTECS trial). Arch Dis Child Fetal Neonatal Ed 2013;98(3):F195–200.

40. Levin HI, Ananth CV, Benjamin-Boamah C, et al. Clinical indication and timing of antenatal corticosteroid administration at a single centre. BJOG 2016;123(3): 409–14.

41. Adams TM, Kinzler WL, Chavez MR, et al. The timing of administration of antenatal corticosteroids in women with indicated preterm birth. Am J Obstet Gynecol 2015;212(5):645.e1-4.

42. Crowley PA. Antenatal corticosteroid therapy: a meta-analysis of the randomized trials, 1972 to 1994. Am J Obstet Gynecol 1995;173(1):322–35.

43. Waters TP, Mercer B. Impact of timing of antenatal corticosteroid exposure on neonatal outcomes. J Matern Fetal Neonatal Med 2009;22(4):311–4.

44. Melamed N, Shah J, Soraisham A, et al. Association between antenatal cortico-steroid administration-to-birth interval and outcomes of preterm neonates. Obstet Gynecol 2015;125(6):1377–84.
45. Norman M, Piedvache A, Borch K, et al. Association of short antenatal cortico-steroid administration-to-birth intervals with survival and morbidity among very preterm infants: results from the EPICE cohort. JAMA Pediatr 2017;171(7): 678–86.
46. Elimian A, Figueroa R, Spitzer AR, et al. Antenatal corticosteroids: are incomplete courses beneficial? Obstet Gynecol 2003;102(2):352–5.
47. Wilms FF, Vis JY, Pattinaja DA, et al. Relationship between the time interval from antenatal corticosteroid administration until preterm birth and the occurrence of respiratory morbidity. Am J Obstet Gynecol 2011;205(1):49.e1-7.
48. Ring AM, Garland JS, Stafeil BR, et al. The effect of a prolonged time interval between antenatal corticosteroid administration and delivery on outcomes in preterm neonates: a cohort study. Am J Obstet Gynecol 2007;196(5):457.e1-6.
49. Peaceman AM, Bajaj K, Kumar P, et al. The interval between a single course of antenatal steroids and delivery and its association with neonatal outcomes. Am J Obstet Gynecol 2005;193(3 Pt 2):1165–9.
50. Costa S, Zecca E, De Luca D, et al. Efficacy of a single dose of antenatal corticosteroids on morbidity and mortality of preterm infants. Eur J Obstet Gynecol Reprod Biol 2007;131(2):154–7.
51. Sehdev HM, Abbasi S, Robertson P, et al. The effects of the time interval from antenatal corticosteroid exposure to delivery on neonatal outcome of very low birth weight infants. Am J Obstet Gynecol 2004;191(4):1409–13.
52. Bonanno C, Wapner RJ. Antenatal corticosteroids in the management of preterm birth: are we back where we started? Obstet Gynecol Clin North Am 2012;39(1):47–63.
53. Brownfoot FC, Gagliardi DI, Bain E, et al. Different corticosteroids and regimens for accelerating fetal lung maturation for women at risk of preterm birth. Cochrane Database Syst Rev 2013;(8):CD006764.
54. Lee BH, Stoll BJ, McDonald SA, et al. Neurodevelopmental outcomes of extremely low birth weight infants exposed prenatally to dexamethasone versus betamethasone. Pediatrics 2008;121(2):289–96.
55. American College of Obstetricians and Gynecologists' Committee on Practice Bulletins—Obstetrics. Practice bulletin no. 171: management of preterm labor. Obstet Gynecol 2016;128(4):e155–64.
56. Crowther CA, McKinlay CJ, Middleton P, et al. Repeat doses of prenatal corticosteroids for women at risk of preterm birth for improving neonatal health outcomes. Cochrane Database Syst Rev 2015;(7):CD003935.
57. Amorim MM, Santos LC, Faundes A. Corticosteroid therapy for prevention of respiratory distress syndrome in severe preeclampsia. Am J Obstet Gynecol 1999;180(5):1283–8.
58. Mastrobattista JM, Patel N, Monga M. Betamethasone alteration of the one-hour glucose challenge test in pregnancy. J Reprod Med 2001;46(2):83–6.
59. Vaisbuch E, Levy R, Hagay Z. The effect of betamethasone administration to pregnant women on maternal serum indicators of infection. J Perinat Med 2002;30(4):287–91.
60. Kadanali S, Ingec M, Kucukozkan T, et al. Changes in leukocyte, granulocyte and lymphocyte counts following antenatal betamethasone administration to pregnant women. Int J Gynaecol Obstet 1997;58(3):269–74.

61. Subtil D, Tiberghien P, Devos P, et al. Immediate and delayed effects of antenatal corticosteroids on fetal heart rate: a randomized trial that compares betamethasone acetate and phosphate, betamethasone phosphate, and dexamethasone. Am J Obstet Gynecol 2003;188(2):524–31.

62. Rotmensch S, Liberati M, Vishne TH, et al. The effect of betamethasone and dexamethasone on fetal heart rate patterns and biophysical activities. A prospective randomized trial. Acta Obstet Gynecol Scand 1999;78(6):493–500.

63. Kelly MK, Schneider EP, Petrikovsky BM, et al. Effect of antenatal steroid administration on the fetal biophysical profile. J Clin Ultrasound 2000;28(5):224–6.

64. Katz M, Meizner I, Holcberg G, et al. Reduction or cessation of fetal movements after administration of steroids for enhancement of lung maturation. I. Clinical evaluation. Isr J Med Sci 1988;24(1):5–9.

65. Derks JB, Mulder EJ, Visser GH. The effects of maternal betamethasone administration on the fetus. Br J Obstet Gynaecol 1995;102(1):40–6.

66. Edwards A, Baker LS, Wallace EM. Changes in umbilical artery flow velocity waveforms following maternal administration of betamethasone. Placenta 2003;24(1):12–6.

67. Wallace EM, Baker LS. Effect of antenatal betamethasone administration on placental vascular resistance. Lancet 1999;353(9162):1404–7.

68. Sawady J, Mercer BM, Wapner RJ, et al, National Institute of Child Health and Human Development Maternal Fetal Medicine Units Network. The National Institute of Child Health and Human Development Maternal-Fetal Medicine Units Network beneficial effects of antenatal repeated steroids study: impact of repeated doses of antenatal corticosteroids on placental growth and histologic findings. Am J Obstet Gynecol 2007;197(3):281.e1-8.

69. Crowther CA, Haslam RR, Hiller JE, et al. Neonatal respiratory distress syndrome after repeat exposure to antenatal corticosteroids: a randomised controlled trial. Lancet 2006;367(9526):1913–9.

70. Crowther CA, Harding JE. Repeat doses of prenatal corticosteroids for women at risk of preterm birth for preventing neonatal respiratory disease. Cochrane Database Syst Rev 2007;(3):CD003935.

71. Murphy KE, Hannah ME, Willan AR, et al. Multiple courses of antenatal corticosteroids for preterm birth (MACS): a randomised controlled trial. Lancet 2008; 372(9656):2143–51.

72. Wapner RJ, Sorokin Y, Thom EA, et al. Single versus weekly courses of antenatal corticosteroids: evaluation of safety and efficacy. Am J Obstet Gynecol 2006; 195(3):633–42.

73. Vermillion ST, Soper DE, Newman RB. Neonatal sepsis and death after multiple courses of antenatal betamethasone therapy. Am J Obstet Gynecol 2000; 183(4):810–4.

74. Wapner RJ, Sorokin Y, Mele L, et al. Long-term outcomes after repeat doses of antenatal corticosteroids. N Engl J Med 2007;357(12):1190–8.

75. Asztalos EV, Murphy KE, Hannah ME, et al. Multiple courses of antenatal corticosteroids for preterm birth study: 2-year outcomes. Pediatrics 2010;126(5): e1045–1055.

76. Asztalos EV, Murphy KE, Willan AR, et al. Multiple courses of antenatal corticosteroids for preterm birth study: outcomes in children at 5 years of age (MACS-5). JAMA Pediatr 2013;167(12):1102–10.

77. Duvanel CB, Fawer CL, Cotting J, et al. Long-term effects of neonatal hypoglycemia on brain growth and psychomotor development in small-for-gestational-age preterm infants. J Pediatr 1999;134(4):492–8.

78. Battista L, Winovitch KC, Rumney PJ, et al. A case-control comparison of the effectiveness of betamethasone to prevent neonatal morbidity and mortality in preterm twin and singleton pregnancies. Am J Perinatol 2008;25(7): 449–53.

79. Gyamfi C, Mele L, Wapner RJ, et al. The effect of plurality and obesity on betamethasone concentrations in women at risk for preterm delivery. Am J Obstet Gynecol 2010;203(3):219.e1-5.

80. de Divitiis O, Fazio S, Petitto M, et al. Obesity and cardiac function. Circulation 1981;64(3):477–82.

81. Claire L, Vieux R. Efficacy of antenatal corticosteroids according to maternal and perinatal factors: a retrospective cohort study. Am J Perinatol 2015; 32(11):1070–7.

82. Hashima JN, Lai Y, Wapner RJ, et al. The effect of maternal body mass index on neonatal outcome in women receiving a single course of antenatal corticosteroids. Am J Obstet Gynecol 2010;202(3):263.e1-5.

83. Viteri OA, Blackwell SC, Chauhan SP, et al. Antenatal corticosteroids for the prevention of respiratory distress syndrome in premature twins. Obstet Gynecol 2016;128(3):583–91.

84. Boghossian NS, McDonald SA, Bell EF, et al. Association of antenatal corticosteroids with mortality, morbidity, and neurodevelopmental outcomes in extremely preterm multiple gestation infants. JAMA Pediatr 2016;170(6):593–601.

85. Melamed N, Shah J, Yoon EW, et al. The role of antenatal corticosteroids in twin pregnancies complicated by preterm birth. Am J Obstet Gynecol 2016;215(4): 482.e1-9.

86. Kuk JY, An JJ, Cha HH, et al. Optimal time interval between a single course of antenatal corticosteroids and delivery for reduction of respiratory distress syndrome in preterm twins. Am J Obstet Gynecol 2013;209(3):256.e1-7.

87. Kosinska-Kaczynska K, Szymusik I, Urban P, et al. Relation between time interval from antenatal corticosteroids administration to delivery and neonatal outcome in twins. J Obstet Gynaecol Res 2016;42(6):625–31.

88. Bibbo C, Deluca L, Gibbs KA, et al. Rescue corticosteroids in twin pregnancies and short-term neonatal outcomes. BJOG 2013;120(1):58–63.

89. Amiya RM, Mlunde LB, Ota E, et al. Antenatal corticosteroids for reducing adverse maternal and child outcomes in special populations of women at risk of imminent preterm birth: a systematic review and meta-analysis. PLoS One 2016;11(2):e0147604.

90. Miracle X, Di Renzo GC, Stark A, et al. Guideline for the use of antenatal corticosteroids for fetal maturation. J Perinat Med 2008;36(3):191–6.

91. Jolley JA, Rajan PV, Petersen R, et al. Effect of antenatal betamethasone on blood glucose levels in women with and without diabetes. Diabetes Res Clin Pract 2016;118:98–104.

92. Refuerzo JS, Garg A, Rech B, et al. Continuous glucose monitoring in diabetic women following antenatal corticosteroid therapy: a pilot study. Am J Perinatol 2012;29(5):335–8.

93. Itoh A, Saisho Y, Miyakoshi K, et al. Time-dependent changes in insulin requirement for maternal glycemic control during antenatal corticosteroid therapy in women with gestational diabetes: a retrospective study. Endocr J 2016;63(1): 101–4.

94. Kaushal K, Gibson JM, Railton A, et al. A protocol for improved glycaemic control following corticosteroid therapy in diabetic pregnancies. Diabet Med 2003; 20(1):73–5.

95. Kalra S, Kalra B, Gupta Y. Glycemic management after antenatal corticosteroid therapy. N Am J Med Sci 2014;6(2):71–6.
96. Mathiesen ER, Christensen AB, Hellmuth E, et al. Insulin dose during glucocorticoid treatment for fetal lung maturation in diabetic pregnancy: test of an algorithm [correction of an algoritm]. Acta Obstet Gynecol Scand 2002;81(9):835–9.
97. Vidaeff AC, Ramin SM. Antenatal corticosteroids after preterm premature rupture of membranes. Clin Obstet Gynecol 2011;54(2):337–43.
98. Harding JE, Pang J, Knight DB, et al. Do antenatal corticosteroids help in the setting of preterm rupture of membranes? Am J Obstet Gynecol 2001;184(2):131–9.
99. Chapman SJ, Hauth JC, Bottoms SF, et al. Benefits of maternal corticosteroid therapy in infants weighing ≤1000 grams at birth after preterm rupture of the amnion. Am J Obstet Gynecol 1999;180(3 Pt 1):677–82.
100. American College of Obstetricians and Gynecologists' Committee on Practice Bulletins—Obstetrics. Practice bulletin no. 172: premature rupture of membranes. Obstet Gynecol 2016;128(4):e165–177.
101. Diebel ND, Parsons MT, Spellacy WN. The effects of Betamethasone on white blood cells during pregnancy with PPROM. J Perinat Med 1998;26(3):204–7.
102. Sheibani L, Fong A, Henry DE, et al. Maternal and neonatal outcomes after antenatal corticosteroid administration for PPROM at 32 to 33 6/7 weeks gestational age. J Matern Fetal Neonatal Med 2017;30(14):1676–80.
103. Been JV, Degraeuwe PL, Kramer BW, et al. Antenatal steroids and neonatal outcome after chorioamnionitis: a meta-analysis. BJOG 2011;118(2):113–22.
104. Elimian A, Verma U, Beneck D, et al. Histologic chorioamnionitis, antenatal steroids, and perinatal outcomes. Obstet Gynecol 2000;96(3):333–6.
105. Brookfield KF, El-Sayed YY, Chao L, et al. Antenatal corticosteroids for preterm premature rupture of membranes: single or repeat course? Am J Perinatol 2015;32(6):537–44.
106. Gyamfi-Bannerman C, Son M. Preterm premature rupture of membranes and the rate of neonatal sepsis after two courses of antenatal corticosteroids. Obstet Gynecol 2014;124(5):999–1003.

Delivery at Term
When, How, and Why

Kate F. Walker, PhD, MRCOG*, Jim G. Thornton, MD, FRCOG

KEYWORDS

- Term • Induction of labor • Cesarean delivery • Antepartum stillbirth

KEY POINTS

- The optimal timing of delivery for the baby is 39 weeks, avoiding the morbidity associated with early term birth and reducing the risk of antepartum stillbirth.
- There is compelling evidence that among high-risk pregnancies and in settings where cesarean rates are high (>20%), induction of labor at 37 to 40 weeks does not, as previously thought, result in a further increased risk of cesarean delivery.
- The only advantage to planned cesarean delivery over induction of labor is the avoidance of the morbidity associated with emergency cesarean delivery; controversy exists on the other reported benefits.
- There is a growing number of well-conducted randomized controlled trials that provide some support for induction of labor shortly before term for a variety of indications (hypertensive disorders, gestational diabetes, suspected growth restriction, macrosomia, and advanced maternal age).

INTRODUCTION

A young, healthy primiparous woman attends your antenatal clinic requesting delivery at 39 weeks. There is no indication for delivery before 41 weeks' gestation. How do you counsel her? What is the optimal timing (when), method (how), and reason (why) for delivery at term? In this article, the authors aim to provide you with a summary of the relevant information to help you counsel this woman and help her to reach an informed decision about her care. When should we offer delivery? What gestation represents the optimal timing for delivery at term? As with all decisions in maternity care, optimal timing may be different for the mother than the baby and a balance must be sought. The authors examine how the timing of delivery across the gestational

Conflict of Interest Disclosures: Dr K.F. Walker has no conflicts of interest to declare. Dr J.G. Thornton reports personal fees and nonfinancial support from Ferring Pharmaceuticals.
Division of Child Health, Obstetrics, and Gynaecology, Maternity Department, School of Medicine, University of Nottingham, Nottingham City Hospital, Nottingham University Hospitals NHS Trust, Hucknall Road, Nottingham NG5 1PB, UK
* Corresponding author.
E-mail address: kate.walker@nottingham.ac.uk

Clin Perinatol 45 (2018) 199–211
https://doi.org/10.1016/j.clp.2018.01.004
0095-5108/18/© 2018 Elsevier Inc. All rights reserved.

weeks (37–42 weeks) may influence the risk of complications for the mother and for the baby.

OPTIMAL DELIVERY TIMING
Baby

Antepartum risks
Risk of antepartum stillbirth Stillbirth accounts for two-thirds of perinatal deaths, and early neonatal deaths account for 33%.[1] Intrapartum causes of stillbirth account for just 8.8% of all stillbirths. Excluding intrapartum causes, antepartum stillbirth accounts for 61% of all perinatal deaths.[1] Twenty-eight percent of antepartum stillbirths are unexplained.[1] Antepartum stillbirth is by far the most common cause of perinatal death at term.[2] Six percent of stillbirths are due to congenital abnormalities, and 35% of stillbirths occur at 37 to 42 weeks (the most common gestation for stillbirths to occur). Term, singleton, normally formed, antepartum stillbirth (ie, potentially preventable stillbirths) made up one-third of all stillbirths (1039 [32%] out of 3286) in the United Kingdom in 2013.

Choosing the correct denominator The risk of perinatal death at gestational ages near term is often expressed as the number of all perinatal deaths at each week divided by the total number of births. However, near term a baby cannot be stillborn once it has been delivered. Thus, the risk of remaining undelivered at each gestational age is better expressed as the risk per 100 babies undelivered at that time point, termed the *perinatal risk index*. Although the perinatal mortality rate is lowest at 41 weeks, the gestational age associated with the lowest cumulative risk of perinatal death is 38 weeks.[2]

Neonatal risks
Risk of respiratory morbidity Most elective cesarean deliveries are performed at or after $39^{0/7}$ weeks' gestation.[3] The timing of this is advised because the risk of neonatal respiratory morbidity decreases with advancing gestation until $40^{0/7}$ weeks. The risk of respiratory morbidity in infants delivered by elective cesarean at $37^{0/7}$ weeks is 4-fold higher than infants delivered at 40 weeks, 3-fold higher compared with those delivered at 38 weeks, and 2-fold higher than those delivered at 39 weeks. The risk of developing neonatal respiratory symptoms for babies born by vaginal delivery decreases from a probability of 0.07 at 37 weeks to 0.04 at 39 weeks and thereafter plateaus.[4] Thus, induction of labor at 39 weeks is the optimal balance between the risk of respiratory morbidity for the neonate and the risk of antepartum stillbirth for the fetus.

Hyperbilirubinaemia There have been reports of an association between the use of oxytocin in labor and neonatal hyperbilirubinaemia.[5] However, it is difficult to disentangle possible confounding by the earlier gestational age of babies who were delivered following induction of labor. Although Cochrane reviews of high versus low doses of oxytocin[6] and early versus late use[7] do not report jaundice, at least one trial showed no effect.[8] Gestational age of less than 38 weeks is a risk factor for the development of significant hyperbilirubinaemia.[9] In an observational study comparing outcomes for low-risk singleton term newborns by gestational age, delivery at less than 38 weeks was an independent risk factor for the development of unexplained jaundice (odds ratio [OR] = 2.1, 95% confidence interval [CI] 1.7–2.5).[10] The DAME trial, a randomized controlled trial (RCT) of induction of labor at 37 to 38 weeks' gestation versus expectant management for suspected large-for-gestational-age babies, found higher rates of hyperbilirubinaemia requiring phototherapy in the induction group compared with the expectantly managed group.[11]

Other neonatal outcomes Gestational age less than 38 weeks is also an independent risk factor for the development of neonatal hypoglycemia (OR = 2.5, 95% CI 1.5–4.3).[10] Perhaps unsurprisingly given the increased risk of respiratory morbidity, jaundice, and hypoglycemia associated with delivery at 37 weeks' gestation, the rates of admission to neonatal intensive care are also inversely proportional to delivery gestational age.[12]

Observational studies have also suggested an increased risk of neonatal encephalopathy in children with cerebral palsy associated with delivery at 41 weeks or greater versus less than 41 weeks.[13]

Thus, the current data suggest that 39 weeks' gestation is the optimal gestational age for delivery for the baby, as it avoids the morbidity associated with early term birth and reduces the risk of antepartum stillbirth post term.

Maternal

Risk of cesarean delivery

Observational data suggest that induction of labor results in an increased risk of cesarean delivery.[14–16] For example, in England from 2010 to 2011, cesarean rates were 11% among women who labored spontaneously and 23% among those who were induced. Rates of operative vaginal delivery followed similar trends (12% and 17%, respectively).[17] However, there is significant confounding by delivery indication, as the reasons for induction (eg, postdates pregnancy, fetal growth restriction, reduced fetal movements) are also established risk factors for operative delivery. When observational studies choose the correct comparison group (ie, induction of labor vs expectant management), studies have shown no difference in cesarean delivery rates at term,[18] irrespective of whether delivery occurs during the early or late-term time period.

Randomized trials of induction near term provide unbiased evidence. There have now been at least 38 such trials and at least 3 systematic reviews.[19–21] These data show that induction of labor at term is not associated with an elevated rate of cesarean or instrumental delivery (**Table 1**). Despite the compelling evidence, this remains a contentious issue among health care professionals and women. Many of the trials included in the systematic reviews are for induction in postdate pregnancies or high-risk groups (eg, hypertensive disorders) rather than low-risk women. The ARRIVE trial, an RCT of induction of labor at 39 weeks versus expectant

Table 1
Rates of cesarean delivery and instrumental delivery in prospective randomized studies and systematic reviews of induction of labor at term

Study	Gestational Age (y)	Cesarean Delivery OR/RR	95% CI	Instrumental Delivery OR/RR	95% CI
Wood et al,[20] 2013	37–42	0.83	0.76, 0.92	1.09	0.98, 1.22
Saccone & Berghella,[21] 2015	39–40	1.25	0.75, 2.08	1.22	0.83, 1.81
Stock et al,[18] 2012	37	1.02	0.89, 1.17	0.93	0.81, 1.06
	38	1.03	0.94, 1.13	0.95	0.87, 1.04
	39	1.08	1.00, 1.16	0.98	0.91, 1.05
	40	0.83	0.79, 0.88	0.85	0.82, 0.89
	41	0.66	0.63, 0.69	0.78	0.74, 0.81
Mishanina et al,[19] 2014	37–41	0.87	0.82–0.92	Not applicable	Not applicable

Abbreviation: RR, relative risk.

management for over 6000 low-risk nulliparous women has shown that induction of labor is associated with a significant reduction in cesarean delivery (18% vs 22%, RR 0.84, 95% CI 0.76 - 0.93).[22]

Are there other maternal risks you can mention briefly? They are discussed briefly later but are worth mentioning here in this context, such as the risk of preeclampsia and so forth, which increases at term, and whether or not expectant management versus a plan to outright deliver at 39 weeks might be associated with an elevated risk for preeclampsia, eclampsia, and so forth.

HOW SHOULD WE DELIVER?

Now that the authors have considered when to deliver at term, they explore the mode of delivery. The choice that exists is not elective cesarean versus vaginal birth. It is elective cesarean versus *trial* of vaginal birth, as the latter may or may not succeed. A planned trial of vaginal birth is accomplished either by induction of labor or expectant management (ie, waiting until the spontaneous onset of labor or until the development of a medical problem that mandated induction). First, the authors explore the risks of induction of labor itself (not the method used).

Induction of Labor

The authors have already examined induction of labor versus expectant management in terms of risk of cesarean delivery, but induction of labor is associated with other potential complications for the mother and her fetus. Risks to the mother during induction include failed induction, cord prolapse during amniotomy due to a poorly engaged presenting part, maternal pain, placental abruption due to rapid decompression of the uterine cavity at amniotomy, and uterine hyperstimulation. Fortunately, these complications are uncommon.

Cord prolapse

Umbilical cord prolapse complicates 1.25 to 2.1 per 1000 deliveries.[23,24] In one retrospective study of 57 cases over a 10-year period, cord prolapse occurred with amniotomy in 42% of cases.[23] However, does amniotomy increase the risk of cord prolapse? A retrospective case control study of 37 patients of intrapartum umbilical cord prolapse and 74 matched control patients with intact membranes found that the use of amniotomy in patients who had a cord prolapse was similar between groups.[25] A larger retrospective case control study in which 80 patients of umbilical cord prolapse were matched with 800 controls found that amniotomy was not associated with umbilical cord prolapse; in contrast, there was a 9-fold increased risk of umbilical cord prolapse associated with spontaneous rupture of membranes.[26] Umbilical cord prolapse is associated with significant morbidity to both the mother and the fetus, as emergent cesarean delivery is indicated as soon as possible after detection.

Uterine hyperstimulation

Uterine hyperstimulation is generally defined as more than 5 contractions in 10 minutes or contractions lasting more than 2 minutes. This complication arises in approximately 1% to 5% of cases whereby pharmacologic agents are used to induce labor[27] and may also occur in spontaneous labor. It may occur with or without fetal heart rate changes. During uterine contractions, blood flow to the intervillous space (where oxygen exchange between the mother and the fetus occurs) is interrupted.[28] Between contractions, in the relaxation phase, blood flow, and, thus, oxygen exchange, is restored. If the interval between contractions is reduced, or if the duration of the contractions increase, then a critical point may be reached whereby fetal hypoxemia ensues. Simpson and James[28] found that uterine hyperstimulation was associated with significant fetal oxygen desaturation and nonreassuring fetal heart rate changes.

Maternal pain
There is evidence that induced labor is more painful than spontaneous labor. UK data on analgesia in labor reveal that women who deliver vaginally who have an induced labor are more than twice as likely to request epidural anesthesia as women in spontaneous labor (21% vs 8%[17]). One small study (n = 61) by Capogna and colleagues[29] found that the minimum effective analgesic dosage of sufentanil (a synthetic opioid) given via an epidural for women with an induced labor was 1.3 times greater than in women with a spontaneous onset of labor (P = .0014). In the authors' RCT of 195 primiparous women aged 35 years or older comparing labor induction at 39 weeks of gestation versus expectant management, they observed a higher rate of epidural usage in women in the induction arm (35%) than the expectant management arm (29%), though this failed to reach statistical significance (P = .11).[30]

Labor duration
It is difficult to perform meaningful comparisons of the duration of labor between induced and spontaneous labor even in randomized trials. Women undergoing induction of labor have a clear time of onset (eg, the time of insertion of prostaglandin, a balloon catheter, or amniotomy). In contrast, the time of onset for women in spontaneous labor is difficult to define. In a large retrospective observational study of low-risk women comparing approximately 10,000 women who labored spontaneously with 1000 women who underwent labor induction for no apparent medical indication, induction was not associated with a prolonged labor. However, induction was associated with a longer admission-to-delivery interval and the maternal total length of stay was 0.34 days longer with induction compared with spontaneous labor (P≤.0001).[14] Findings were similar in a retrospective study of 2681 low-risk multiparous women, whereby women who were induced had a significantly shorter labor than those who labored spontaneously (99 minutes vs 161 minutes, P≤.001).[31]

MODE OF DELIVERY
Cesarean Delivery

To avoid these complications of induction of labor, should we offer elective cesarean delivery? In 2013, the National Institute for Health and Clinical Excellence introduced new guidance on maternal requests for cesarean delivery stating that "if after discussion and offer of support, a vaginal birth is still not an acceptable option, offer a planned [cesarean section] CS."[32] Rates of cesarean delivery performed primarily for maternal request vary by country. In the United Kingdom in 2001, 7% of all cesareans were elective for maternal request.[33] Although there is a paucity of data in the literature to know whether these rates have recently increased, overall cesarean delivery rates in the United Kingdom have remained stable (2012 25.5%, 2015 26.5%). It is imperative that the comparison groups are carefully examined when evaluating observational data on vaginal delivery versus planned cesarean. The best comparison is planned cesarean delivery versus planned vaginal delivery (ie, an intention-to-treat approach). Some women in the planned vaginal delivery group will deliver by unplanned cesarean delivery.

Benefits to cesarean delivery
Avoidance of perineal trauma An elective cesarean delivery avoids the risk of perineal trauma associated with vaginal delivery. Perineal trauma of varying degrees occurs in 85% of women who give birth vaginally in the United Kingdom. Obstetric anal

sphincter injury, composed of third- and fourth-degree tears, is diagnosed in 3.0% of primiparous women and 0.8% of multiparous women following a vaginal delivery, though its true incidence is likely to be 11.0%.[34] One randomized study with clear unbiased data (the Twin Birth study) had no cases (0%) of obstetric anal sphincter injury in the planned cesarean delivery group and 4 cases (0.3%) in the planned vaginal delivery group.[35]

Reduction in urinary and fecal incontinence and pelvic organ prolapse There is less certainty when it comes to the matter of long-term urogynecologic outcomes, including urinary and fecal incontinence and pelvic organ prolapse.[34] In the case of stress urinary incontinence, any protection offered by a planned cesarean delivery is reduced by advancing age, multiple cesarean deliveries (no protection if ≥3), cesarean deliveries performed in labor and future vaginal births. Even women with all deliveries by cesarean delivery are not immune to developing these complications. Vaginal delivery may lead to an impairment in anal function in 2 ways: obstetric anal sphincter injury and pudendal neuropathy. This latter mechanism may explain why, although planned cesarean delivery has been shown to be protective against obstetric anal sphincter injury,[36] it may not be completely protective against anal dysfunction. In a questionnaire study of 1336 women aged 40 to 60 years, there was no association between vaginal delivery (as opposed to cesarean delivery) and self-reporting of symptoms of anal dysfunction.[37]

The Term Breech Trial found lower rates of urinary incontinence at 3 months post partum among women in the planned cesarean delivery group (36 of 798 women in the cesarean group [4.5%] and 58 out of 797 women in the planned vaginal delivery [7.3%]; relative risk [RR] 0.62; 95% CI 0.41–0.93),[38] but at 2 years post partum, the rates of urinary incontinence were not significantly different between groups (81 of 457 women in the cesarean group [17.8%] and 100 of 460 women in the planned vaginal delivery [21.8%]; RR 0.81; 95% CI 0.63–1.06).[39] The Term Breech Trial found no significant difference in self-reported rates of fecal or flatus incontinence between groups at 3 months or 2 years.[38,39] Thus, there is insufficient evidence to recommend a planned cesarean delivery to reduce the risk of stress urinary incontinence.

A large observational study looking at the risk factors for pelvic organ prolapse found that parity was the most significant independent risk factor and the risk increases with each successive baby (**Fig. 1**).[40]

Although parity has a significant role in the risk of pelvic organ prolapse, is planned cesarean delivery protective? A large questionnaire study of more than 4000 women measured self-reported pelvic organ prolapse and found there was no significant

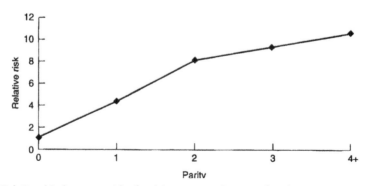

Fig. 1. Relationship between risk of pelvic organ prolapse and parity.

difference in the rate of prolapse between nulliparous women and parous women who had delivered by cesarean. However, the risk was increased in parous women who had delivered vaginally. When comparing parous women who had delivered by cesarean versus parous women who had delivered vaginally, the adjusted OR (aOR) was 1.82 (CI 1.04–3.19). When comparing parous women who had delivered vaginally versus nulliparous women, the aOR was 3.21 (CI 1.96–5.26). The findings were similar in another large questionnaire study of 2000 women, whereby the OR increased with increasing numbers of vaginal births (cesarean only OR 1.6 [0.4–6.4], 1 vaginal birth OR 2.8 [1.1–7.2], 2 vaginal births OR 4.1 [1.8–9.5], 3 or more vaginal births OR 5.3 [2.3–12.5]). From the observational data, there seems to be an association between vaginal delivery and self-reporting of pelvic organ prolapse.

Risks of cesarean delivery
Cesarean delivery constitutes major abdominal surgery and carries both short- and long-term risks, summarized in **Table 2**.

Lilford and colleagues[41] explored the risks of maternal mortality associated with vaginal delivery, elective cesarean, and emergency cesarean excluding women with medical or life-threatening antenatal complications. They found that the risk of maternal mortality for cesarean versus vaginal delivery was 5:1 and emergency cesarean versus elective cesarean was 1.5:1. The main reason vaginal delivery is safer than cesarean delivery is not the comparison between the first cesarean delivery and first vaginal birth but the exponential increase in risks associated with subsequent cesarean deliveries summarized with the phrase "the first cut is not the deepest."

Placenta previa and the morbidly adherent placenta The maternal and neonatal morbidity and mortality associated with placenta previa and placenta accrete are considerable. Rates of both conditions are increasing because of the increasing cesarean delivery rate and increasing maternal age. This increase is because the placenta is less likely to migrate upward with the development of the lower uterine segment if there is a scar in it. Placenta previa is associated with an increased risk of major obstetric hemorrhage (≥1000 mL blood loss; OR 13.1, 95% CI 7.47–23.0),[42] massive obstetric hemorrhage (≥1500 mL blood loss) (21%),[43] need for blood

Table 2
Summary of short- and longer-term risks of cesarean delivery versus vaginal delivery

Studies Suggest May be Reduced by Vaginal Delivery	Studies Give Conflicting Evidence	Studies Suggest No Difference	Studies Suggest May be Reduced by Cesarean Delivery
• Length of maternal hospital stay • Peripartum hysterectomy due to postpartum hemorrhage • Cardiac arrest	• Maternal death • Deep vein thrombosis • Blood transfusion • Infection • Hysterectomy • Anesthetic complications	• Perineal and abdominal pain at 4 mo post partum • Injury to urinary tract • Injury to cervix • Iatrogenic surgical injury • Pulmonary embolism • Wound infection • Intraoperative trauma • Uterine trauma • Assisted ventilation or intubation • Acute renal failure	• Perineal and abdominal pain during birth and at 3 d post partum • Vaginal trauma • Early postpartum hemorrhage • Obstetric shock

transfusion, and need for peripartum hysterectomy (11%). The risks with placenta accreta are profound. Women with the placenta accrete spectrum are at high risk for an indicated preterm delivery, which most commonly occurs by planned cesarean hysterectomy, and are at risk for major or massive obstetric hemorrhage, urologic (bladder, ureteral) injury, and other complications. Risks of placenta accrete spectrum increase exponentially with the number of prior cesarean deliveries and are highest among women with multiple prior cesarean deliveries and placenta previa.

Uterine scar dehiscence or rupture Uterine rupture is associated with maternal and perinatal morbidity and mortality. A landmark observational study by Landon and colleagues[44] examined the maternal and perinatal outcomes of vaginal birth after cesarean delivery versus elective repeat cesarean delivery and showed that the risk of uterine rupture associated with vaginal birth after one cesarean delivery was 0.7%. Twelve babies whose mothers had a trial of vaginal birth developed hypoxic ischemic encephalopathy (0.08%); of those 12 cases, 7 were associated with uterine rupture. Thirty-five women (0.2%) had a hysterectomy (5 cases were performed for irreparable rupture), and 3 women (0.02%) died (of which no cases were associated with uterine rupture). In a large observational study of 159 cases of uterine rupture in the United Kingdom from 2009 to 10, 2 women (1.3%) died and 18 perinatal deaths associated with uterine rupture occurred (12.0%).[45]

Antepartum stillbirth in subsequent pregnancy There is an association between cesarean delivery in the first pregnancy and unexplained antepartum stillbirth in the second pregnancy. Smith and colleagues[46] found that the risk of unexplained antepartum stillbirth at 39 weeks' or greater gestation was 1.1 per 1000 women who had had a previous cesarean delivery versus 0.5 per 1000 women in those who had delivered vaginally. The investigators postulate this association may be due to impaired uterine vasculature due to previous surgery, abnormal placentation, and subsequent uteroplacental dysfunction.

WHY SHOULD WE DELIVER?
Specific Indications for Delivery at Term

Reduced fetal movements and stillbirth prevention
Raised awareness of reduced fetal movements is one of the 4 key elements of the Saving Babies Lives care bundle implemented across the United Kingdom to try to reduce antepartum stillbirths.[47] In the confidential inquiry into term antepartum stillbirths, in just less than half of a random sample of stillbirths reviewed by an expert panel women reported decreased fetal movement.[48] In a third of those stillbirths, a major failure of care was identified; in the remaining cases, there were also lesser deficiencies in care identified. In a retrospective cohort study in New Zealand comparing fetal movement data from women with late stillbirth with women with ongoing pregnancies at the same gestational age as the stillbirth had occurred, decreased fetal movement was associated with an increased risk of late stillbirth (aOR 2.37, 95% CI 1.29–4.35).[49] The results of this study must be interpreted with caution, as the study is limited by recall bias. Although the association between decreased and antepartum stillbirth is clear, complaints of reduced fetal movements are common and subjective; it is uncertain how to differentiate pathologic decreased movements from a more transient situation. One Norwegian quality-improvement study implemented a policy of (1) providing written information about reduced fetal movements, (2) an invitation to monitor fetal movement, and (3) a guideline for health professionals on the management of reduced fetal movement across 14 hospitals.[50] They found a reduction in

the stillbirth rate among women with reduced fetal movement during the intervention (4.2% versus 2.4%; OR 0.51 95%, CI 0.32–0.81) and an overall reduction in the stillbirth rate in the whole study population 3.0 per 1000 versus 2.0 per 1000 (OR 0.67, 95% CI 0.48–0.93). What is remarkable was that this was achieved with a reduction in the number of inductions of labor and no change in the rate of cesarean deliveries.

Hypertensive disorders

Hypertensive disorders in pregnancy are common and cause considerable maternal and fetal morbidity and mortality. The Hypertension and Preeclampsia Intervention Trial At Term (HYPITAT), an RCT of induction of labor within 48 hours versus expectant management for women with pregnancy-induced hypertension or mild preeclampsia between 36^{+0} and 41^{+0} weeks found that induction of labor was associated with a reduction in the primary outcome (a composite of poor maternal outcomes).[51] These investigators concluded that induction of labor should be advised at 37 weeks' gestation for women with pregnancy-induced hypertension or mild preeclampsia. However, it is notable that the only individual component of the composite that was statistically significantly increased in the control group versus the induction group was the occurrence of severe hypertension and subsequent need for antihypertensive medication, though the study was likely underpowered to detect less common individual outcomes, such as eclampsia.

Gestational diabetes

The association between pregestational diabetes and stillbirth is widely known.[52] The perinatal mortality rate for women with preexisting diabetes (type 1 or 2) is 32 per 1000, compared with 9 per 1000 in the general population. The guidelines from the United Kingdom National Institute for Health and Care Excellence and the American College of Obstetricians and Gynecologists both recommend that pregnant women with pregestational diabetes be offered medically indicated delivery from 38 weeks.[53] Notably, however, in a retrospective audit of 25 cases of stillbirth in women with type I diabetes mellitus in Denmark, the median gestational age at the time the stillbirth was diagnosed was 35 weeks.[54]

Advanced maternal age

The average age at childbirth in industrialized nations has been steadily increasing for about 30 years.[55] Between 1996 and 2006, births to women older than 35 years have increased from 12% to 20% of all births. In the same year, 5.6% of live births were to nulliparous women older than 35 years.[56] Women older than 35 years are at a higher risk of antepartum and intrapartum stillbirths and neonatal deaths, hypertensive disease, gestational diabetes, placenta previa, and placental abruption.[1,55,57] Further, they are at an increased risk of preterm labor and of bearing macrosomic (>3999 g) or low-birth-weight infants (<2500 g). The women themselves typically think that their age puts their infant at increased risk.[57] Unsurprisingly, they have higher rates of obstetric intervention.

The cesarean delivery rate for nulliparous women older than 35 years in the United Kingdom is 38% and 50% in women older than 40 years.[57] In nulliparous women, the relationship between maternal age and delivery by emergency cesarean is linear.[58]

Stillbirth is an important risk to mitigate among women 35 years old or older because older women are relatively less likely to have future pregnancies. Induction at or before term may be beneficial because 38 weeks is the gestational age of delivery associated with the lowest cumulative risk of perinatal death.[2] Nulliparous women have a higher risk of stillbirth than multiparous women for all maternal age groups.[59,60] It is recognized by obstetricians that older women reach the 41- to 42-week stillbirth risk at which induction is currently offered to all women[27,61] at earlier gestational ages[59]; but as discussed, stillbirth risk is only one risk to consider.

Some obstetricians induce older pregnant women at the due date (40 weeks) (39% women aged 40–44 years, 58% women aged more than 45 years); but of those who do not, one-third are reluctant to offer it for fear of increasing the risk of cesarean despite thinking it will improve perinatal outcomes.[30] The authors conducted an RCT of 619 primiparous women 35 years old or older. Women were randomly assigned to labor induction at 39^{+0} to 39^{+6} weeks' gestation or to expectant management. The primary outcome was cesarean delivery. In an intention-to-treat analysis, there were no significant between-group differences in the percentage of women who underwent a cesarean delivery (98 of 304 women in the induction group [32%] and 103 of 314 women in the expectant-management group [33%]; RR 0.99; 95% CI 0.87–1.14) or in the percentage of women who had a vaginal delivery with the use of forceps or vacuum (115 of 304 women [38%] and 104 of 314 women [33%], respectively; RR 1.30; 95% CI 0.96–1.77). There were no maternal or infant deaths and no significant between-group differences in the women's experience of childbirth or in the frequency of adverse maternal or neonatal outcomes.

In conclusion, the optimal timing of delivery for the baby is 39 weeks, avoiding the morbidity associated with early term birth and reducing the risk of antepartum stillbirth.

There is compelling evidence that among high-risk pregnancies and in settings where cesarean rates are high (>20%), induction of labor at 37 to 40 weeks does not, as previously thought, result in a further increased risk of cesarean delivery. The only advantage to planned cesarean delivery over induction of labor is the avoidance of the morbidity associated with emergency cesarean delivery; controversy exists on the other reported benefits. There is a growing number of well-conducted RCTs that provide some support for induction of labor shortly before term for a variety of indications (hypertensive disorders, gestational diabetes, suspected growth restriction, macrosomia, and advanced maternal age).

REFERENCES

1. CMACE. Centre for Maternal and Child Enquiries (CMACE) perinatal mortality 2009. London: CMACE; 2011.
2. Smith GCS. Life-table analysis of the risk of perinatal death at term and post term in singleton pregnancies. Am J Obstet Gynecol 2001;184(3):489–96.
3. Excellence NIfHaC. Caesarean section. London: National Institute for Health and Care Excellence; 2011. Report no.
4. Heinzmann A, Brugger M, Engels C, et al. Risk factors of neonatal respiratory distress following vaginal delivery and caesarean section in the German population. Acta Paediatr 2009;98(1):25–30.
5. Gundur NM, Kumar P, Sundaram V, et al. Natural history and predictive risk factors of prolonged unconjugated jaundice in the newborn. Pediatr Int 2010;52(5):769–72.
6. Budden A, Chen LJY, Henry A. High-dose versus low-dose oxytocin infusion regimens for induction of labour at term. Cochrane Database Syst Rev 2014;(10):CD009701.
7. Bugg GJ, Siddiqui F, Thornton JG. Oxytocin versus no treatment or delayed treatment for slow progress in the first stage of spontaneous labour. Cochrane Database Syst Rev 2013;(6):CD007123.
8. Shennan AH, Smith R, Browne D, et al. The elective use of oxytocin infusion during labour in nulliparous women using epidural analgesia: a randomised double-blind placebo-controlled trial. Int J Obstet Anesth 1995;4(2):78–81.

9. National Institute for Health and Care Excellence. Jaundice in newborn babies under 28 days. London: National Institute for Health and Care Excellence; 2010.
10. Linder N, Hiersch L, Fridman E, et al. The effect of gestational age on neonatal outcome in low-risk singleton term deliveries. J Matern Fetal Neonatal Med 2015;28(3):297–302.
11. Boulvain M, Senat MV, Perrotin F, et al. Induction of labour versus expectant management for large-for-date fetuses: a randomised controlled trial. Lancet 2015; 385(9987):2600–5.
12. Parikh L, Singh J, Timofeev J, et al. Timing and consequences of early term and late term deliveries. J Matern Fetal Neonatal Med 2014;27(11):1158–62.
13. Frank R, Garfinkle J, Oskoui M, et al. Clinical profile of children with cerebral palsy born term compared with late- and post-term: a retrospective cohort study. BJOG 2017;124(11):1738–45.
14. Glantz JC. Elective induction vs. spontaneous labor. J Reprod Med 2005;50(4): 235–40.
15. Luthy DA, Malmgren JA, Zingheim RW. Cesarean delivery after elective induction in nulliparous women: the physician effect. Am J Obstet Gynecol 2004;191(5): 1511–5.
16. Seyb ST, Berka RJ, Socol ML, et al. Risk of cesarean delivery with elective induction of labor at term in nulliparous women. Obstet Gynecol 1999;94(4):600–7.
17. Hospital Episode Statistics. NHS maternity statistics, 2010-11. London: NHS Digital; 2011.
18. Stock SJ, Ferguson E, Duffy A, et al. Outcomes of elective induction of labour compared with expectant management: population based study. BMJ 2012; 344:e2838.
19. Mishanina E, Rogozinska E, Thatthi T, et al. Use of labour induction and risk of cesarean delivery: a systematic review and meta-analysis. CMAJ 2014;186(9):665–73.
20. Wood S, Cooper S, Ross S. Does induction of labour increase the risk of caesarean section? A systematic review and meta-analysis of trials in women with intact membranes. BJOG 2013;121(6):674–85 [discussion: 685].
21. Saccone G, Berghella V. Induction of labor at full term in uncomplicated singleton gestations: a systematic review and meta-analysis of randomized controlled trials. Am J Obstet Gynecol 2015;213(5):629–36.
22. Grobman W. A randomized trial of elective induction of labor at 39 weeks compared with expectant management of low-risk nulliparous women. Am J Obstet Gynecol 2018;218(1):S601.
23. Alouini S, Mesnard L, Megier P, et al. Management of umbilical cord prolapse and neonatal outcomes. J Gynecol Obstet Biol Reprod (Paris) 2010;39(6):471–7.
24. Dufour P, Vinatier D, Bennani S, et al. Cord prolapse. Review of the literature. A series of 50 cases. J Gynecol Obstet Biol Reprod (Paris) 1996;25(8):841–5 [in French].
25. Roberts WE, Martin RW, Roach HH, et al. Are obstetric interventions such as cervical ripening, induction of labor, amnioinfusion, or amniotomy associated with umbilical cord prolapse? Am J Obstet Gynecol 1997;176(6):1181–3.
26. Dilbaz B, Ozturkoglu E, Dilbaz S, et al. Risk factors and perinatal outcomes associated with umbilical cord prolapse. Arch Gynecol Obstet 2006;274(2):104–7.
27. National Institute for Health and Care Excellence. Induction of labour. London: National Institue for Health and Clinical Excellence; 2008.
28. Simpson KR, James DC. Effects of oxytocin-induced uterine hyperstimulation during labor on fetal oxygen status and fetal heart rate patterns. Am J Obstet Gynecol 2008;199(1):34.e1-5.

29. Capogna G, Parpaglioni R, Lyons G, et al. Minimum analgesic dose of epidural sufentanil for first-stage labor analgesia: a comparison between spontaneous and prostaglandin-induced labors in nulliparous women. Anesthesiology 2001; 94(5):740–4.
30. Walker KF, Bugg GJ, Macpherson M, et al. Induction of labour at term for women over 35 years old: a survey of the views of women and obstetricians. Eur J Obstet Gynecol Reprod Biol 2012;162(2):144–8.
31. Hoffman MK, Vahratian A, Sciscione AC, et al. Comparison of Labor progression between induced and noninduced multiparous women. Obstet Gynecol 2006; 107(5):1029–34.
32. National Institute for Health and Care Excellence. Caesarean section (update). London: National Institute for Health and Care Excellence; 2011. Contract No: CG132.
33. Unit RCES. The national sentinel caesarean section audit report. London: RCOG Press; 2001.
34. Dolan L. An update on damage to the pelvic floor in childbirth. Obstetrician and Gynaecologist 2009;11:157–62.
35. Barrett JFR. A randomized trial of planned cesarean or vaginal delivery for twin pregnancy. N Engl J Med 2013;369(24):1295.
36. Sultan AH, Kamm MA, Hudson CN, et al. Anal-sphincter disruption during vaginal delivery. N Engl J Med 1993;329(26):1905–11.
37. Uustal Fornell E, Wingren G, Kjølhede P. Factors associated with pelvic floor dysfunction with emphasis on urinary and fecal incontinence and genital prolapse: an epidemiological study. Acta Obstet Gynecol Scand 2004;83(4):383–9.
38. Hannah ME, Hannah WJ, Hodnett ED, et al. Outcomes at 3 months after planned cesarean vs planned vaginal delivery for breech presentation at term - the international randomized Term Breech Trial. JAMA 2002;287(14):1822–31.
39. Hannah ME, Whyte H, Hannah WJ, et al. Maternal outcomes at 2 years after planned cesarean section versus planned vaginal birth for breech presentation at term: the international randomized Term Breech Trial. Am J Obstet Gynecol 2004;191(3):917–27.
40. Mant J, Painter R, Vessey M. Epidemiology of genital prolapse: observations from the Oxford family planning association study. Br J Obstet Gynaecol 1997;104(5): 579–85.
41. Lilford RJ, Degroot HAV, Moore PJ, et al. The relative risks of cesarean-section (intrapartum and elective) and vaginal delivery - a detailed analysis to exclude the effects of medical disorders and other acute preexisting physiological disturbances. Br J Obstet Gynaecol 1990;97(10):883–92.
42. Stones R, Paterson C, Saunders N. Risk factors for major obstetric haemorrhage. Eur J Obstet Gynecol Reprod Biol 1993;48(1):15–8.
43. Royal College of Obstetricians and Gynaecologists. Caesarean section for placenta praevia. London: Royal College of Obstetricians and Gynaecologists; 2010.
44. Landon MB, Spong CY, Thom E, et al. Risk of uterine rupture with a trial of labor in women with multiple and single prior cesarean delivery. Obstet Gynecol 2006; 108(1):12–20.
45. Fitzpatrick KE, Kurinczuk JJ, Alfirevic Z, et al. Uterine rupture by intended mode of delivery in the UK: a national case-control study. PLoS Med 2012;9(3): e1001184.
46. Smith GCS, Pell JP, Dobbie R. Caesarean section and risk of unexplained stillbirth in subsequent pregnancy. Lancet 2003;362(9398):1779–84.

47. NHS England. Saving babies' lives: a care bundle for reducing stillbirth. Leeds (UK): NHS England; 2016.
48. Mothers and Babies: Reducing Risk through Audits and Confidential Enquiries across the UK (MBRRACE-UK collaboration). Term, singleton, normally-formed, antepartum stillbirth. Leicester (UK): University of Leicester; 2015.
49. Stacey T, Thompson JMD, Mitchell EA, et al. Maternal perception of fetal activity and late stillbirth risk: findings from the Auckland stillbirth study. Birth 2011;38(4): 311–6.
50. Tveit JVH, Saastad E, Stray-Pedersen B, et al. Reduction of late stillbirth with the introduction of fetal movement information and guidelines - a clinical quality improvement. BMC Pregnancy Childbirth 2009;9:32.
51. Koopmans CM, Bijlenga D, Groen H, et al. Induction of labor versus expectant monitoring for gestational hypertension or mild preeclampsia after 36 weeks' gestation (HYPITAT): a multicentre, open-label randomized controlled trial EDITORIAL COMMENT. Obstet Gynecol Surv 2009;64(12):776–8.
52. Mathiesen ER, Ringholm L, Damm P. Stillbirth in diabetic pregnancies. Best Pract Res Clin Obstet Gynaecol 2011;25(1):105–11.
53. National Institute for Health and Care Excellence. Diabetes in pregnancy: management of diabetes and its complications from pre-conception to the postnatal period. London: National Institute for Health and Care Excellence; 2008.
54. Lauenborg J, Mathiesen E, Ovesen P, et al. Audit on stillbirths in women with pre-gestational type 1 diabetes. Diabetes Care 2003;26(5):1385–9.
55. Jacobsson B, Ladfors L, Milsom I. Advanced maternal age and adverse perinatal outcome. Obstet Gynecol 2004;104(4):727–33.
56. Office for National Statistics. Data on first births. In: Walker K, editor. Fertility analysis unit. London: ONS Centre for Demography; 2006.
57. Joseph KS, Allen AC, Dodds L, et al. The perinatal effects of delayed childbearing. Obstet Gynecol 2005;105(6):1410–8.
58. Smith GCS, Cordeaux Y, White IR, et al. The effect of delaying childbirth on primary cesarean section rates. PLoS Med 2008;5(7):1123–32.
59. Reddy UM, Ko CW, Willinger M. Maternal age and the risk of stillbirth throughout pregnancy in the United States. Am J Obstet Gynecol 2006;195(3):764–70.
60. Raymond EG, Cnattingius S, Kiely JL. Effects of maternal age, parity, and smoking on the risk of stillbirth. Br J Obstet Gynaecol 1994;101(4):301–6.
61. Gulmezoglu AM, Crowther CA, Middleton P. Induction of labour for improving birth outcomes for women at or beyond term. Cochrane Database Syst Rev 2006;(4):CD004945.

Perinatal Care of Infants with Congenital Birth Defects

Elizabeth K. Sewell, MD, MPH, Sarah Keene, MD*

KEYWORDS

- Congenital anomalies • Congenital heart disease • CDH • Perinatal management
- Resuscitation

KEY POINTS

- Prenatal imaging has allowed for in utero diagnosis of congenital anomalies.
- Most neonates with congenital anomalies need only standard resuscitation, but the availability of advanced care is crucial.
- In utero intervention and specialized delivery are indicated for a small proportion of patients.
- Standardization of care using clinical algorithms might be beneficial to neonatal outcomes.

INTRODUCTION

Perinatal care for infants with congenital birth defects has changed dramatically over the past century. Previously, infants with congenital anomalies presented at birth if defect(s) were obvious on physical examination, and in the neonatal period or childhood if the defect or defects were more subtle. Delayed diagnosis is associated with worse outcomes for certain anomalies, but this is dependent on the type and severity of the anomaly and which outcome is being evaluated.[1,2] Prenatal diagnosis allows for changes in perinatal management to benefit the newborn, including increased monitoring, counseling, changes in the mode and timing of delivery, fetal intervention, and planning for postnatal care.[1] However, definitive data are rare and documented improvement is limited to a few diagnoses.[2–4] In the last decade, interventions aimed at preventing mortality have transitioned to those aimed at improving quality of life, complicating the ethical concerns regarding maternal well-being and autonomy, as well as research and innovation.[5,6]

Disclosure Statement: The authors have no relevant financial disclosures.
Emory Children's Center Neonatology Offices, 2015 Uppergate Drive-3rd floor, Atlanta, GA 30322, USA
* Corresponding author.
E-mail address: skeene@emory.edu

Clin Perinatol 45 (2018) 213–230
https://doi.org/10.1016/j.clp.2018.01.007
0095-5108/18/© 2018 Elsevier Inc. All rights reserved.

PRENATAL DIAGNOSIS AND MANAGEMENT
Prenatal Imaging and Diagnosis

Prenatal obstetric management changed dramatically with the application of ultrasound technology in the 1960s, and subsequently, Doppler sonography and 3-dimensional ultrasound.[1,7] Incorporation of ultrasound into routine pregnancy management allows for dating, detection of multiples, evaluation of growth, monitoring of well-being, and diagnosis of congenital anomalies and aneuploidy. Although widely available and cost-effective, ultrasound is limited by gestational age, maternal body habitus, amniotic fluid volume, image resolution, and fetal positioning.[1] The development of fetal MRI has helped overcome some of these limitations and allows for more detailed visualization. However, fetal MRI is not routinely used except for in limited circumstances when a fetal anomaly is known or strongly suspected, but further visualization beyond that which can be obtained with ultrasound is needed. More widespread use of fetal MRI is limited because of concerns regarding cost, access to equipment, and lack of trained personnel to acquire and interpret images.[1,8]

Referrals

Infants with an anomaly diagnosed as likely to impact the neonatal period should be referred to perinatology (maternal-fetal medicine).[6] Perinatologists provide counseling, follow-up, and further referral to consultation with neonatology, pediatric subspecialists, or a fetal care center as appropriate. Fetal care centers evolved through a collaborative approach between subspecialties; referral is typically indicated if the fetus is a candidate for fetal intervention or if immediate postdelivery care will be required. Centers vary in the services offered: some are multidisciplinary clinics offering diagnostic services and prenatal consultation, whereas others also offer pregnancy management, fetoscopic interventions, or open surgeries.[9]

Anticipatory Guidance and Counseling

Prenatal diagnosis of an anomaly allows for education of the family, including anticipatory guidance and likely decisions on care. Providers should attempt to present options with minimal bias, which may include prenatal intervention, postnatal treatment, palliative care, or termination of pregnancy.[6] Perinatologists and obstetricians, pediatric subspecialists, pediatric surgeons, and neonatologists can all provide unique and area-specific counseling and recommendations.[10] Counseling varies among and within different specialties; thus, it is important to ensure a coordinated approach.[10,11] Social workers, genetic counselors, and palliative care services also provide support to families. Evidence is limited regarding whether parental stress is lower if the diagnosis is made in the prenatal compared with postnatal time period, but studies have demonstrated that comprehensive, multidisciplinary counseling on fetal anomalies after diagnosis can decrease maternal anxiety.[1,2,10]

Maternal and Fetal Monitoring

Close fetal surveillance with ultrasound, nonstress testing, and potentially advanced imaging can provide updates on evolution of the disease process and fetal well-being.[2] Development or progression of intrauterine growth restriction or hydrops is a common complication of some congenital anomalies that may prompt early delivery. It is also important to monitor for maternal "mirror syndrome" with hydrops.[8] If fetal intervention occurs, the mother should be monitored closely for complications, such as uterine dehiscence or premature rupture of membranes.

FETAL INTERVENTIONS
Fetal Transfusions and Maternal Medications

The first successful fetal intervention was the intraperitoneal fetal transfusion by Sir William Liley in 1963.[12,13] Improved survival has been achieved with the development of intravascular fetal transfusions and a staged approach to correct severe fetal anemia. Fetal anemia remains one of the most common and successful conditions able to be corrected by fetal interventions in the United States.[12] Fetal arrhythmias lend themselves to noninvasive treatment options. For example, administration of maternal antiarrhythmics that cross the placenta (such as flecainide or digoxin) can be used to treat fetal tachyarrhythmias. Success has been demonstrated with conversion to sinus rhythm in most cases and even reversal of hydrops fetalis, with limited maternal risk.[14,15] Treatment of fetal anemia and arrhythmia remain archetypal examples but have not been duplicated for other diseases.

Open and Endoscopic Fetal Surgery

Initial fetal surgical interventions were open procedures that required a hysterotomy, causing substantial risks for the mother, and a high risk for preterm delivery.[5,16] Recognition of this risk-benefit balance shifted fetal interventions toward minimally invasive techniques.[10] Requirements for fetal intervention include accurate and timely diagnosis, known natural history of the disease with a reasonable probability of benefit with intervention, and a technically feasible fetal procedure.[13,17,18] Significant progress in prenatal imaging, molecular diagnosis, and postnatal management has influenced the risks and benefits of fetal intervention.[13,17] When preterm delivery is indicated, antenatal betamethasone and magnesium sulfate, and postnatal surfactant reduce the risks of prematurity-related complications.[13] In addition, the challenges of recruiting patients for randomized controlled trials targeting specific fetal anomalies frequently limit the evidence for the effect on postnatal outcome.[2] Common prenatal diagnoses and fetal interventions are listed in **Table 1**.

DELIVERY PLANNING

For most, spontaneous vaginal delivery is the goal because of the lower maternal morbidity and mortality.[8] Cases where preterm delivery is recommended are rare given the risks of prematurity, the most likely indication is declining fetal status.[1,67] Planned induction may be beneficial if the patient lives far from a tertiary care center.[8] Cesarean section is generally indicated where there is concern for dystocia, bleeding, or disruption of a protective sac. Examples include giant omphaloceles, severe hydrocephalus, large myelomeningocele, and teratomas. Ex utero intrapartum treatment (EXIT) may be offered for complex airway masses but carries much higher maternal risk than a cesarean section.[1,27] Finally, the location is important: it is typically safest to transport the mother before delivery to a hospital with the needed level of care, because neonatal transport has inherent risk.

Facilities now exist that provide delivery services and comprehensive care, including neonatal surgery, such as delivery units contained within a children's hospital. For a very select, very high-risk group of patients who need immediate treatment at delivery, this may have a significant benefit, such as a planned EXIT or need for an immediate Rashkind procedure.[56,64] Such facilities decrease risks of neonatal transport and lessen maternal child separation, but are not always available.[90] The vast majority of infants can be safely cared for in a tertiary center: All infants with prenatally diagnosed anomalies expected to cause symptoms in the neonatal period should be delivered at a center experienced in caring for these patients.[2,8]

Table 1
Perinatal management of specific congenital anomalies

Congenital Anomaly	Fetal Management & Intervention	Delivery Timing & Mode	Delivery Room Management & Stabilization	Alteration of Perinatal Management due to Prenatal Diagnosis	Alteration of Neonatal Outcome due to Prenatal Diagnosis
Abdominal Wall Defects					
• Omphalocele • Gastroschisis	• No fetal intervention • Monitor for intrauterine growth restriction, oligohydramnios, & evidence of bowel dilation or suspected necrosis • Fetal echocardiogram & karyotype in omphalocele due to association with other anomalies[8,19,20]	• Cesarean delivery frequently recommended for large omphaloceles to prevent dystocia or sac rupture. Bowel injury can occur in either delivery modality • Vaginal delivery is safe for gastroschisis • Early delivery rarely indicated; consider early term delivery in gastroschisis due to risk of stillbirth[8,19,21-25]	• Immediate gastric decompression, consideration of early intubation especially for giant omphaloceles • Saline-soaked gauze & plastic bag/wrap available to cover defect • Attention to fluid loss and thermoregulation • Peripheral intravenous line, avoid umbilical catheters • Pediatric surgery assessment soon after delivery[8,19,23]	• Yes. Delivery mode & preparedness	• Unknown. Dilated bowel associated with worse outcome but no studies demonstrating improved outcome with earlier delivery[25]
Airway Masses and Malformations					
• Teratomas • Lymphangiomas • Micrognathia • Congenital high airway obstruction	• Monitoring and advanced imaging • Evaluation for evidence of hydrops • Signs of significant airway compromise (anatomy scans, polyhydramnios) may require specialized delivery[26,27]	• Cesarean delivery with EXIT procedure for significant concern for airway obstruction, usually at 34-37 wk[27,28]	• EXIT procedure for intubation, resection, or tracheostomy in selected cases[26-28] • Otolaryngology available for some deliveries if EXIT not appropriate[29]	• Yes. Delivery location, & preparedness, including otolaryngology presence & EXIT in select cases	• Yes. Multiple infants have survived typically lethal anomalies (eg, congenital high airway obstruction syndrome) with EXIT, consensus opinion; trials not considered appropriate[26,27,30]

Diaphragm Abnormalities

• Congenital diaphragmatic hernia (CDH)	• No prenatal interventions universally recommended, betamethasone for premature infants only[31] • Increasing evidence for fetal endoscopic tracheal occlusion (FETO) in severe, isolated left CDH (typically LHR <1, O/E <25%)[32,33] • Consider karyotype particularly in nonisolated CDH • Imaging provides prognosis based on suspected degree of pulmonary hypoplasia	• Delivery at term if possible, prematurity is a risk factor for mortality • No specific delivery mode[34,35] • Delivery at a tertiary care center with standardized protocol recommended, consider planned delivery/induction at >39 wk[36,37] • EXIT to extracorporeal membrane oxygenation offered at some centers in severe cases, of unclear benefit[38]	• Consensus expert opinion recommends immediate intubation and gastric decompression[37,39] • Standardized treatment protocol strongly recommended typically including gentle ventilation, judicious oxygen administration (target saturation 85%–95%), and avoiding paralysis[37,40,41] • Conventional ventilation superior to HFOV[42]	• Yes. Delivery preparedness & location. Potential role for fetal intervention	• Yes. Multiple cohort studies have shown increased survival with standardized protocol.[37,40] • Potentially. One RCT & cohort studies with improved survival with FETO in most severe patients, but high risk of complications[32,33]

Esophageal Abnormalities

• Esophageal atresia • Tracheoesophageal fistula (TEF)	• TEF difficult to diagnose accurately prenatally by US; fetal MR can aid in diagnosis • No fetal interventions offered for TEF[43,44]	• No evidence to support change in delivery timing or management with prenatal diagnosis of TEF without additional anomalies	• A suction catheter is placed into esophageal pouch • Avoid initiation of oral feedings in infants with known TEF, potentially reducing the risk of aspiration[45–47]	• Potentially. Change in neonatal management with avoidance of oral feedings	• Unknown. No studies demonstrating improved outcome with prenatal diagnosis of TEF[46,48]

(continued on next page)

Table 1
(continued)

Heart Disease: Fetal Arrhythmias

Congenital Anomaly	Fetal Management & Intervention	Delivery Timing & Mode	Delivery Room Management & Stabilization	Alteration of Perinatal Management due to Prenatal Diagnosis	Alteration of Neonatal Outcome due to Prenatal Diagnosis
• Supraventricular tachycardia (SVT) • Atrial flutter (AF) • Congenital heart block (CHB) (maternal autoimmune disease most common)	• Maternal administration of digoxin, sotalol, or flecainide if persistent, second-line dual therapy in SVT/AF[14,15] • Monitoring of PR interval in antibody-positive mothers; dexamethasone *may* slow progression in 1st- or 2nd-degree CHB[49,50] • No efficacious treatments for 3rd-degree CHB, close monitoring[51,52]	• Term delivery unless there are indicators of significant fetal compromise[53] • Early delivery may be indicated for refractory SVT with hydrops[53] • CHB: HR <55 is a risk factor for fetal death[54,55] • Delivery may be indicated for development of dilated cardiomyopathy or hydrops fetalis[52,54]	• Routine delivery room care sufficient unless heart failure or hydrops • Medication or direct conversion for symptomatic infant[53] • Central access for monitoring, supportive care • In severe cases of CHB (HR <50 or concurrent CHD) cardiologist present for initiation of transepicardial pacing[54,56]	• Yes. Maternal treatment as well as delivery location & preparedness	• Yes. Conversion to sinus rhythm in >70% of medically treated infants with reversal of hydrops fetalis in cases[14,15] • Unknown. Conflicting data for maternal dexamethasone.[49,50] Case reports of success of pacing[57]; mortality remains high[55]

Heart Disease: Structural Defects

• Hypoplastic left heart (HLHS) • Transposition of the great arteries (TGA) • Total anomalous pulmonary venous return (TAPVR) • Tetralogy of Fallot (TOF)/pulmonary stenosis (PS) • Coarctation of the aorta (CoA) • Ventricular septal defect (VSD) • Atrioventricular canal (AVC)	• Fetal echo/monitoring, including markers predictive of need for immediate intervention[58,59] • Fetal cardiac intervention (typically US-guided balloon dilation) offered in some cases (severe valvular disease, HLHS with restrictive atrial septum)[60]	• Vaginal delivery at term if possible as prematurity and low birth weight risk factors for death[59,61] • Low-risk lesions (VSD, AVC) can deliver at local centers • Delivery at a tertiary care center for patients likely to need neonatal intervention, consider planned delivery/induction at term[59,62] • Delivery at a center with surgical capabilities if available if immediate treatment required (TAPVR, TGA, TOF/APV)[56]	• Supportive care and central access depending on diagnosis, availability of pediatric cardiology[59] • Prostaglandin (PGE) infusion started just after birth for known or suspected PGE-dependent pulmonary or systemic blood flow (HLHS, PS, CoA) • Immediate transfer for intervention/surgery in selected patients[56] • Elective intubation due to PGE infusion not recommended[63]	• Yes. Delivery location & preparedness	• Yes. Echo 47%–70% predictive of need for immediate intervention.[64] Improved neurologic outcomes, mortality with prenatal diagnosis in select patients (TGA, HLHS)[4,65] • Potentially. Case series with improved survival following emergent intervention[56] and fetal intervention with HLHS/RAS[60]

(continued on next page)

Table 1
(continued)

Congenital Anomaly	Fetal Management & Intervention	Delivery Timing & Mode	Delivery Room Management & Stabilization	Alteration of Perinatal Management due to Prenatal Diagnosis	Alteration of Neonatal Outcome due to Prenatal Diagnosis
Hydrops Fetalis					
• Identifiable cause (eg, SVT, anemia, congenital pulmonary airway malformation [CPAM]) • Idiopathic	• Prenatal intervention indicated if treatable cause is identified[66] • Monitoring middle cerebral artery Dopplers for those at risk of anemia, intrauterine transfusion (IUT) for severe anemia[67] • Genetic testing. No indication/evidence for intervention for idiopathic hydrops[68]	• Anemia: Consider late preterm or early term (35+ wk) delivery if further IUT planned, balance risks of prematurity with risk of IUT[67] • Delivery at term if possible, consider cesarean delivery for severe ascites	• Team should be available for advanced resuscitation. • Intubation and aggressive support typically required • Pleurocentesis or paracentesis may be attempted; success depends on underlying disease and degree of pulmonary hypoplasia[66,68]	• Potentially. Delivery location & preparedness	• Yes. Reversal of hydrops described and >90% survival for IUT in severe anemia, some increased ND disability[3] • No. Aggressive intervention does not improve survival in idiopathic cases,[68] high mortality[66,69]
Intestinal Atresias					
• Duodenal atresia • Jejunal atresia • Ileal atresia • Colonic atresia	• Prenatal diagnosis of proximal atresias easier than distal[47] • No fetal interventions	• No evidence to support change in delivery timing or management[47]	• A suction catheter in the stomach • Gastric decompression and avoidance of oral feedings	• Potentially. Change in neonatal management with avoidance of oral feedings	• Unknown. No studies demonstrating improved outcome

Lung Abnormalities

Defect				
• CPAM • Bronchopulmonary Sequestration (BPS) *(may present prenatally with effusion)* • Fetal hydrothorax (FH) *(chylothorax most common)*	• CPAM: Monitoring of lesion, cyst volume ratio (CVR), some spontaneous regression[70,71] • Maternal betamethasone for large microcystic CPAM, CVR >1.6, very rarely fetal resection for hydrops[71-73] • Macrocystic CPAM or BPS with pleural effusion; consider fetal thoracoamniotic (TA) shunting if large or hydrops[26,71,72,74] • TA shunt in FH for severity/hydrops[75] • Genetic testing	• Term delivery in most cases of CPAM/BPS, no specific mode • Low CVR (<1.0) standard delivery at regional center[73] • Consider planned induction for severe cases • Delivery at specialized center for severe cases (polyhydramnios, hydrops); EXIT to resection offered for some[70-72] • Delivery at term in FH, delivery <32 wk higher mortality[77]	• Standard care, 90% CPAM asymptomatic[73] • Avoidance of positive pressure if possible, macrocystic CPAMs may air trap, worsen with intubation[71] • Rapid transfer for definitive treatment in sick infants[72] • Consider intrauterine drainage just before delivery for severe hydrothorax[75] • Despite TA shunt, many FH will need postnatal drainage[77]	• Yes. Maternal treatment in some cases of severe CPAM & TA shunt or intrauterine drain in FH	• Yes. Improvement in CPAM lesion size and hydrops seen in >70% of patients given betamethasone[71,72] • Potentially. Large case series with reversal of hydrops with TA shunting in both CPAM and hydrothorax; however risk of respiratory morbidity & mortality remains high[75-77]

Lower Urinary Tract Obstructions

Defect				
• Posterior urethral valves	• Majority are managed expectantly, serial ultrasounds • Fetal intervention with vesicoamniotic shunting (VAS) & fetal cystoscopy/ablation in specific cases (oligohydramnios and preserved renal function) • Palliative care in extreme cases with associated anomalies or pulmonary hypoplasia[1,78]	• Some consideration for early delivery in fetuses with oligohydramnios and documented lung maturity but no evidence of long-term benefits, especially in setting showing increased neonatal morbidity in early term and late preterm infants[78] • No specific delivery mode	• If severe oligohydramnios is present, infant may require extensive resuscitation due to pulmonary hypoplasia	• Yes. Fetal intervention	• Potentially. VAS seems to improve survival & pulmonary function. Survival with normal renal function unlikely regardless of fetal intervention[5,78-80] • Potential improvement in renal function with fetal cystoscopy compared with VAS[81]

(continued on next page)

Table 1
(continued)

Congenital Anomaly	Fetal Management & Intervention	Delivery Timing & Mode	Delivery Room Management & Stabilization	Alteration of Perinatal Management due to Prenatal Diagnosis	Alteration of Neonatal Outcome due to Prenatal Diagnosis
Neural Tube Defects					
• Myelomeningocele	• Open fetal surgery or fetoscopic surgery in some cases[16,82,83] • Consideration for termination or palliative care in extreme cases[1,8]	• Frequently cesarean delivery to prevent sac rupture and infection if large myelomeningocele (although lack of evidence demonstrating improved outcome) or to prevent dystocia if severe associated hydrocephalus[1,8,84]	• Sterile saline-soaked gauze & plastic bag/ wrap available immediately to cover defect • Use of latex-free materials • Empiric antibiotics frequently started • Cranial & spinal imaging and NS consultation soon after delivery[8,84]	• Yes. Delivery mode & preparedness	• Potentially. For open fetal surgery, decreased need for shunting and improved motor outcomes at 30 mo but increased premature birth and maternal risk[5,82,85,86]
Vascular Masses					
• Sacrococcygeal teratomas	• Monitoring: High output heart failure. May occur in large vascular masses • Rarely fetal intervention (laser ablation/surgery) when mortality is imminent[5,87]	• Cesarean delivery recommended to prevent sac rupture; hemorrhage • Early delivery for surgery may be considered depending on gestational age[87,88]	• Delivery at specialized center with surgeon available, blood available for transfusion[88,89]	• Yes. Delivery preparation, with rare fetal intervention consideration	• Potentially. Case series with survival after fetal intervention when death expected, but continued mortality and risk of prematurity[5,87]

Abbreviations: HR, heart rate; LHR, lung area to head circumference ratio; NS, neurosurgery; O/E, observed LHR/expected LHR; RAS, restrictive atrial septum.

SPECIALIZED POSTNATAL CARE
Delivery Room Management

Postnatal care in the delivery room and neonatal intensive care unit varies depending on the specific anomaly and the presentation of the infant.[1] For example, early intubation and gastric decompression are recommended with congenital diaphragmatic hernia and some abdominal wall defects.[8,37,40] A selected number of specific congenital anomalies are presented in **Table 1**. Unexpected anomalies from lack of prenatal care or missed on standard screening can present without warning in the delivery room. In these cases, providers should proceed with resuscitation via standard algorithms until special equipment or personnel is obtained.

STABILIZATION AND TRANSPORT

Although there are now a few children's hospitals that host delivery services, most neonates with congenital anomalies who need immediate postpartum intervention need to be transferred to a specialized center.

Maternal Bonding

Even for significant congenital anomalies, those who truly need immediate care and resuscitation are few.[2] Most neonates with congenital heart disease or bowel malformations will be well at delivery and for hours and even days after. This period may also be the only time for the next several weeks that a family is able to hold their child, and this is even more important for an infant with a life-limiting anomaly.

Transport Stabilization

Transportation requires moving the infant several times and an ambulance ride with no access to additional staff or equipment. Maternal transport is always preferable but often impossible.[91] Risks of transport include dislodgement of lines or tubes, hypothermia, and unexpected worsening of clinical condition. The ideal transport team functions as a mobile intensive care unit with all that is required.[92] Infants should be stabilized as possible; invasive devices should be secured, and additional support devices may be added. A specialized team with experience caring for sick neonates is essential, and, because most neonatal arrests are respiratory, should include a respiratory therapist or someone with advanced airway management skills.[91,92] The development of a regional perinatal system, effective communication system, standardized transport procedures, and provision of skilled attendants has been shown to decrease mortality for transported infants.[92,93]

OUTCOMES

The effect of prenatal diagnosis on neonatal outcome remains unclear; several factors make establishing this association difficult. Part of the improvement in perinatal mortality from prenatal diagnosis is due to increased early termination rates.[1,2] There is selection bias because more severe cases tend to be detected prenatally.[2] The specific anomaly being evaluated is important—few anomalies explicitly influence the fetal transition after birth. Anomalies where there is a documented benefit to prenatal diagnosis are detailed in **Table 1**. Although assessing mortality is relatively straightforward, assessing neonatal morbidity, especially neurodevelopmental morbidity, is more convoluted.[94]

   Thus, it is not surprising that there is limited evidence demonstrating improved neonatal outcome because of prenatal diagnosis. There is some evidence in certain circumstances, including cases of specific congenital heart defects, fetal anemia, and twin-to-twin transfusion syndrome.[2,3] Intrauterine repair of myelomeningocele has also shown some benefit; however, side effects such as maternal morbidity and premature birth remain confounding factors.[2,85] Gebb and colleagues[94] demonstrate that with the exception of twin-to-twin transfusion syndrome, there is limited evidence on long-term neurologic outcomes after fetal interventions.

ETHICAL CONSIDERATIONS

Families with prenatally diagnosed anomalies are challenged with several decisions, including whether to continue the pregnancy, and then potentially, whether to proceed with offered fetal interventions or advanced resuscitation at delivery.[94] It is also vital to recognize that although the offer of fetal therapies originates from a desire for benef-icence, they cannot be undertaken without the informed consent of the pregnant woman, including risks and benefits of any procedure. Careful explanation of the con-flicting and limited data regarding the risks and benefits to prenatal versus postnatal interventions is essential. A distinction should be made between goals of medicine versus research, and safeguards such as research subject advocates should be put in place to protect pregnant women considering fetal research.[6]

SUMMARY

Prenatally diagnosed anomalies encompass a broad spectrum from those that will never impact the health of the infant to those severe enough that fetal intervention is considered. The best care can be provided when diagnosis is timely, appropriate referrals are made when indicated, and consideration for the health of both mother and baby is given when determining treatment. Care decisions and delivery planning should be individualized based on prenatal diagnosis and family. Although most infants with anomalies will be well immediately after delivery, a select portion will require immediate intervention. Delivery should occur at a center adept at dealing with complex care needs and prepared for

---

Best Practices

What is the current practice?

Prenatal diagnosis and referral are varied. Not all patients are referred to specialists, and not all infants with anomalies are delivered at experienced centers.

What changes in current practice are likely to improve outcomes?

Consistency in referrals and availability of advanced imaging and counseling should be accessible to all regardless of cost. Infants with significant anomalies that present in the neonatal period should be delivered at an experienced center. Clinical algorithms for referral and care should be developed with consensus and widely available.

Is there a clinical algorithm?

Individual centers have algorithms, but care is variable between centers, and families have access to different options depending on location. Specific care varies by diagnosis.

Rating for the strength of the evidence

Most of the evidence is in the form of cohort studies and expert opinion. There are very limited data from randomized trials, especially on improved outcomes.

Summary statement

Prenatal diagnosis has allowed preparation and advanced perinatal care, and there is evidence for improved outcomes in specific congenital anomalies. However, variation in the access to and application of prenatal care limits the benefit to the overall population.

the unexpected. Although evidence is limited in many cases, mortality and morbidity benefit from advanced, targeted perinatal management in specific circumstances.

REFERENCES

1. Cass DL. Impact of prenatal diagnosis and therapy on neonatal surgery. Semin Fetal Neonatal Med 2011;16(3):130–8.
2. Kermorvant-Duchemin E, Ville Y. Prenatal diagnosis of congenital malformations for the better and for the worse. J Matern Fetal Neonatal Med 2017;30(12): 1402–6.
3. Lindenburg IT, van Klink JM, Smits-Wintjens VE, et al. Long-term neurodevelopmental and cardiovascular outcome after intrauterine transfusions for fetal anaemia: a review. Prenatal Diagn 2013;33(9):815–22.
4. Peyvandi S, De Santiago V, Chakkarapani E, et al. Association of prenatal diagnosis of critical congenital heart disease with postnatal brain development and the risk of brain injury. JAMA Pediatr 2016;170(4):e154450.
5. Kitagawa H, Pringle KC. Fetal surgery: a critical review. Pediatr Surg Int 2017; 33(4):421–33.
6. American College of Obstetricians and Gynecologists, Committee on Ethics; American Academy of Pediatrics, Committee on Bioethics. Maternal-fetal intervention and fetal care centers. Pediatrics 2011;128(2):e473–8.
7. Luks FI. New and/or improved aspects of fetal surgery. Prenatal Diagn 2011; 31(3):252–8.
8. Colby CE, Carey WA, Blumenfeld YJ, et al. Infants with prenatally diagnosed anomalies: special approaches to preparation and resuscitation. Clin Perinatol 2012;39(4):871–87.
9. Davis AS, Chock VY, Hintz SR. Fetal centers and the role of the neonatologist in complex fetal care. Am J Perinatol 2014;31(7):549–56.
10. Chock VY, Davis AS, Hintz SR. The roles and responsibilities of the neonatologist in complex fetal medicine: providing a continuum of care. Neoreviews 2015;16: e9–15.
11. Brown SD, Donelan K, Martins Y, et al. Differing attitudes toward fetal care by pediatric and maternal-fetal medicine specialists. Pediatrics 2012;130(6):e1534–40.
12. Moise KJ Jr. The history of fetal therapy. Am J Perinatol 2014;31(7):557–66.
13. Wenstrom KD, Carr SR. Fetal surgery: principles, indications, and evidence. Obstet Gynecol 2014;124(4):817–35.
14. Jaeggi ET, Carvalho JS, De Groot E, et al. Comparison of transplacental treatment of fetal supraventricular tachyarrhythmias with digoxin, flecainide, and sotalol: results of a nonrandomized multicenter study. Circulation 2011;124(16):1747–54.
15. van der Heijden LB, Oudijk MA, Manten GT, et al. Sotalol as first-line treatment for fetal tachycardia and neonatal follow-up. Ultrasound Obstet Gynecol 2013;42(3): 285–93.
16. Araujo Junior E, Eggink AJ, van den Dobbelsteen J, et al. Procedure-related complications of open vs endoscopic fetal surgery for treatment of spina bifida in an era of intrauterine myelomeningocele repair: systematic review and meta-analysis. Ultrasound Obstet Gynecol 2016;48(2):151–60.
17. Vrecenak JD, Flake AW. Fetal surgical intervention: progress and perspectives. Pediatr Surg Int 2013;29(5):407–17.
18. Sudhakaran N, Sothinathan U, Patel S. Best practice guidelines: fetal surgery. Early Hum Dev 2012;88(1):15–9.

19. Ledbetter DJ. Congenital abdominal wall defects and reconstruction in pediatric surgery: gastroschisis and omphalocele. Surg Clin North Am 2012;92(3): 713–27, x.
20. Fratelli N, Papageorghiou AT, Bhide A, et al. Outcome of antenatally diagnosed abdominal wall defects. Ultrasound Obstet Gynecol 2007;30(3):266–70.
21. Gamba P, Midrio P. Abdominal wall defects: prenatal diagnosis, newborn management, and long-term outcomes. Semin Pediatr Surg 2014;23(5):283–90.
22. Grant NH, Dorling J, Thornton JG. Elective preterm birth for fetal gastroschisis. Cochrane Database Syst Rev 2013;(6):CD009394.
23. Prefumo F, Izzi C. Fetal abdominal wall defects. Best Pract Res Clin Obstet Gynaecol 2014;28(3):391–402.
24. Kleinrouweler CE, Kuijper CF, van Zalen-Sprock MM, et al. Characteristics and outcome and the omphalocele circumference/abdominal circumference ratio in prenatally diagnosed fetal omphalocele. Fetal Diagn Ther 2011;30(1):60–9.
25. Christison-Lagay ER, Kelleher CM, Langer JC. Neonatal abdominal wall defects. Semin Fetal Neonatal Med 2011;16(3):164–72.
26. Ryan G, Somme S, Crombleholme TM. Airway compromise in the fetus and neonate: prenatal assessment and perinatal management. Semin Fetal Neonatal Med 2016;21(4):230–9.
27. Walz PC, Schroeder JW Jr. Prenatal diagnosis of obstructive head and neck masses and perinatal airway management: the ex utero intrapartum treatment procedure. Otolaryngol Clin North Am 2015;48(1):191–207.
28. Neidich MJ, Prager JD, Clark SL, et al. Comprehensive airway management of neonatal head and neck teratomas. Otolaryngol Head Neck Surg 2011;144(2): 257–61.
29. Diercks GR, Hartnick CJ, Bates SV. Management of the critical airway when an EXIT procedure is not an option: a case report. Int J Pediatr Otorhinolaryngol 2015;79(12):2433–7.
30. Saadai P, Jelin EB, Nijagal A, et al. Long-term outcomes after fetal therapy for congenital high airway obstructive syndrome. J Pediatr Surg 2012;47(6): 1095–100.
31. Grivell RM, Andersen C, Dodd JM. Prenatal interventions for congenital diaphragmatic hernia for improving outcomes. Cochrane Database Syst Rev 2015;(11):CD008925.
32. Al-Maary J, Eastwood MP, Russo FM, et al. Fetal tracheal occlusion for severe pulmonary hypoplasia in isolated congenital diaphragmatic hernia: a systematic review and meta-analysis of survival. Ann Surg 2016;264(6):929–33.
33. Araujo Junior E, Tonni G, Martins WP, et al. Procedure-related complications and survival following fetoscopic endotracheal occlusion (FETO) for severe congenital diaphragmatic hernia: systematic review and meta-analysis in the FETO Era. Eur J Pediatr Surg 2017;27(4):297–305.
34. Burgos CM, Frenckner B, Luco M, et al. Prenatally diagnosed congenital diaphragmatic hernia: optimal mode of delivery? J Perinatol 2017;37(2):134–8.
35. Safavi A, Lin Y, Skarsgard ED, Canadian Pediatric Surgery Network. Perinatal management of congenital diaphragmatic hernia: when and how should babies be delivered? Results from the Canadian Pediatric Surgery Network. J Pediatr Surg 2010;45(12):2334–9.
36. Nasr A, Langer JC, Canadian Pediatric Surgery Network. Influence of location of delivery on outcome in neonates with congenital diaphragmatic hernia. J Pediatr Surg 2011;46(5):814–6.

37. Snoek KG, Reiss IK, Greenough A, et al. Standardized postnatal management of infants with congenital diaphragmatic hernia in Europe: the CDH EURO Consortium Consensus - 2015 update. Neonatology 2016;110(1):66–74.

38. Stoffan AP, Wilson JM, Jennings RW, et al. Does the ex utero intrapartum treatment to extracorporeal membrane oxygenation procedure change outcomes for high-risk patients with congenital diaphragmatic hernia? J Pediatr Surg 2012;47(6):1053–7.

39. Logan JW, Rice HE, Goldberg RN, et al. Congenital diaphragmatic hernia: a systematic review and summary of best-evidence practice strategies. J Perinatol 2007;27(9):535–49.

40. van den Hout L, Schaible T, Cohen-Overbeek TE, et al. Actual outcome in infants with congenital diaphragmatic hernia: the role of a standardized postnatal treatment protocol. Fetal Diagn Ther 2011;29(1):55–63.

41. Bojanic K, Pritisanac E, Luetic T, et al. Survival of outborns with congenital diaphragmatic hernia: the role of protective ventilation, early presentation and transport distance: a retrospective cohort study. BMC Pediatr 2015;15:155.

42. Snoek KG, Capolupo I, van Rosmalen J, et al. Conventional mechanical ventilation versus high-frequency oscillatory ventilation for congenital diaphragmatic hernia: a randomized clinical trial (The VICI-trial). Ann Surg 2016;263(5):867–74.

43. de Jong EM, de Haan MA, Gischler SJ, et al. Pre- and postnatal diagnosis and outcome of fetuses and neonates with esophageal atresia and tracheoesophageal fistula. Prenatal Diagn 2010;30(3):274–9.

44. Ethun CG, Fallon SC, Cassady CI, et al. Fetal MRI improves diagnostic accuracy in patients referred to a fetal center for suspected esophageal atresia. J Pediatr Surg 2014;49(5):712–5.

45. Houben CH, Curry JI. Current status of prenatal diagnosis, operative management and outcome of esophageal atresia/tracheo-esophageal fistula. Prenatal Diagn 2008;28(7):667–75.

46. Kalish RB, Chasen ST, Rosenzweig L, et al. Esophageal atresia and tracheoesophageal fistula: the impact of prenatal suspicion on neonatal outcome in a tertiary care center. J Perinat Med 2003;31:111–4.

47. Morris G, Kennedy A Jr, Cochran W. Small bowel congenital anomalies: a review and update. Curr Gastroenterol Rep 2016;18(4):16.

48. Garabedian C, Sfeir R, Langlois C, et al. Does prenatal diagnosis modify neonatal treatment and early outcome of children with esophageal atresia? Am J Obstet Gynecol 2015;212(3):340.e1–7.

49. Friedman DM, Kim MY, Copel JA, et al. Prospective evaluation of fetuses with autoimmune-associated congenital heart block followed in the PR Interval and Dexamethasone Evaluation (PRIDE) Study. Am J Cardiol 2009;103(8):1102–6.

50. Gleicher N, Elkayam U. Preventing congenital neonatal heart block in offspring of mothers with anti-SSA/Ro and SSB/La antibodies: a review of published literature and registered clinical trials. Autoimmun Rev 2013;12(11):1039–45.

51. Friedman DM, Llanos C, Izmirly PM, et al. Evaluation of fetuses in a study of intravenous immunoglobulin as preventive therapy for congenital heart block: results of a multicenter, prospective, open-label clinical trial. Arthritis Rheum 2010;62(4):1138–46.

52. Levesque K, Morel N, Maltret A, et al. Description of 214 cases of autoimmune congenital heart block: results of the French neonatal lupus syndrome. Autoimmun Rev 2015;14(12):1154–60.

53. Hinkle KA, Peyvandi S, Stiver C, et al. Postnatal outcomes of fetal supraventricular tachycardia: a multicenter study. Pediatr Cardiol 2017;38(7):1317–23.

54. Yildirim A, Tunaoolu FS, Karaaoac AT. Neonatal congenital heart block. Indian Pediatr 2013;50(5):483–8.

55. Izmirly PM, Saxena A, Kim MY, et al. Maternal and fetal factors associated with mortality and morbidity in a multi-racial/ethnic registry of anti-SSA/Ro-associated cardiac neonatal lupus. Circulation 2011;124(18):1927–35.

56. Donofrio MT, Levy RJ, Schuette JJ, et al. Specialized delivery room planning for fetuses with critical congenital heart disease. Am J Cardiol 2013;111(5):737–47.

57. Glatz AC, Gaynor JW, Rhodes LA, et al. Outcome of high-risk neonates with congenital complete heart block paced in the first 24 hours after birth. J Thorac Cardiovasc Surg 2008;136(3):767–73.

58. Donofrio MT, Skurow-Todd K, Berger JT, et al. Risk-stratified postnatal care of newborns with congenital heart disease determined by fetal echocardiography. J Am Soc Echocardiogr 2015;28(11):1339–49.

59. Sanapo L, Moon-Grady AJ, Donofrio MT. Perinatal and delivery management of infants with congenital heart disease. Clin Perinatol 2016;43(1):55–71.

60. Jaeggi E, Renaud C, Ryan G, et al. Intrauterine therapy for structural congenital heart disease: contemporary results and Canadian experience. Trends Cardiovasc Med 2016;26(7):639–46.

61. Chu PY, Li JS, Kosinski AS, et al. Congenital heart disease in premature infants 25-32 weeks' gestational age. J Pediatr 2017;181:37–41.e31.

62. Bensemlali M, Bajolle F, Laux D, et al. Neonatal management and outcomes of prenatally diagnosed CHDs. Cardiol Young 2017;27(2):344–53.

63. Meckler GD, Lowe C. To intubate or not to intubate? Transporting infants on prostaglandin E1. Pediatrics 2009;123(1):e25–30.

64. Bensemlali M, Stirnemann J, Le Bidois J, et al. Discordances between pre-natal and post-natal diagnoses of congenital heart diseases and impact on care strategies. J Am Coll Cardiol 2016;68(9):921–30.

65. Colaco SM, Karande T, Bobhate PR, et al. Neonates with critical congenital heart defects: impact of fetal diagnosis on immediate and short-term outcomes. Ann Pediatr Cardiol 2017;10(2):126–30.

66. Ota S, Sahara J, Mabuchi A, et al. Perinatal and one-year outcomes of non-immune hydrops fetalis by etiology and age at diagnosis. J Obstet Gynaecol Res 2016;42(4):385–91.

67. Lindenburg IT, van Kamp IL, Oepkes D. Intrauterine blood transfusion: current indications and associated risks. Fetal Diagn Ther 2014;36(4):263–71.

68. Nassr AA, Ness A, Hosseinzadeh P, et al. Outcome and treatment of antenatally diagnosed nonimmune hydrops fetalis. Fetal Diagn Ther 2018;43:123–8.

69. Randenberg AL. Nonimmune hydrops fetalis part II: does etiology influence mortality? Neonatal Netw 2010;29(6):367–80.

70. Peranteau WH, Boelig MM, Khalek N, et al. Effect of single and multiple courses of maternal betamethasone on prenatal congenital lung lesion growth and fetal survival. J Pediatr Surg 2016;51(1):28–32.

71. Macardle CA, Kunisaki SM. Management of perinatal lung malformations. Minerva Ginecol 2015;67(1):81–94.

72. Baird R, Puligandla PS, Laberge JM. Congenital lung malformations: informing best practice. Semin Pediatr Surg 2014;23(5):270–7.

73. Macardle CA, Ehrenberg-Buchner S, Smith EA, et al. Surveillance of fetal lung lesions using the congenital pulmonary airway malformation volume ratio: natural history and outcomes. Prenatal Diagn 2016;36(3):282–9.

74. Degenhardt J, Kohl T, Enzensberger C, et al. Review on current management and outcome data of echogenic lung lesions and hydrothorax of the fetus. Z Geburtshilfe Neonatol 2013;217(6):204–10.

75. Mallmann MR, Graham V, Rosing B, et al. Thoracoamniotic shunting for fetal hydrothorax: predictors of intrauterine course and postnatal outcome. Fetal Diagn Ther 2017;41(1):58–65.

76. Attar MA, Donn SM. Congenital chylothorax. Semin Fetal Neonatal Med 2017; 22(4):234–9.

77. Witlox R, Klumper F, Te Pas AB, et al. Neonatal management and outcome after thoracoamniotic shunt placement for fetal hydrothorax. Arch Dis Child Fetal Neonatal Ed 2017. [Epub ahead of print].

78. Liu DB, Armstrong WR 3rd, Maizels M. Hydronephrosis: prenatal and postnatal evaluation and management. Clin Perinatol 2014;41(3):661–78.

79. Morris RK, Malin GL, Quinlan-Jones E, et al. Percutaneous vesicoamniotic shunting versus conservative management for fetal lower urinary tract obstruction (PLUTO): a randomised trial. Lancet 2013;382(9903):1496–506.

80. Nassr AA, Shazly SAM, Abdelmagied AM, et al. Effectiveness of vesicoamniotic shunt in fetuses with congenital lower urinary tract obstruction: an updated systematic review and meta-analysis. Ultrasound Obstet Gynecol 2017;49(6): 696–703.

81. Ruano R, Sananes N, Sangi-Haghpeykar H, et al. Fetal intervention for severe lower urinary tract obstruction: a multicenter case-control study comparing fetal cystoscopy with vesicoamniotic shunting. Ultrasound Obstet Gynecol 2015; 45(4):452–8.

82. Adzick NS, Thom EA, Spong CY, et al. A randomized trial of prenatal versus postnatal repair of myelomeningocele. N Engl J Med 2011;364(11):993–1004.

83. Joyeux L, Engels AC, Russo FM, et al. Fetoscopic versus open repair for spina bifida aperta: a systematic review of outcomes. Fetal Diagn Ther 2016;39(3): 161–71.

84. Thompson DN. Postnatal management and outcome for neural tube defects including spina bifida and encephalocoeles. Prenatal Diagn 2009;29(4):412–9.

85. Grivell RM, Andersen C, Dodd JM. Prenatal versus postnatal repair procedures for spina bifida for improving infant and maternal outcomes. Cochrane Database Syst Rev 2014;(10):CD008825.

86. Johnson MP, Bennett KA, Rand L, et al. The Management of Myelomeningocele Study: obstetrical outcomes and risk factors for obstetrical complications following prenatal surgery. Am J Obstet Gynecol 2016;215(6):778.e1–9.

87. Van Mieghem T, Al-Ibrahim A, Deprest J, et al. Minimally invasive therapy for fetal sacrococcygeal teratoma: case series and systematic review of the literature. Ultrasound Obstet Gynecol 2014;43(6):611–9.

88. Roybal JL, Moldenhauer JS, Khalek N, et al. Early delivery as an alternative management strategy for selected high-risk fetal sacrococcygeal teratomas. J Pediatr Surg 2011;46(7):1325–32.

89. Usui N, Kitano Y, Sago H, et al. Outcomes of prenatally diagnosed sacrococcygeal teratomas: the results of a Japanese nationwide survey. J Pediatr Surg 2012; 47(3):441–7.

90. Jegatheeswaran A, Oliveira C, Batsos C, et al. Costs of prenatal detection of congenital heart disease. Am J Cardiol 2011;108(12):1808–14.

91. Whyte HE, Jefferies AL, Canadian Paediatric Society, Fetus and Newborn Committee. The interfacility transport of critically ill newborns. Paediatr Child Health 2015;20(5):265–75.

92. Stroud MH, Trautman MS, Meyer K, et al. Pediatric and neonatal interfacility transport: results from a national consensus conference. Pediatrics 2013;132(2): 359–66.
93. Kong XY, Liu XX, Hong XY, et al. Improved outcomes of transported neonates in Beijing: the impact of strategic changes in perinatal and regional neonatal transport network services. World J Pediatr 2014;10(3):251–5.
94. Gebb J, Dar P, Rosner M, et al. Long-term neurologic outcomes after common fetal interventions. Am J Obstet Gynecol 2015;212(4):527.e1–9.

Prognosis as an Intervention

Matthew A. Rysavy, MD, PhD

KEYWORDS

• Prognosis • Neonatal outcomes • Prediction • NICU

KEY POINTS

- Prognostication can be conceived of as a perinatal intervention that should be evaluated, like other clinical interventions, for its effects on important outcomes.
- Several studies have examined the effect of communicating prognoses on parental anxiety and understanding, although further research on specific methods and approaches is needed in this area. Less is known about how communicating prognoses might affect patient clinical outcomes.
- Clinicians should be aware of the potential hazards of self-fulfilling prognoses (for example, evidence where the practice of resuscitation is based on outdated survival statistics and, in turn, perpetuates these statistics) and expectancy effects (whereby expectation of certain outcomes may make the outcomes more likely through subtle changes in practice). Such effects of prognostication on clinical outcomes deserve further study.

Although prognostication is classically 1 of 3 aspects of medicine (the others being diagnosis and therapy[1]), there are reasons to consider prognostication an intervention in itself, maybe even a therapy. What are the effects of prognostication—For the clinician? For the patient? Does establishing and communicating a prognosis affect patient outcomes?

Like all medical interventions, the details of prognosis matter: What sort is made? To whom? How? In what quantities? And under what circumstances? In this light, the effect of prognosis on outcomes might be understood in the same way that effects of other neonatal interventions—like surfactant, antenatal corticosteroids, and oxygen—are understood.

Neonatology and perinatology were early adopters of the rigorous methods of evidence-based medicine. Yet, although prognostication is practiced daily in both fields, its effects remain poorly understood. The intent of this article is to elaborate on how neonatologists and perinatologists might conceive of prognosis as an intervention—with outcomes relevant to patients, families, and society at large—and to highlight aspects of this important area of practice that require further study.

Disclosure Statement: No disclosures.
Department of Pediatrics, University of Iowa Stead Family Children's Hospital, 200 Hawkins Drive, Iowa City, IA 52242, USA
E-mail address: matthew-rysavy@uiowa.edu

WHAT IS PROGNOSIS?

Prognosis, literally translated from its Greek roots, means "foreknowing."[2] It can be described as "what to expect" regarding a patient's health.

Prognostication has deep roots in medical tradition. A volume on prognosis attributed to Hippocrates, from 400 BC, begins: "It appears to me a most excellent thing for the physician to cultivate Prognosis; ... he will manage the cure best who has foreseen what is to happen from the present state of matters. ... Thus a man will be the more esteemed to be a good physician, for he will be the better able to treat those aright who can be saved, having long anticipated everything; and by seeing and announcing beforehand those who will live and those who will die, he will thus escape censure."[3]

Modern neonatologists and perinatologists continue to focus some part of their medical practice on "seeing and announcing beforehand those who will live and those who will die." Antenatal consults, where such information is discussed with a family expecting a complicated birth, have become standard practice[4] and integral to training in these specialties.[5] Moreover, recommendations for antenatal consultation and other forms of prognostication elaborate the need to convey information about conditions besides mortality.[6] There is more to life than death.[7] For many conditions in neonatal and perinatal medicine, researchers and clinicians have focused on understanding and conveying information about specific impairments, usually sensory, motor, or cognitive, that are sometimes equated with poor "quality of life" or states "worse than death."[8] In this way, the word *prognosis*, as used in common parlance among neonatologists, perinatologists, and the families they care for—in phrases, such as "a poor prognosis" or "a good prognosis"—may be synonymous with the risk for mortality or severe life-altering impairment.[9]

Notwithstanding that death and severe impairments receive the most attention, neonatologists and perinatologists are called on to make predictions about what to expect regarding all variety of outcomes: How long will the infant be in the hospital? How much will the medical care cost? What sort of medical care will this child need after leaving the neonatal intensive care unit (NICU)? How will this illness affect these parents' work, relationship, and family? In this way, prognosis can be conceptualized more broadly.[10,11]

Classically, knowledge of prognosis links diagnosis and therapy so that, by understanding what to expect after a diagnosis, an appropriate course of intervention can be determined. In modern circumstances, understanding prognosis is intimately linked with notions of informed consent and shared decision making.[12]

FIRST, FORMULATE EVIDENCE-BASED PROGNOSES

There are 2 key aspects to approaching prognosis as an evidence-based intervention: how to formulate an accurate prognosis and what to do with that prognosis.[13] This section focuses on the former: When a prognosis is made, what supports that claim?

Doctors have long understood that questions about prognosis for an individual patient can be answered in terms of what has happened to other similar patients. As William Farr, one of the earliest medical statisticians, recognized: "In prognosis, patients may be considered in two lights: in collective masses, when general results can be predicted with certainty; or separately, when the question becomes one of probability. If 7000 of 10,000 cases of fever terminate fatally, it may be predicted that the same proportion will die in another series of cases; and experience has proved that the prediction will be verified, or so nearly verified as to leave no room for cavil or skepticism. The recovery or death of one of the cases is a mere matter of probability."[14]

Farr's formulation clarifies an important point: When looked at in large groups under stable circumstances, prognosis is a consistent, measurable phenomenon. The rate of an outcome for a group under stable conditions varies randomly around a true mean (as quantified by statistical concepts, such as the confidence interval) and can be predicted with relative certainty. In contrast, the outcome for a specific patient may be much more difficult to know, even under stable circumstances. In Farr's example, the probability of death for an individual patient would be 0.7, or 70%. In reality, however, the patient will survive or will die—the rate of death will be 0 or 1. The application of a probability like 70% becomes merely a tool to assist with what Farr called "the Art of guessing."[14]

The best evidence-based prognostic tools for binary outcomes, such as mortality, have positive predictive values or negative predictive values approaching 100%. They show that in large generalizable groups of patients, where a specific characteristic—for example, a finding on the history or physical examination, from a blood test, or on imaging—is present or absent, nearly all infants have the outcome. (Note that the positive and negative predictive values need not both approach 100%. For example, consider that the positive predictive value of birth at 20 weeks' gestation for perinatal mortality is 100%. Many births at later gestations result in perinatal mortality for various reasons, making the negative predictive value of this characteristic poor; yet the utility of this previable gestational age for prognosticating mortality remains excellent.)

The tools available for prognostication in neonatology and perinatology are numerous. For premature births, for example, prognosis of "viability" was historically based on birthweight. More recently, with the development of improved gestational age-estimation methods, prognostic studies have used the duration of gestation as a primary criterion for prognosis.[15] Similarly, individual aspects of the physical examination, such as the presence of fused eyelids, were historically used to determine whether a premature infant could survive.[16,17] More recently, computer-based multivariable models have been developed to predict premature infant mortality. These models take into account multiple characteristics, such as gestational age; infant gender and race; the presence or absence of congenital malformations; the receipt of prenatal interventions, such as antenatal corticosteroids; and findings on examination, including the Apgar score and infant's body temperature and respiratory status. A 2011 systematic review identified 41 such models in the peer-reviewed literature.[18]

Beyond these methods of predicting mortality and survival, various technologies have been used to predict impairments and developmental outcomes after premature birth. These include head ultrasound examinations, term-equivalent MRI, amplitude-integrated electroencephalography, and whole-exome sequencing.[19] Less work has been done to prognosticate other important outcomes, although there is growing interest in doing so.[19,20]

Although the advantages and limitations of individual prognostic tools are beyond the scope of this review, suffice to say that many do not approach 100% positive or negative predictive values for clinically important outcomes, as described previously.

Pitfalls in Formulating Prognoses

Excellent prognostic guides for neonatal and perinatal medicine are difficult to develop for several reasons, including

1. Many commonly used functional outcomes in neonatal and perinatal medicine—such as bronchopulmonary dysplasia, neurodevelopmental impairment, cerebral palsy, blindness, and deafness—may be categorized as binary (ie, present or not

present) outcomes for the convenience of researchers and clinicians. In reality, however, they are better understood on a spectrum.[19] Where dichotomies are made, similar patients may fall marginally along one side or the other of a threshold despite no meaningful differences in outcomes. Dichotomizing continuous variables in this way affects both research (by increasing noise and decreasing predictive values) and clinical interpretation (by making dichotomized descriptions less relevant to patients, families, and clinicians).

2. Even clearly binary outcomes, such as mortality, may be measured at various points in time and for different denominators. One recent study of outcomes used in neonatal clinical trials found 17 different time periods used to assess mortality across studies.[21] In a review of studies presenting survival statistics after premature birth, differences in the denominator used to define the study cohort (eg, all births, only live births, or only infants admitted to the NICU) had a substantial impact on outcome rates.[22] Similarly, it has been shown that the use of data for infants born at a tertiary institution should not be used to infer the probability of survival for any particular infant born in the surrounding area who may not present to such an institution.[23]

3. Some prognostic indicators may self-perpetuate their own associations and reinforce a *self-fulfilling prognosis*.[24] A self-fulfilling prognosis occurs where clinicians use historical information about an outcome (eg, mortality) to inform decisions about interventions that affect that outcome (electing whether to resuscitate, continue treatment, perform surgery, and so forth), leading to further studies that show similar rates of the same outcome.[12] In neonatology, this phenomenon has been written about regarding extremely preterm birth,[25] hypoxic-ischemic encephalopathy,[26] and cardiac surgery for patients with trisomy 21.[27]

4. Many conditions and circumstances in neonatal-perinatal medicine are rare. Small sample sizes may preclude precise prognostication and some studies omit measures of uncertainty, including confidence intervals, that convey this.[28]

5. Prognosis may change substantially over time. A stay in a NICU may last for weeks or months, and new events and new information can have large effects on prognosis. Some researchers have developed tools to model outcome trajectories to account for these changes.[29]

Issues with defining measurements and populations, as well as the potential for self-fulfilling prognoses, statistical imprecision, and variation over the clinical course, may lead to difficulties in reporting and interpretation of prognostic research.[28] Moreover, it is not always clear how to overcome such issues. Despite the improvement of scientific methods in several areas of medicine during recent decades, such as with randomized controlled trials for neonatal and perinatal therapies, some investigators have argued that methods to support prognosis research remain poorly implemented and understood.[30,31]

Nonetheless, producing an evidence-based prognosis is worth striving for. Many groups are working to improve the conduct and reporting of prognosis research to improve its clinical utility.[32–34] New techniques, such as decision curve analysis, provide clinically relevant methods to compare imperfect prognostic tools.[35,36] Even with a solid evidence base for accurate prognostication, however, important questions remain: What is prognosis for? Does it actually achieve what it is intended to?

SECOND, LEARN WHAT TO DO WITH AN ACCURATE PROGNOSIS

Why prognosticate? Hippocrates identified that prognostication assisted with determining the appropriate course of action (and, if correct, he added, it might make a physician look better). But other important potential outcomes exist. Today, prognostication may contribute to meaningful shared decision making. Accurate prognostic information may be particularly useful in areas of neonatal-perinatal medicine where physicians have inaccurate intuition[37,38] and where families and physicians have discordant expectations.[39] Even in the absence of making treatment decisions, prognosis may be useful for setting expectations. Prognosis may also provide a sense of comfort to patients or families in distress, reducing anxiety or increasing acceptance of a given clinical course.

Any of these ends should be considered outcomes for potential studies of prognosis: having an impact on care decisions, enabling shared decision making, allowing families and others to prepare, reducing stress and anxiety, and providing comfort. Existing studies of prognostication on these outcomes are elaborated later.

Of note, although it is possible to prognosticate for large groups—for example, to make predictions about the resources required to care for a population and to identify expected population-level needs warranting further research—this article highlights several aspects of implementing prognoses for individual patients.

Content

In a broad review of comparative effectiveness studies, mostly randomized, for methods used to convey prognostic information, Zipkin and colleagues[40] showed that several strategies of presenting information were more effective at improving understanding and satisfaction. Based on their synthesis, the investigators recommended expressing probabilities as event rates (percentages) or natural frequencies (numerators/denominators as whole numbers) versus using qualitative risk descriptors (such as "very high risk") alone and placing patient risks in context by comparing them to other events.

Heuristics

Heuristics may also play an important role in how people use prognostic information. Haward and Janvier[41] summarized how aspects of presenting prognostic information may affect decisions made with that information, such as through anchoring, framing, order effects, and loss aversion. For example, in a study where participants received a hypothetical vignette of a threatened extremely preterm delivery with the outcome randomly framed as a gain (eg, "25 of 100 babies will survive if provided intensive care; of the 25 who survive, 15 will not have severe developmental disabilities.") or a loss (eg, "75 of 100 babies will die even if provided intensive care; of the 25 who do not die, 10 will have severe developmental disabilities."), respondents with the prognostic information framed as a gain were more likely to elect for resuscitation.[42]

Context

Context also matters. Irrelevant or incomprehensible information may confuse or distress families.[43] In a qualitative study of interviews with women who received antenatal counseling during pregnancies affected with congenital anomalies, receiving conflicting information from physicians was shown to increase anxiety and erode confidence in prognostic information.[44] The same study noted that patients were more satisfied with the prognostic information when physicians provided adequate time for the discussion and demonstrated sensitivity to the circumstances.

Auxiliary Materials

Several studies have evaluated the use of materials for conveying neonatal and perinatal prognostic information. Cope and colleagues[45] performed a randomized controlled trial of providing letters and audiotapes to supplement prenatal diagnostic consultation and found that 2 weeks after the consultation, women with either or both of these materials reported less anxiety, although recall was no different across groups. Others have studied the use of decision aids. In a descriptive study, Guillen and colleagues[46] showed that a decision aid conveying prognostic information about extremely preterm birth may increase parental recall of certain prognostic facts and may improve satisfaction with the care provided.[47] A clinical trial of a decision aid for extremely preterm birth is currently listed on ClinicalTrials.gov as enrolling patients; its primary outcome is "decisional conflict," whereby the parents sense uncertainty about the course of action to take with regards to resuscitation.[48]

Stories

Less well understood, but potentially important in neonatal-perinatal prognostication, are the roles of stories and of social media. In other fields of medicine, the inclusion of stories with decision aids has been shown to improve recall and affect judgments and decisions.[49] Stories may convey a richness of detail and, perhaps, meaning about a prognosis that statistics cannot. They may be limited in their generalizability, however, in the same way that case studies in the medical literature are. Stories, among other information, are also widely available to families on the Internet, in a way that they had not been during previous decades. Many families, such as those having children with trisomy 13 or 18, have joined communities on social media where they actively share stories and advice with each other.[50] The best ways to integrate this growing source of information into the clinical provision of prognosis deserve further attention.

CAN PROGNOSIS MODIFY CLINICAL OUTCOMES?

One of the most salient questions about prognostication—but also among the most difficult to answer—is whether it might have an impact on patients' clinical outcomes.

The largest clinical trial to evaluate this question to date was the Study to Understand Prognoses and Preferences for Outcomes and Risks of Treatments (SUPPORT) trial.[51] In the early 1990s, this study randomized nearly 5000 adult patients with life-threatening conditions to either a control group (standard care) or an intervention where physicians received information on expected survival and caregiver goals. The study evaluated the impact of providing physicians with objective estimates of 6-month survival (using survival curves) based on several easily measured factors that were included in a computer-based multivariable model.[52] The model estimates were placed in the patients' charts or given to physicians directly. The study found that the intervention did not affect whether a do-not-resuscitate (DNR) agreement was made, the time to the DNR agreement, the patient's pain, days spent on mechanical ventilation, or medical resource use.

The approach, however, had several limitations. The intervention did not explicitly define whether or how such estimates should be communicated with patients or caregivers.[53] Nurses in the study were to elicit clinical goals and preferences as well as patient or caregiver understanding of prognosis. But in a majority of cases (60%), patients and surrogates did not discuss prognosis directly with the physician. Many physicians (>40%) did not consider the estimates in their own decision making.

In considering the relevance of the study to modern practice, it should also be noted that methods used to present prognostic information, as well as the standard of care to which the intervention was compared, were particular to the circumstances of the era. Physicians today may be more familiar with using statistical models. Since the early 1990s, evidence-based medicine has become a standard part of medical school curricula[54] and statistical models are more widely used in many areas of clinical practice. Moreover, paradigms for decision making have shifted over the past decades, with further empowerment of patients and surrogates in defining their medical care.[55]

Regardless, the study set a high evidentiary bar for an important question: Can providing prognostic information modify clinical outcomes? I am unaware of similarly robust studies in neonatal-perinatal medicine—but, given the prominence of prognostication in certain aspects of the field, such studies may be warranted.

The SUPPORT study in adult patients, as discussed previously, was limited in large part due to clinician utilization (and perhaps understanding or acceptance) of prognostic information. But it is worth considering whether expectation of certain prognostic outcomes might also have more subtle influences on outcomes. The notion of an *expectancy effect* has been well demonstrated in studies of education.[56] When teachers were told that students—who were selected entirely at random and with no evidence of prior success—would excel intellectually, these students later demonstrated higher scores on IQ and other tests. To evaluate whether the same phenomenon might occur in the medical setting, Learman and colleagues conducted a randomized controlled trial to test the effects of caregiver expectations on clinical outcomes of nursing home residents. Residents were randomly assigned "high-expectancy" (ie, in comparison with other residents, were expected to do better in their rehabilitation) and "low-expectancy" prognoses, which were communicated with their nurses. Three months later, high-expectancy residents were less likely to be admitted to the hospital and less likely to be depressed.[57]

In a NICU, do nurses, doctors, or parents spend more time with or pay more attention to infants they think will do well? Are they more careful with these infants? Are dozens of daily small decisions made slightly differently for infants with "good" prognoses versus "bad" ones, and do such decisions affect infant outcomes? Whether such an expectancy effect applies to this field should also be further considered.

NEXT STEPS

Prognosis has a key role in neonatal-perinatal medicine. Methods for formulating accurate and meaningful prognoses are improving. Many questions remain, however, about the best ways to use prognostic information. Clinicians and researchers should consider evaluating, prognosis as an intervention—like other neonatal interventions, with outcomes relevant to patients, families, and the public at large.

REFERENCES

1. Chauffard A. Medical prognosis: its methods, its evolution, its limitations. BMJ 1913;2:286–90.

2. Banay GL. An introduction to medical terminology I. Greek and Latin derivations. Bull Med Libr Assoc 1948;36:1–27.

3. Hippocrates (translated by Francis Adams). The Internet Classics Archive | The Book of Prognostics by Hippocrates. Available at: http://classics.mit.edu/Hippocrates/prognost.html. Accessed August 1, 2017.

4. Halamek LP. The advantages of prenatal consultation by a neonatologist. J Perinatol 2001;21:116–20.

5. Arzuaga BH, Cummings CL. Practices and education surrounding anticipated periviable deliveries among neonatal-perinatal medicine and maternal-fetal medicine fellowship programs. J Perinatol 2016;36:699–703.

6. Bell EF, American Academy of Pediatrics Committee on Fetus and Newborn. Noninitiation or withdrawal of intensive care for high-risk newborns. Pediatrics 2007;119:401–3.

7. Hartzband P, Groopman J. There is more to life than death. N Engl J Med 2012; 367:987–9.

8. Saigal S, Stoskopf BL, Burrows E, et al. Stability of maternal preferences for pediatric health states in the perinatal period and 1 year later. Arch Pediatr Adolesc Med 2003;157:261–9.

9. Suresh GK. Newborn baby is borderline; should the doctor resuscitate? Washington Post 2013. Available at: https://www.washingtonpost.com/national/health-science/newborn-baby-is-borderline-should-the-doctor-resuscitate/2013/11/04/e35d58aa-2b92-11e3-8ade-a1f23cda135e_story.html. Accessed August 1, 2017.

10. Rysavy MA, Colaizy TT, Bann CM, et al. Expanding the frame–outcomes following extremely preterm birth beyond neurodevelopmental impairment. Acta Paediatr 2017;106(Suppl 469):8–9.

11. Janvier A. Pepperoni pizza and sex. Curr Probl Pediatr Adolesc Health Care 2011;41:106–8.

12. Rysavy MA, Tyson JE. The problem and promise of prognosis research. JAMA Pediatr 2016;170:411–2.

13. Christakis NA, Sacks GA. The role of prognosis in clinical decision making. J Gen Intern Med 1996;11:422–5.

14. Farr W. "On prognosis" by William Farr (British Medical Almanack 1838; supplement 199–216) part 1 (pages 199–208). Soz Praventivmed 2003;48:219–24.

15. Arnold CC, Kramer MS, Hobbs CA, et al. Very low birth weight: a problematic cohort for epidemiologic studies of very small or immature neonates. Am J Epidemiol 1991;134:604–13.

16. Cross G, Becker M, Congdon P. Prognosis for babies born with fused eyelids. Arch Dis Child 1985;60:479–80.

17. Stephano JL, Morales M. Fused eyelids in the extremely premature infant: multivariate analysis of survival and outcome. Am J Perinatol 1992;9:84–6.

18. Medlock S, Ravelli ACJ, Tamminga P, et al. Prediction of mortality in very premature infants: a systematic review of prediction models. PLoS One 2011;6:e23441.

19. Janvier A, Farlow B, Baardsnes J, et al. Measuring and communicating meaningful outcomes in neonatology: a family perspective. Semin Perinatol 2016;40: 571–7.

20. McCormick M, Litt JS. The outcomes of very preterm infants: is it time to ask different questions? Pediatrics 2017;139:e20161694.

21. Webbe J, Brunton G, Ali S, et al. Core outcomes in neonatology (COIN): a core outcome set based on routinely collected data. Core Outcome Measures in Effectiveness Trials (COMET) Conference. Amsterdam (Netherlands), November 10–11, 2016. Available at: http://neoepoch.com/presentations/. Accessed August 1, 2017.

22. Guillen U, DeMauro S, Ma L, et al. Survival rates in extremely low birthweight infants depend on the denominator: avoiding potential for bias by specifying denominators. Am J Obstet Gynecol 2011;205:329.e1–7.

23. Harrison MR, Bjoardl R, Langmark F, et al. Congenital diaphragmatic hernia: the hidden mortality. J Pediatr Surg 1978;13:227–30.

24. Wilkinson D. The self-fulfilling prophecy in intensive care. Theor Med Bioeth 2009; 30:401–10.

25. Rysavy MA, Li L, Bell EF, et al. Between-hospital variation in treatment and outcomes in extremely preterm infants. N Engl J Med 2015;372:1801–11.

26. Wilkinson D. MRI and Withdrawal of life support from newborn infants with hypoxic-ischemic encephalopathy. Pediatrics 2010;126:e451–8.
27. Feingold M. Down's syndrome and heart surgery. Pediatrics 1978;61:331.
28. Rysavy MA, Marlow N, Doyle LW, et al. Reporting outcomes of extremely preterm births. Pediatrics 2016;138:e20160689.
29. Ambalavanan N, Carlo WA, Tyson JE, et al. Outcome trajectories in extremely preterm infants. Pediatrics 2012;130:e115–25.
30. Hemingway H. Prognosis research: why is Dr Lydgate still waiting? J Clin Epidemiol 2006;59:1229–38.
31. Hemingway H, Riley RD, Altman DG. Ten steps towards improving prognosis research. BMJ 2009;339:b4184.
32. Scope of our work. Cochrane methods prognosis. Available at: http://prognosismethods.cochrane.org/scope-our-work. Accessed August 1, 2017.
33. PROGRESS Group. Prognosis research strategy (PROGRESS) 1: a framework for researching clinical outcomes. BMJ 2013;346:e5595.
34. Collins GS, Reitsma JB, Altman DG, et al. Transparent Reporting of a multivariable prediction model for individual prognosis or diagnosis (TRIPOD): the TRIPOD statement. Ann Intern Med 2015;162:55–63.
35. Vickers AJ, Elkin EB. Decision curve analysis: a novel method for evaluating prediction models. Med Decis Making 2006;26:565–74.
36. Fitzgerald M, Saville BR, Lewis RJ. Decision curve analysis. JAMA 2015;313:409–10.
37. Morse SB, Haywood JL, Goldenberg RL, et al. Estimation of neonatal outcome and perinatal therapy use. Pediatrics 2000;105:1046–50.
38. Blanco F, Suresh G, Howard D, et al. Ensuring accurate knowledge of prematurity outcomes for prenatal counseling. Pediatrics 2005;115:e478–87.
39. White DB, Ernecoff N, Buddadhumaruk P, et al. Prevalence of and factors related to discordance about prognosis between physicians and surrogate decision makers of critically ill patients. JAMA 2016;315:2086–94.
40. Zipkin DA, Umscheid CA, Keating NL, et al. Evidence-based risk communication: a systematic review. Ann Intern Med 2014;161:270–80.
41. Haward MF, Janvier A. An introduction to behavioural decision-making theories for paediatricians. Acta Paediatr 2015;104:340–5.
42. Haward MF, Murphy RO, Lorenz JM. Message framing and perinatal decisions. Pediatrics 2008;122:109–18.
43. Schenker Y, Meisel A. Informed consent in clinical care: practical considerations in the effort to achieve ethical goals. JAMA 2011;305:1130–1.
44. Miquel-Verges F, Woods SL, Aucott SW, et al. Prenatal consultation with a neonatologist for congenital anomalies: parental perceptions. Pediatrics 2009;124:e573–9.
45. Cope CD, Lyons AC, Donovan V, et al. Providing letters and audiotapes to supplement a prenatal diagnostic consultation: effects on later distress and recall. Prenat Diagn 2003;23:1060–7.
46. Guillen U, Suh S, Munson D, et al. Development and pretesting of a decision-aid to use when counseling parents facing imminent extreme premature delivery. J Pediatr 2012;160:382–7.
47. Kakkilaya V, Groome LJ, Platt D, et al. Use of a visual aid to improve counseling at the threshold of viability. Pediatrics 2011;128:e1511–9.
48. Utility of a clinically relevant decision aid, for parents facing extremely premature delivery. ClinicalTrials.gov. Accessed at: https://clinicaltrials.gov/ct2/show/NCT01713894. Accessed August 1, 2017.

49. Bekker HL, Winterbottom AE, Butow P, et al. Do personal stories make patient decision aids more effective? A critical review of theory and evidence. BMC Med Inform Decis Mak 2013;13(Suppl 2):S9.
50. Janvier A, Farlow B, Barrington K. Parental hopes, interventions, and survival of neonates with trisomy 13 and trisomy 18. Am J Med Genet C Semin Med Genet 2016;172:279–87.
51. The SUPPORT Principal Investigators. A controlled trial to improve care for seriously ill hospitalized patients. The study to understand prognoses and preferences for outcomes and risks of treatments (SUPPORT). JAMA 1995;274:1591–8.
52. Knaus WA, Harrell FE, Lynn J, et al. The SUPPORT prognostic model: objective estimates of survival for seriously ill hospitalized adults. Ann Intern Med 1995; 122:191–203.
53. Bellamy PE. Why did prognosis presentation not work in the SUPPORT study? Curr Opin Crit Care 1997;3:188–91.
54. Rysavy M. Evidence-based medicine: a science of uncertainty and an art of probability. Virtual Mentor 2013;15:4–8.
55. Hoffman TC, Montori VM, Del Mar C. The connection between evidence-based medicine and shared decision making. JAMA 2014;312:1295–6.
56. Rosenthal R, Jacobson L. Teachers' expectancies: determinants of pupils' IQ gains. Psychol Rep 1966;19:115–8.
57. Learman LA, Avorn J, Everitt DE, et al. Pygmalion in the nursing home: the effects of caregiver expectations on patient outcomes. J Am Geriatr Soc 1990;38(7): 797–803.

Therapeutic Hypothermia
How Can We Optimize This Therapy to Further Improve Outcomes?

Girija Natarajan, MD[a], Abbot Laptook, MD[b],
Seetha Shankaran, MD[a],*

KEYWORDS

- Hypoxic-ischemic encephalopathy • Cooling • Neonate

KEY POINTS

- Therapeutic hypothermia to 33.0°C to 34.0°C for moderate to severe hypoxic-ischemic encephalopathy has been demonstrated to be safe and efficacious in reducing death and disability.
- In addition to the biochemical criteria, evidence of moderate or severe encephalopathy on neurologic examination is a prerequisite to cooling; serial examinations have prognostic utility.
- Avoidance of hypocarbia, hyperoxia, and glucose derangements and detection and control of seizures during cooling are important to optimize outcomes in neonatal encephalopathy.

CURRENT RATES OF MORTALITY AND DISABILITY FOLLOWING HYPOTHERMIA THERAPY

Neonatal encephalopathy is a condition of disordered neonatal brain function and is associated with many risk factors. The incidence of neonatal encephalopathy is estimated to be 3.0 per 1000 live births. Neonatal encephalopathy due to hypoxic-ischemic events is a subset of neonatal encephalopathy and occurs in 1.5 per 1000 livebirths. About 15% to 20% of affected newborns die in the postnatal period, and

Funding: Funded by NIH: U10 HD 21385; U10 HD 27904.
Disclosures: The authors have no relationship with any commercial company that has a direct financial interest in subject matter or materials discussed in the article or with a company making a competing product.
[a] Department of Pediatrics, Division of Neonatology, Wayne State University, Children's Hospital of Michigan and Hutzel Women's Hospital, 3901 Beaubien Boulevard, Detroit, MI 48201, USA; [b] Department of Pediatrics, Division of Neonatology, Women and Infants Hospital of Rhode Island, Brown University, 101 Dudley Street, Providence, RI 02905, USA
* Corresponding author.
E-mail address: sshankar@med.wayne.edu

Clin Perinatol 45 (2018) 241–255
https://doi.org/10.1016/j.clp.2018.01.010
0095-5108/18/© 2018 Elsevier Inc. All rights reserved.

perinatology.theclinics.com

an additional 25% will sustain childhood disabilities.[1] Six randomized clinical trials of induced therapeutic hypothermia (TH) at 33.0°C to 34.0°C for 72 hours for neonatal moderate or severe hypoxic-ischemic encephalopathy (HIE) have demonstrated a decrease in death or disability up to 24 months of age.[2–7] This neuroprotection continues to childhood.[8–10] TH is currently the standard of care for term neonates with encephalopathy due to hypoxia-ischemia.[11] The rate of death or disability in the cooled group ranged from 44% to 55% in these clinical trials. In the most recent Eunice Kennedy Shriver National Institute of Child Health and Human Development Neonatal Research Network's (NICHD NRN) randomized clinical trial of standard cooling at 33.0°C to 34.0°C for 72 hours compared with deeper or longer cooling, the rate of death or disability in the usual care group following neonatal moderate or severe HIE was 29%.[12] This lower rate may be due to fewer infants with severe HIE in the recent trial (23% compared with 38% in the cooled group of the first NICHD NRN trial[3]), lower acuity of neonates, and earlier initiation of cooling.

HOW EFFECTIVE IS THERAPEUTIC HYPOTHERMIA?

TH is an effective therapy to reduce death or disability at 18 months of age after moderate or severe neonatal HIE (typical relative risk [RR] 0.75, 95% confidence interval [CI] 0.68–0.83).[11] TH was also associated with significant reduction in mortality and in disability in survivors.[11] The number needed to treat (NNT) to prevent one case of death or disability is 7,[11] much lower than the NNT of adults receiving statins to prevent cardiovascular disease (n = 72)[13] or that of neonates receiving surfactant to prevent complications of respiratory distress syndrome (n = 25)[14]; thus, TH for moderate or severe HIE is a very robust therapy.

SELECTION OF NEONATES FOR THERAPEUTIC HYPOTHERMIA

It is important to select the appropriate neonates for hypothermia therapy; the safety and efficacy of this therapy has been demonstrated only for neonates with moderate or severe HIE.[11,15] All the clinical trials have had a 2-step process of selection, initially with biochemical evidence of hypoxia-ischemia followed by evolving moderate or severe encephalopathy. In the NICHD NRN trials,[3,12] acidosis was required at birth on cord pH or the first blood gas within 1 hour of age (pH <7.0 or base deficit >16 mmol/L). If a blood gas was not available or the pH was between 7.01 and 7.15 and the base deficit was between 10.0 and 15.9 mmol/L, additional criteria were required, including a history of an acute perinatal event and either a 10-minute Apgar score of 5 or less or assisted ventilation initiated at birth and continued for at least 10 minutes. The second parameter was evidence of moderate or severe encephalopathy on the neurologic examination.

THE NEUROLOGIC EXAMINATION FOR MODERATE OR SEVERE ENCEPHALOPATHY

The clinical trials of hypothermia for neonatal HIE have required 3 or more out of 6 abnormalities in the moderate or severe categories of the neurologic examination or clinical seizures within 6 hours of age for trial eligibility. The CoolCap and TOBY (Total Body Hypothermia for Neonatal Encephalopathy) trials mandated that one of the abnormal categories of the neurologic examination needed to be level of consciousness, and they both also required an abnormal amplitude integrated electroencephalogram (aEEG).[2,4] The NICHD NRN has standardized the examination to minimize examiner variability and promote enrollment of appropriate infants. The examination is challenging because it is subjective and the one performed within 6 hours of age (the therapeutic window for initiation of cooling) may be influenced by the delivery process and/or maternal anesthesia or analgesia. The examination findings are dynamic and may change based on the neonates' compensatory response to the hypoxic-ischemic insult and the timing and severity of the insult. The most important characteristic is that there can be a mix of findings in the normal or mild as well as moderate or severe encephalopathy stage of the modified Sarnat examination (**Table 1**). This examination has 6 categories; each category contributes one point. Primitive reflexes (suck and Moro) and the autonomic nervous system (pupils, heart rate, and respiration) have multiple signs, but these contribute only one point; when multiple signs within a category are moderate or severe, the higher severity of encephalopathy is noted; that is, if suck is moderate and Moro is severe, severe encephalopathy is selected for the primitive reflexes category. The neurologic examination should be conducted in 2 phases. The first phase is the observation phase (assessment of spontaneous activity, posture, heart rate, and respiration); the second phase is the active manipulation phase (assessment of level of consciousness, tone, suck, Moro, and pupils) whereby the least noxious part should be performed first, leaving the pupils for the last part of the examination. The infant should be assessed in the awake state and when stimuli are applied to assess activity; the examiner should start with a mild stimulus before proceeding to a more severe one.

The following definitions have been developed for the NICHD NRN examination: under level of consciousness, *lethargic* is delayed but a complete response to external stimuli, whereas *stupor or coma* is not arousable and nonresponsive or a delayed incomplete response to external stimuli. For the assessment of spontaneous activity, if the infant is sedated, clinical judgment needs to be used to decide whether the examination is reliable; paralysis of the infant will preclude a meaningful examination. Under moderate encephalopathy, *posture* is strong distal flexion, complete extension, or a frog-legged position; *decerebrate* means the legs and arms are extended, the wrists flexed, and the hands fisted. If posture is abnormal but does not fit either the moderate or severe category, the infant should be coded as moderate. For assessment of tone, the extremities, neck, and trunk should be assessed and the

Table 1
Components of neurologic examination for categorization as moderate or severe hypoxic-ischemic encephalopathy

Category	Moderate HIE	Severe HIE
Level of consciousness	Lethargic	Stupor/coma
Spontaneous activity	Decreased activity	No activity
Posture	Distal flexion, complete extension	Decerebrate
Tone	Hypotonia, focal or general Hypertonia	Flaccid Rigid
Primitive reflexes		
Suck	Weak or has bite	Absent
Moro	Incomplete	Absent
Autonomic nervous system		
Pupils	Constricted	Deviation/dilated/nonreactive to light
Heart rate	Bradycardia	Variable heart rate
Respirations	Periodic breathing	On ventilator with or without spontaneous breaths

predominant tone should be categorized. Abnormalities may be either an increase or decrease in tone. *Hypotonia* is floppy, either focal or generalized, and can be assessed in ventral suspension; *flaccid* resembles a rag doll; in the severe category of hypertonia, *rigid* is stiffness or inflexibility. The *Moro* reflex can be elicited in an intubated infant by gently raising and lowering the head. If the infant has brachial plexus injury or fracture of the clavicle, the other extremity should be assessed. Under autonomic nervous system, *bradycardia* is a heart rate less than 100/min with only occasional increases to greater than 120/min, a *variable* heart rate is not constant and varies widely between less than 100/min and greater than 120/min. It should be noted that the heart rate may be influenced by the phase of cooling and should not be part of the evaluation if cooling has been initiated. *Periodic breathing*, whether associated with desaturations, and with or without supplemental oxygen, is categorized as moderate; an intubated infant is categorized as severe encephalopathy because it cannot be ascertained whether the infant could sustain spontaneous respirations without ventilator support. Asymmetric or nonreactive pupils should be coded as severe encephalopathy. The classification as moderate or severe HIE is based on the predominant number of categories that are moderate or severe; if the number of moderate and severe categories are equal, the infant should be assigned the stage of HIE based on the level of consciousness. Clinical seizures can be subtle; the infant may have ocular deviations, sucking, lip smacking, rowing, swimming, or bicycling movements. In addition, seizures can be tonic/clonic, localized, multifocal, or generalized. An infant with clinical seizures (documented by a neonatal nurse clinician or neonatologist) is coded as moderate HIE whether the neurologic examination for eligibility is moderate or normal/mild. Increased tone in the neurologic examination for eligibility was infrequent, but decerebrate posture was noted in the eligibility criteria of the first NICHD NRN trial.[3]

The additional components of the neurologic examination that are added to the assessment of the stage of HIE during serial and discharge assessments are clonus, fisted hand, abnormal movements, gag reflex, and asymmetric tonic neck reflex (ATNR). *Clonus* is defined as more than 4 to 5 beats; *fisted hand* is the thumb across the palm or cortical thumb; *abnormal movements* are tremulous, excessive movements, either jerky, involuntary, bicycling, or myotonic. The *ATNR* is assessed with the infant supine and head rotated to either side. A normal tonic neck reflex is extension of arm and leg to the side to which the face is turned with flexion of the arm and leg of the opposite side (fencing position). Infant should spontaneously (within 30 seconds) terminate this position. For the NICHD NRN hypothermia trials,[3,12] the site or trial principal investigator (PI) was the gold standard examiner and reviewed the training slides developed by 2 trial PIs (S.S. and A.L.) with all site physicians. Physician examiners at each clinical site performed 2 examinations with the gold standard examiner, within an hour of each other. Examination findings were reviewed for concordance by the trial PIs (S.S. and A.L.); agreement of at least 5 of 6 categories was needed for certification and allows investigators to independently evaluate infants for inclusion in trials. An annual refresher course using training slides was conducted. The NICHD certification process is currently used for ongoing BABYBAC II: A Phase II Multi-site Study of Autologous Cord Blood Cells for Hypoxic-Ischemic Encephalopathy funded by Duke University and the Robertson Foundation and the Hypothermia for Encephalopathy in Low- and Middle-Income Countries trial. The performance of serial examinations, daily during hypothermia therapy and at discharge, is important for prognosis; the persistence of severe HIE at 72 hours increased the risk of death or disability at 18 months of age after controlling for the treatment group, with an odds ratio (OR) (95% CI) of 60 (15–246). An increased risk of death or disability was also associated with abnormal findings in the extended neurologic examination (OR 2.7 [1.1–6.7]).

Gavage tube or gastrostomy feedings at discharge also increased the risk of death or disability (OR 8.6 [2.7–26.8]).[16] Therefore, careful neurologic examinations before initiation, following TH, and at discharge should be part of clinical practice.

TIME TO INITIATION OF COOLING AND TRANSPORT COOLING

In both the NICHD NRN and TOBY trials, neither time to initiation of cooling nor location of birth (inborn vs out-born) impacted outcome, although enrollment heavily clustered around 3 to 4 hours.[4,15,17] However, in the most recent NICHD NRN trial of usual cooling compared with longer and deeper cooling, the mortality and disability rates were lower in the usual care cooled group; time to initiation of cooling was earlier in spite of more out-born infants when compared with the first NICHD NRN trial.[12]

The NICHD workshop in 2011 identified targeted temperature management before arrival at a cooling center as a knowledge gap.[18] Passive cooling during transport and active cooling without a servo-controlled device are associated with risks of temperature overshoot and rapid fluctuations, with infants with severe HIE being at the greatest risk.[19,20] Following these reports, studies have shown that active cooling with servo-controlled devices and continuous core temperature monitoring achieve target temperatures in less time and have less variability and greater efficacy in maintaining temperatures within a target range, compared with passive cooling during transport.[21–23] In situations whereby transport distances are long, transport cooling with servo-controlled devices and careful temperature monitoring may be important to ensure its initiation within the window of 6 hours.

DELIVERY ROOM MANAGEMENT

A persistently low Apgar score at 10 minutes is associated with death or moderate/severe disability at 18 months and also at 6 to 7 years of age.[24,25] However, not all infants with a 10-minute Apgar score of 3 or less had a uniformly poor outcome; 20% of children with a score of 0 at 10 minutes survived without disability at school age.[25]

OPTIMUM DURATION OF COOLING

Early discontinuation of cooling due to clinical improvement has been reported in registry data[26]; this practice should be discouraged, as evidence of brain injury has been noted with incomplete cooling following mild encephalopathy.[27]

MANAGEMENT OF ELEVATED TEMPERATURE

Elevated temperature in the control group of the NICHD NRN and CoolCap trials was associated with higher risk of death or disability compared with noncooled infants without elevated temperatures after controlling for stage of encephalopathy, race, and sex.[28,29] In the NICHD NRN childhood follow-up data, the association with elevated temperature and death or IQ less than 70 was still present.[30] Brain temperature measured with magnetic resonance spectroscopy reveals a higher temperature among cooled infants with brain injury on MRI compared with cooled infants without brain injury on MRI.[31] Therefore, it is important to avoid and treat elevations of temperature before and after TH.

HEMODYNAMIC STABILITY DURING THERAPEUTIC HYPOTHERMIA

The link between cerebral ischemia and cardiac dysfunction is unclear; but HIE is associated with multi-organ dysfunction, including myocardial dysfunction.[15,32]

Cooling may exacerbate blood pressure and temperature instability, especially in smaller sicker infants during induction and maintenance of cooling,[33] hence, the need to provide hemodynamic support during cooling and rewarming.[34]

HYPOCARBIA DURING THERAPEUTIC HYPOTHERMIA

The cumulative exposure to hypocarbia in the early phase of TH was linked with a higher risk of death or disability at 18 months of age in the NICHD NRN's first randomized controlled trial (RCT).[35] The CoolCap data noted that Pco_2 during the 72 hours of TH was inversely related to an unfavorable outcome after adjustment for HIE severity and other confounding variables.[36] Low carbon dioxide levels may impact cerebral perfusion, thus, exacerbating the risk of brain injury. Thus, it is essential to maintain Pco_2 in the normal range during TH. This effort may be challenging if an infant is hyperventilating from metabolic acidosis or the hyperventilation is centrally driven because of possible brainstem dysfunction.

HYPEROXEMIA DURING THERAPEUTIC HYPOTHERMIA

In an evaluation of infants with birth acidosis, hyperoxemia during the first hour of life was associated with a higher incidence of encephalopathy; among infants with HIE who had a brain MRI, there was a higher incidence of brain injury.[37] An association between an increased inspired oxygen concentration during the first 6 hours of life and an adverse outcome (death or Bayley II Mental Developmental Index or Psychomotor Index <70) was noted in another study, although no association was found between hypocarbia and adverse outcomes.[38] Neonates are susceptible to an increase in free radical production and oxidative stress immediately after birth. Therefore, hyperoxemia should be avoided in high-risk infants during TH.

HYPOGLYCEMIA AND HYPERGLYCEMIA DURING THERAPEUTIC HYPOTHERMIA

In a single-center study conducted between 1994 and 2010, 15 of 94 (16%) neonates with neonatal encephalopathy and early brain imaging studies had hypoglycemia (glucose values <46 mg/dL) in the first 24 hours after birth. TH was provided for 10 infants in the no-hypoglycemia group (n = 79) and one infant in the hypoglycemia group. Among all infants, hypoglycemia was associated with an increased risk of corticospinal tract injury on brain MRI imaging and lower Bayley II Psychomotor Developmental and Mental Developmental Index or Bayley III cognitive and language scores at 1 year of age, after adjusting for perinatal distress and need for resuscitation.[39] The CoolCap study examined the association of hypoglycemia (≤40 mg/dL) and hyperglycemia (>150 mg/dL) among trial participants and outcomes.[40] Among 234 infants enrolled, 121 had abnormal plasma glucose values within the first 12 hours and an unfavorable outcome was noted among 160 infants. Death or neurodevelopmental disability at 18 months of age was more common among infants with hypoglycemia (81%), hyperglycemia (67%), or any glucose derangement (67%) during the first 12 hours, compared with 48% among normoglycemic infants, after controlling for stage of encephalopathy, birth weight, Apgar score, pH, and intervention. The impact on death or disability separately is not presented. The investigators suggested that the data confirm pathophysiologic observations of deranged glucose metabolism in the preclinical models of hypoxia-ischemia. Maintaining glucose levels in the normal range should be the goal during TH for neonatal HIE.

SEIZURES DURING THERAPEUTIC HYPOTHERMIA

In the NICHD NRN RCT, 127 of 208 neonates had clinical seizures at less than 6 hours of age. In the univariate analysis, death or disability at 18 months of age was associated with seizures and severe HIE; on multivariate analysis, seizures no longer had an independent effect on outcomes.[41] It should be noted that clinical seizures may not always represent electrographic seizures and instead may be abnormal movements. In another study in 47 neonates with HIE who underwent continuous electroencephalography, 62% had electrographic seizures.[42] Seizures per se were not associated with an abnormal outcome, but the risk of an abnormal outcome at 24 to 48 months of age increased more than 9-fold if the total seizure burden was more than 40 minutes or the maximum hourly seizure burden was more than 13 minutes per hour.[42] TH decreases seizure burden, as noted on electroencephalography.[43] The administration of phenobarbital before initiation of TH may cause lower temperatures during the induction phase of cooling.[44] During TH, continuous video electroencephalogram (EEG) monitoring and treatment of clinical seizures confirmed by EEG or amplitude-integrated EEG should be considered, although definitive data justifying the treatment of electrographic seizures are lacking.

CEREBRAL FUNCTIONING MONITORING AT LESS THAN 6 HOURS OF AGE

Both the CoolCap and TOBY trials had an abnormal aEEG as an eligibility criterion, in addition to birth acidosis or need for resuscitation and moderate or severe encephalopathy.[2,4] Death or disability was lower among infants who had a less severely abnormal background aEEG pattern, and an absence of seizures on the aEEG was associated with a better outcome in the CoolCap trial.[2] The effect of cooling did not vary according to the severity of the abnormality on the aEEG.[29] In an observational study comparing cooled infants with a prior noncooled cohort, the positive predictive value of an abnormal aEEG at 3 to 6 hours of age was 84% for infants not cooled and lower (59%) in cooled infants.[45] The recovery to normal of the background pattern of the aEEG was the best predictor of outcome; infants with a good outcome normalized by 24 hours if they were not cooled and in 48 hours if undergoing TH. The NICHD NRN aEEG study, which included infants from the first NRN TH trial as well as those following the trial, demonstrated that severe HIE and an abnormal aEEG pattern at less than 9 hours of age were related to poor outcomes in the univariate analysis. Severe HIE alone persisted as a predictor in the multivariate analysis, and the addition of the aEEG to HIE stage did not add to the predictive value (area under the curve increased from 0.72 to 0.75).[46] The TOBY trial noted that the positive predictive values of a severely abnormal aEEG assessed by voltage and pattern before study intervention for an adverse outcome at 18 months of age were 0.63 and 0.59, respectively, in the noncooled infants and 0.55 and 0.51 in the cooled infants with the lower effect in cooled infants related to the neuroprotective effect of cooling.[47] The positive predictive value of an abnormal aEEG for abnormal outcome in the NICHD NRN study was 0.56, whereas that of severe HIE by examination was 0.81 and moderate HIE by examination was 0.32; thus, the predictive value of the aEEG to identify infants who will subsequently manifest brain injury is limited.

USE OF SEDATION-ANALGESIA DURING THERAPEUTIC HYPOTHERMIA

The administration of sedation, analgesia, and neuromuscular blockade during TH for neonatal HIE is determined by center and clinician preferences and may be a surrogate of the severity of illness. Of the neonatal trials of TH, only the neo.nEURO.network hypothermia randomized controlled trial treated all infants with morphine (0.1 mg/kg) or an equivalent dose of fentanyl every 4 hours or by continuous infusion.[5] In the TOBY trial, all infants underwent sedation with morphine infusions or with chloral hydrate if they "appeared to be distressed."[4] In multiple studies in animals, adults, and older children, mild to moderate TH has been shown to decrease the systemic clearance of cytochrome P450 metabolized drugs between approximately 7% and 22% per degree Celsius less than 37°C.[48] In a small study in neonates, serum morphine concentrations at 6, 12, 24, 48, and 72 hours after birth were higher and clearance lower in infants who underwent TH, compared with normothermia, at similar morphine infusion rates and cumulative doses.[49] In addition, sedation, analgesia, and neuromuscular blockade used during TH may affect the neurologic examinations, seizure detection and the results of EEGs, duration of mechanical ventilation, and hemodynamic status. The effects of sedation, analgesia, and neuromuscular blockade on long-term neurodevelopment are unclear. There is insufficient evidence for routine use of these agents during TH; therefore, careful use to achieve a desired level of sedation seems prudent.[50,51]

ASSESSMENT OF SERUM BIOMARKERS

The assessment of the utility of serum biomarkers in HIE is an area of active research. Two markers, ubiquitin carboxyl-terminal esterase Li (UCHL1), known to be released from neurons following cardiac arrest, and glial fibrillary acidic protein (GFAP), released from astrocytes following possible hypoxia during extracorporeal oxygenation, were measured in neonates with HIE undergoing cooling. The markers were elevated at differing time points; infants with brain injury on MRI had higher UCHL1 at initiation and end of cooling, whereas GFAP was higher at 24 and 72 hours.[52] In another observational study, elevated GFAP and inflammatory cytokines were associated with an abnormal neurologic outcome at 15 to 18 months.[53] Elevated cardiac troponin 1 levels have been noted to be correlated with reduced fractional shortening and severity of tricuspid regurgitation on echocardiogram and also with the risk of a poor neurodevelopmental outcome at 18 months in an observational study.[54] Another observational study provided the cutoff values (<0.22 ng/mL for normothermic and <0.15 ng/mL for hypothermic infants) of cardiac troponin 1 at less than 24 hours of age that were predictive of a good outcome in infancy.[55]

HEART RATE VARIABILITY

Monitoring of heart rate variability is a useful adjunct tool to assess the severity of HIE in infants undergoing TH.[56] Depressed heart rate variability (the normalized RR interval also known as the NN interval) correlates well with the EEG and the neurodevelopmental outcome; a lower NN value is seen with a more severe EEG grade of HIE and with an abnormal neurodevelopmental outcome at 2 years.[57,58]

NEUROIMAGING FOR NEONATES UNDERGOING THERAPEUTIC HYPOTHERMIA

The MRI findings among 131 of 325 infants who participated in the TOBY trial, performed at a mean age of 8 days, demonstrated that TH reduced injury in the basal ganglia and thalamus (BGT) (OR [95% CI] 0.36 [0.15–0.84]), the posterior limb of the internal capsule (PLIC) (0.38 [0.17–0.85]), and white matter (WM), (0.30 [0.12–0.77]) among cooled infants compared with the noncooled group. There was no reduction of signal abnormalities in the cortex. Cooled infants were more likely to have normal scans, and the brain injury on the scans were predictive of death or disability at 18 months in both cooled and noncooled infants.[59] The NICHD NRN trial evaluated 136 of 208 trial participants at a mean age of 15 days. Normal scans were noted in

38 of 73 infants (52%) in the hypothermia group and 22 of 63 (35%) in the control group (P = .06). Infants in the hypothermia group had fewer areas of infarction (12%) compared with the control group (22%) (P = .02). A brain injury pattern was described with each level reflecting greater involvement of injury: 0, normal; 1A, minimal cerebral lesions only and no involvement of the BGT or anterior limb of the internal capsule (ALIC) or PLIC and no area of watershed (WS) infarction; 1B, more extensive cerebral lesions without BGT, ALIC, PLIC, or WS involvement; 2A, any BGT, ALIC, PLIC, or WS involvement without any other cerebral lesions; 2B, involvement of BGT, ALIC, PLIC, or infarction and additional cerebral lesions; 3, cerebral hemispheric devastation. This categorization of injury correlated with the outcome of death or disability and with disability among survivors at 18 months in both cooled and control groups.[60] Infants with perinatal sentinel events had more BGT lesions on MRI imaging but similar neurodevelopmental outcomes at 18 months than infants without perinatal sentinel events. Outcomes correlated with neonatal MRI findings.[61] The neonatal MRI imaging categorization of brain injury was also a marker of childhood outcomes following the NICHD NRN trial of hypothermia for neonatal HIE. Death or IQ less than 70 was seen in 4 of 50 (8%) children with pattern 0; 1 of 6 (17%) with 1A; 1 of 4 (25%) with 1B; 3 of 8 (38%) with 2A; 32 of 49 (65%) with 2B; and 7 of 7 (100%) with pattern 3 (P<.001). This association was seen within hypothermia and control subgroups.[62] The ICE trial (infant cooling evaluation collaboration) evaluated MRIs from 127 of 221 trial participants obtained at a mean age of 6 days. On T1- and T2-weighted imaging, in the hypothermia group compared with the normothermia group, WM abnormalities (OR 0.28, 95% CI 0 [0.09–0.82]) as well as gray matter (0.41 [0.17–1.00]) abnormalities were reduced. Abnormal MRI predicted an adverse outcome, with diffusion-weighted abnormalities in the BGT and PLIC having the most predictive value.[63] The American College of Obstetrics and Gynecology and the American Academy of Pediatrics have suggested an early MRI between 24 and 96 hours to delineate timing of perinatal cerebral injury (to distinguish injury occurring peripartum and remote from delivery), whereas one obtained at 10 days (between 7 and 21 days) would delineate the full extent of cerebral injury.[64]

WITHDRAWAL OF SUPPORT OR DECISION TO REDIRECT CARE IN THE NEONATAL INTENSIVE CARE UNIT FOLLOWING THERAPEUTIC HYPOTHERMIA

The mortality rate of neonates undergoing TH for moderate/severe HIE in the first NICHD NRN[3] trial was 19% in the cooled arm (72 hours at 33.5°C), whereas the mortality rate in the trial comparing usual depth and duration with longer and deeper cooling was 8 of 92 (9%) in the 33.5°C for 72 hours group.[12] Withdrawal of support occurred among 12 of 24 infants who died in the hypothermia group in the first NICHD NRN trial[3]; in the Optimizing Cooling strategies trial, among the infants assigned to usual care of cooling for 72 hours at 33.5°C, support was withdrawn for 6 of 8 infants who died.[12] A single-center study described characteristics of death in the NICU among neonates with moderate or severe encephalopathy receiving TH and observed that 31 of 229 infants died in a 7-year period and all deaths followed withdrawal of support or redirection of care; for 19 infants, support was withdrawn during TH. Twenty-eight of the infants had severe encephalopathy on examination, and 87% had severely abnormal EEG; the 13 who had MRIs performed had moderate or severe brain injury.[65] Available data suggest that persistence of severe encephalopathy on serial neurologic examinations, lack of improvement in the abnormal background in the aEEG and EEG, and MRI evidence of severe injury may be useful to identify infants at highest risk of severe neurologic sequelae.[16,66]

FOLLOW-UP OF INFANTS WHO RECEIVE THERAPEUTIC HYPOTHERMIA

The major RCTs of TH for neonatal moderate/severe HIE have all reported outcomes at 18 or 24 months.[2–7] The 6- to 7-year outcome of the CoolCap trial was assessed by parent interview with the WeeFIM, a pediatric functional independence measure, among 62 of 135 surviving children; disability rates at 18 months were strongly associated with WeeFIM ratings in childhood, and there was no significant effect of treatment.[8] The NICHD NRN trial evaluated 91% of trial participants at 6 to 7 years of age. The primary outcome was death or IQ less than 70, whereas secondary outcomes focused on disabilities. The primary outcome occurred among 46 of 97 (47%) children in the hypothermia group and 58 of 93 (62%) children in the control group (adjusted risk ratio 0.78 [0.61–1.01]); the mortality rates and death or cerebral palsy (CP) were significantly lower in the hypothermia group. The 18-month outcome correlated well with the outcome in childhood.[9] The primary outcome of the TOBY trial was survival with IQ greater than 85; data were available for 85% of children; 75 of 145 (52%) in the hypothermia group compared with 52 of 132 (39%) in the control group had this outcome (RR 1.31 [1.01–1.71]). Children in the hypothermia group had significantly lower rates of CP and moderate or severe disability compared with the control group.[10] It is imperative that neonates who have undergone TH be evaluated for neuromotor and cognitive disabilities following NICU discharge in a standardized follow-up program.

The extent of neuromotor, cognitive, growth, and functional deficits was examined in the outcomes of children in the NICHD NRN trial because it has been noted in the past that the primary deficits after neonatal HIE was CP. One of the findings was the extent of growth failure among children with severe CP. Compared with those with no CP, those with CP had parameters less than the 10th percentile in weight (57% vs 3%), height (70% vs 2%), and head circumference (82% vs 13%); the growth failure severity increased with increasing age. Gastrostomy feeds were associated with better growth. These findings emphasize the need for early nutritional supplements for children who develop CP following neonatal HIE.[67]

The functional status of the children was evaluated by parental report in another study from the NICHD NRN hypothermia trial cohort.[68] Children with disability, compared with those without disability, had higher rates of severe HIE, public insurance, and Impact on Family Scales and lower mean Functional Status-II (FS-II) independence and general health scores. The FS-II scores were associated with childhood disability. Each unit increase in the FS-II Independence score at 18 months was associated with reduction in disability at 6 to 7 years of age, highlighting the need to make early referrals for special education services for the child and support services for parents.

The trajectory of cognitive outcomes to childhood noted that subnormal IQ was identified in more than 25% of the children at 6 to 7 years of age, almost all surviving children with CP (96%) had an IQ less than 70, 9% of children without CP had an IQ less than 70, and 31% had an IQ of 70 to 84. Children with a mental developmental index less than 70 at 18 months, had, on average an adjusted IQ that was 42 points lower than those with a score greater than 85. However, among the children with an IQ less than 70 who underwent formal testing, 23% had a normal gait, 16% had normal complex motor function and 10% had intact fine motor and coordination skills. Twenty percent of children with normal IQ and 28% of those with IQ of 70 to 84 received special education support services and were held back 1 or more grade levels in school. These findings emphasize cognitive impairment remains a concern for all children with neonatal HIE.[69]

SUMMARY

Based on the evidence presented, to optimize TH for neonatal HIE, cooling should be limited to infants with moderate or severe encephalopathy by following the eligibility criteria of the clinical trials. A careful neurologic examination for eligibility should be performed after the infant has been resuscitated and stabilized after birth. Serial neurologic examinations should be performed during TH and at discharge to assess prognosis. During TH, avoid hypocarbia, hypoxemia, and hyperoxemia and maintain blood sugar in the normal range. Sedation and analgesia should be used with caution. Avoid elevated temperatures before initiation of cooling and following rewarming. Imaging studies (MRI) should be performed at 7 to 10 days of age. Neonates should have neurophysiologic monitoring with aEEG and continuous EEG, if available. Standardized follow-up should be performed on all cooled infants with a focus on optimizing nutritional status of children with CP and referrals to early intervention programs for infants at risk for later disabilities or those with limited access to health care.

REFERENCES

1. Kurinczuk JJ, White-Koning M, Badawi N. Epidemiology of neonatal encephalopathy and hypoxic-ischaemic encephalopathy. Early Hum Dev 2010;86:329–38.
2. Gluckman PD, Wyatt J, Azzopardi DV, et al. Selective head cooling with mild systemic hypothermia after neonatal encephalopathy: multicenter randomised trial. Lancet 2005;365:663–70.
3. Shankaran S, Laptook AR, Ehrenkranz RA, et al. Whole-body hypothermia for neonates with hypoxic-ischemic encephalopathy. N Engl J Med 2005;353:1574–84.
4. Azzopardi DV, Strohm B, Edwards AD, et al. Moderate hypothermia to treat perinatal asphyxial encephalopathy. N Engl J Med 2009;361(14):1349–58.
5. Simbruner G, Mittal RA, Rohlmann F, et al, neo.nEURO.network Trial Participants. Systemic hypothermia after neonatal encephalopathy: outcomes of neo.nEURO.network RCT. Pediatrics 2010;126(4):e771–8.
6. Jacobs SE, Morley CJ, Inder TE, et al. Whole-body hypothermia for term and near term newborns with hypoxic ischemic encephalopathy: a randomized controlled trial. Arch Pediatr Adolesc Med 2011;165(8):692–700.
7. Zhou WH, Cheng GQ, Shao XM, et al. Selective head cooling with mild systemic hypothermia after neonatal hypoxic-ischemic encephalopathy: a multicenter randomized controlled trial in China. J Pediatr 2010;157(3):367–72, 372.e1–3.
8. Guillet R, Edwards AD, Thoresen M, et al. Seven- to eight-year follow-up of the CoolCap trial of head cooling for neonatal encephalopathy. Pediatr Res 2012; 71(2):205–9.
9. Shankaran S, Pappas A, McDonald SA, et al. Childhood outcomes after hypothermia for neonatal encephalopathy. N Engl J Med 2012;366(22):2085–92.
10. Azzopardi D, Strohm B, Marlow N, et al. Effects of hypothermia for perinatal asphyxia on childhood outcomes. N Engl J Med 2014;371(2):140–9.
11. Jacobs SE, Berg M, Hunt R, et al. Cooling for newborns with hypoxic ischaemic encephalopathy. Cochrane Database Syst Rev 2013;1:CD003311.
12. Shankaran S, Laptook AR, Pappas A, et al. Effect of depth and duration of cooling on deaths in the NICU among neonates with hypoxic-ischemic encephalopathy. A randomized clinical trial. JAMA 2014;312(24):1–11.
13. Chou R, Dana T, Blazina I, et al. Statins for prevention of cardiovascular disease in adults: evidence report and systematic review for the U.S Preventive Services Task Force. JAMA 2016;316(19):2008–14.

14. Ardell S, Pfister RH, Soll R. Animal derived surfactant extract versus protein free synthetic surfactant for the prevention and treatment of respiratory distress syndrome. Cochrane Database Syst Rev 2015;8:CD000144.

15. Shankaran S, Pappas A, Laptook AR, et al. Outcomes of safety and effectiveness in a multicenter randomized controlled trial of whole-body hypothermia for neonatal hypoxic-ischemic encephalopathy. Pediatrics 2008;122:e791–8.

16. Shankaran S, Laptook AR, Tyson JE, et al. Evolution of encephalopathy during whole body hypothermia for neonatal hypoxic-ischemic encephalopathy. J Pediatr 2012;160(4):567–72.e3.

17. Natarajan G, Pappas A, Shankaran S, et al. Effect of inborn vs. outborn delivery on neurodevelopmental outcomes in infants with hypoxic-ischemic encephalopathy: secondary analyses of the NICHD whole-body cooling trial. Pediatr Res 2012;72(4):414–9.

18. Higgins RD, Raju T, Edwards AD, et al. Hypothermia and other treatment options for neonatal encephalopathy: an executive summary of the Eunice Kennedy Shriver NICHD workshop. J Pediatr 2011;159(5):851–8.e1.

19. Fairchild K, Sokora D, Scott J, et al. Therapeutic hypothermia on neonatal transport: 4-year experience in a single NICU. J Perinatol 2010;30(5):324–9.

20. Hallberg B, Olson L, Bartocci M, et al. Passive induction of hypothermia during transport of asphyxiated infants: a risk of excessive cooling. Acta Paediatr 2009;98(6):942–6.

21. Stafford TD, Hagan JL, Sitler CG, et al. Therapeutic hypothermia during neonatal transport: active cooling helps reach the target. Ther Hypothermia Tem Manag 2017;7(2):88–94.

22. Goel N, Mohinuddin SM, Ratnavel N, et al. Comparison of passive and servo-controlled active cooling for infants with hypoxic-ischemic encephalopathy during neonatal transfers. Am J Perinatol 2017;34(1):19–25.

23. Akula VP, Joe P, Thusu K, et al. A randomized clinical trial of therapeutic hypothermia mode during transport for neonatal encephalopathy. J Pediatr 2015;166(4):856–61.e1-2.

24. Laptook AR, Shankaran S, Ambalavanan N, et al. Outcome of term infants using Apgar scores at 10 minutes following hypoxic-ischemic encephalopathy. Pediatrics 2009;124(6):1619–26.

25. Natarajan G, Shankaran S, Laptook AR, et al. Apgar scores at 10 min and outcomes at 6-7 years following hypoxic-ischaemic encephalopathy. Arch Dis Child Fetal Neonatal Ed 2011;98(6):F473–9.

26. Mehta S, Joshi A, Bajuk B, et al. Eligibility criteria for therapeutic hypothermia: from trials to clinical practice. J Paediatr Child Health 2017;53(3):295–300.

27. Lally PJ, Montaldo P, Oliveira V, et al. Residual brain injury after early discontinuation of cooling therapy in mild neonatal encephalopathy. Arch Dis Child Fetal Neonatal Ed 2017;0:F1–5.

28. Laptook A, Tyson J, Shankaran S, et al. Elevated temperature after hypoxic-ischemic encephalopathy: a risk factor for adverse outcome. Pediatrics 2008;122(3):491–9.

29. Wyatt JS, Gluckman PD, Liu PY, et al. Determinants of outcomes after head cooling for neonatal encephalopathy. Pediatrics 2007;119:912–21.

30. Laptook AR, McDonald SA, Shankaran S, et al. Elevated temperature and 6- to 7-year outcome of neonatal encephalopathy. Ann Neurol 2013;73(4):520–8.

31. Owji ZP, Gilbert G, Saint-Martin C, et al. Brain temperature is increased during the first days of life in asphyxiated newborns: developing brain injury despite hypothermia treatment. AJNR Am J Neuroradiol 2017;38(11):2180–6.

32. Shankaran S, Laptook AR, McDonald SA, et al. Temperature profile and outcomes of neonates undergoing whole body hypothermia for neonatal hypoxic-ischemic encephalopathy. Pediatr Crit Care Med 2012;13(1):53–9.

33. Liu X, Tooley J, Løberg EM, et al. Immediate hypothermia reduces cardiac troponin I after hypoxic-ischemic encephalopathy in newborn pigs. Pediatr Res 2011;70(4):352–6.

34. Giesinger RE, Bailey LJ, Deshpande P, et al. Hypoxic-ischemic encephalopathy and therapeutic hypothermia: the hemodynamic perspective. J Pediatr 2017;180: 22–30.e2.

35. Pappas A, Shankaran S, Laptook AR, et al. Hypocarbia and adverse outcome in neonatal hypoxic-ischemic encephalopathy. J Pediatr 2011;158(5):752–8.e1.

36. Lingappan K, Kaiser JR, Srinivasan C, et al. Relationship between PCO2 and unfavorable outcome in infants with moderate-to-severe hypoxic ischemic encephalopathy. Pediatr Res 2016;80(2):204–8.

37. Kapadia VS, Chalak LF, DuPont TL, et al. Perinatal asphyxia with hyperoxemia within the first hour of life is associated with moderate to severe hypoxic-ischemic encephalopathy. J Pediatr 2013;163(4):949–54.

38. Sabir H, Jary S, Tooley J, et al. Increased inspired oxygen in the first hours of life is associated with adverse outcome in newborns treated for perinatal asphyxia with therapeutic hypothermia. J Pediatr 2012;161(3):409–16.

39. Tam EW, Haeusslein LA, Bonifacio SL, et al. Hypoglycemia is associated with increased risk for brain injury and adverse neurodevelopmental outcome in neonates at risk for encephalopathy. J Pediatr 2012;161(1):88–93.

40. Basu SK, Kaiser JR, Guffey D, et al, CoolCap Study Group. Hypoglycaemia and hyperglycaemia are associated with unfavourable outcome in infants with hypoxic ischaemic encephalopathy: a post hoc analysis of the CoolCap Study. Arch Dis Child Fetal Neonatal Ed 2016;101(2):F149–55.

41. Kwon JM, Guillet R, Shankaran S, et al. Clinical seizures in neonatal hypoxic-ischemic encephalopathy have no independent impact on neurodevelopmental outcome: secondary analyses of data from the Neonatal Research Network hypothermia trial. J Child Neurol 2011;26(3):322–8.

42. Kharoshankaya L, Stevenson NJ, Livingstone V, et al. Seizure burden and neurodevelopmental outcome in neonates with hypoxic-ischemic encephalopathy. Dev Med Child Neurol 2016;58(12):1242–8.

43. Low E, Boylan GB, Mathieson SR, et al. Cooling and seizure burden in term neonates: an observational study. Arch Dis Child Fetal Neonatal Ed 2012;97: F267–72.

44. Sant'Anna G, Laptook AR, Shankaran S, et al. Phenobarbital and temperature profile during hypothermia for hypoxic-ischemic encephalopathy. J Child Neurol 2012;27(4):451–7.

45. Thoresen M, Hellström-Westas L, Liu X, et al. Effect of hypothermia on amplitude-integrated electroencephalogram in infants with asphyxia. Pediatrics 2010;126: e131–9.

46. Shankaran S, Pappas A, McDonald SA, et al. Predictive value of an early amplitude integrated electroencephalogram and neurologic examination. Pediatrics 2011;128(1):e112–20.

47. Azzopardi D, TOBY Study Group. Predictive value of the amplitude integrated EEG in infants with hypoxic ischaemic encephalopathy: data from a randomised trial of therapeutic hypothermia. Arch Dis Child Fetal Neonatal Ed 2014;99:F80–2.

48. Tortorici MA, Kochanek PM, Poloyac SM. Effects of hypothermia on drug disposition, metabolism, and response: a focus of hypothermia-mediated alterations on the cytochrome P450 enzyme system. Crit Care Med 2007;35(9):2196–204.

49. Róka A, Melinda KT, Vásárhelyi B, et al. Elevated morphine concentrations in neonates treated with morphine and prolonged hypothermia for hypoxic ischemic encephalopathy. Pediatrics 2008;121(4):e844–9.

50. Kapetanakis A, Azzopardi D, Wyatt J, et al. Therapeutic hypothermia for neonatal encephalopathy: a UK survey of opinion, practice and neuro-investigation at the end of 2007. Acta Paediatr 2009;98:631–5.

51. Wassink G, Lear CA, Gunn KC, et al. Analgesics, sedatives, anticonvulsant drugs, and the cooled brain. Semin Fetal Neonatal Med 2015;20(2):109–14.

52. Massaro AN, Jeromin A, Kadom N, et al. Serum biomarkers of MRI brain injury in neonatal hypoxic ischemic encephalopathy treated with whole-body hypothermia: a pilot study. Pediatr Crit Care Med 2013;14(3):310–7.

53. Chalak LF, Sánchez PJ, Adams-Huet B, et al. Biomarkers for severity of neonatal hypoxic-ischemic encephalopathy and outcomes in newborns receiving hypothermia therapy. J Pediatr 2014;164(3):468–74.e1.

54. Montaldo P, Rosso R, Chello G, et al. Cardiac troponin I concentrations as a marker of neurodevelopmental outcome at 18 months in newborns with perinatal asphyxia. J Perinatol 2014;34(4):292–5.

55. Liu X, Chakkarapani E, Stone J, et al. Effect of cardiac compressions and hypothermia treatment on cardiac troponin I in newborns with perinatal asphyxia. Resuscitation 2013;84(11):1562–7.

56. Vergales BD, Zanelli SA, Matsumoto JA, et al. Depressed heart rate variability is associated with abnormal EEG, MRI, and death in neonates with hypoxic ischemic encephalopathy. Am J Perinatol 2014;31(10):855–62.

57. Goulding RM, Stevenson NJ, Murray DM, et al. Heart rate variability in hypoxic ischemic encephalopathy during therapeutic hypothermia. Pediatr Res 2017; 81(4):609–15.

58. Goulding RM, Stevenson NJ, Murray DM, et al. Heart rate variability in hypoxic ischemic encephalopathy: correlation with EEG grade and 2-y neurodevelopmental outcome. Pediatr Res 2015;77(5):681–7.

59. Rutherford M, Ramenghi LA, Edwards AD, et al. Assessment of brain tissue injury after moderate hypothermia in neonates with hypoxic-ischaemic encephalopathy: a nested substudy of a randomised controlled trial. Lancet Neurol 2010; 9(1):39–45.

60. Shankaran S, Barnes PD, Hintz SR, et al. Brain injury following trial of hypothermia for neonatal hypoxic-ischaemic encephalopathy. Arch Dis Child Fetal Neonatal Ed 2012;97(6):F398–404.

61. Shankaran S, Laptook AR, McDonald SA, et al. Acute perinatal sentinel events, neonatal brain injury pattern, and outcome of infants undergoing a trial of hypothermia for neonatal hypoxic-ischemic encephalopathy. J Pediatr 2017;180: 275–8.e2.

62. Shankaran S, McDonald SA, Laptook AR, et al. Neonatal magnetic resonance imaging pattern of brain injury as a biomarker of childhood outcomes following a trial of hypothermia for neonatal hypoxic-ischemic encephalopathy. J Pediatr 2015;167:987–93.

63. Cheong JL, Coleman L, Hunt RW, et al. Prognostic utility of magnetic resonance imaging in neonatal hypoxic-ischemic encephalopathy: sub-study of a randomized trial. Arch Pediatr Adolesc Med 2012;166:634–40.

64. American College of Obstetricians and Gynecologists and the American Academy of Pediatrics. Neonatal encephalopathy and neurologic outcome. 2nd edition. Washington: American College of Obstetrics and Gynecology; 2014.

65. Lemmon ME, Boss RD, Bonifacio SL, et al. Characterization of death in neonatal encephalopathy in the hypothermia era. J Child Neurol 2017;32(4):360–5.

66. Bonifacio SL, deVries LS, Groenendaal F. Impact of hypothermia on predictors of poor outcome: how do we decide to redirect care? Semin Fetal Neonatal Med 2015;20(2):122–7.

67. Vohr BR, Stephens BE, McDonald SA, et al. Cerebral palsy and growth failure at 6 to 7 years. Pediatrics 2013;132(4):e905–14.

68. Natarajan G, Shankaran S, Pappas A, et al. Functional status at 18 months of age as a predictor of childhood disability after neonatal hypoxic-ischemic encephalopathy. Dev Med Child Neurol 2014;56(11):1052–8.

69. Pappas A, Shankaran S, McDonald SA, et al. Cognitive outcomes after neonatal encephalopathy. Pediatrics 2015;135(3):e624–34.

Preventing Continuous Positive Airway Pressure Failure

Evidence-Based and Physiologically Sound Practices from Delivery Room to the Neonatal Intensive Care Unit

Clyde J. Wright, MD[a],*, Laurie G. Sherlock, MD[a],
Rakesh Sahni, MD[b], Richard A. Polin, MD[c]

KEYWORDS

- Continuous positive airway pressure • Bronchopulmonary dysplasia
- Ventilatory-induced lung injury • Sustained lung inflation • INSURE
- Randomized controlled trial • Mechanical ventilation • Infant flow driver

KEY POINTS

- The incidence of bronchopulmonary dysplasia, and the competing outcomes death or bronchopulmonary dysplasia, is decreased with early initiation of nCPAP.
- The best available evidence supports the premise that efforts to minimize CPAP failure start in the delivery room.
- Various modes and interfaces to deliver CPAP exist; although there may be considerable differences in the ability of these various CPAP devices to prevent failure, little data from RCT exist to support this.

Continued

Disclosure Statement: R.A. Polin is a consultant for Discovery Labs and Fisher Paykel and has a grant from Fisher Paykel.
[a] Section of Neonatology, Department of Pediatrics, Children's Hospital Colorado, University of Colorado School of Medicine, Perinatal Research Center, Mail Stop F441, 13243 East 23rd Avenue, Aurora, CO 80045, USA; [b] Department of Pediatrics, NICU, Columbia University College of Physicians and Surgeons, NewYork-Presbyterian Morgan Stanley Children's Hospital, CUMC, 622 West 168th Street, PH 17-112, New York, NY 10032, USA; [c] Department of Pediatrics, Division of Neonatology, Columbia University College of Physicians and Surgeons, NewYork-Presbyterian Morgan Stanley Children's Hospital, 622 West 168th Street, PH 17-110, New York, NY 10032, USA
* Corresponding author.
E-mail address: clyde.wright@ucdenver.edu

Clin Perinatol 45 (2018) 257–271
https://doi.org/10.1016/j.clp.2018.01.011
0095-5108/18/© 2018 Elsevier Inc. All rights reserved.

Continued

- Compared with infant flow driver, bubble CPAP may decrease the risk of postextubation failure in infants less than 30 weeks' gestation who are ventilated ≤14 days.
- Available data demonstrate that the INSURE approach is not superior to use of CPAP without prophylactic surfactant in preventing CPAP failure.
- Sustained lung inflation may increase the rate of CPAP success, but may not decrease the incidence of BPD if positive pressure ventilation is needed.

WHY PREVENT CONTINUOUS POSITIVE AIRWAY PRESSURE FAILURE?

The need to identify safe and effective interventions to prevent bronchopulmonary dysplasia (BPD) has reached a critical point. In the simplest terms, BPD is the most common morbidity affecting a cohort of patients whose survival is increasing at the greatest rate. Data collected by the Neonatal Research Network recently on more than 34,000 infants born at 22 to 28 weeks gestation between 1993 and 2012 demonstrated significant increases in survival among infants born at 23, 24, and 25 weeks' gestational age (GA).[1] Importantly, these tiny babies are at the highest risk of developing BPD, with an incidence of 60% to 80%. In this same cohort of patients, it seems that practice changes over this period did little to improve the incidence of BPD.

An alternative to identifying additional interventions to prevent BPD is improving the interventions clinicians already make to support the highest risk neonates. More than 85% of the 34,000 infants in the Neonatal Research Network cohort were exposed to mechanical ventilation during their neonatal intensive care unit (NICU) stay.[1] Recent clinical data continue to support a direct relationship between exposure to mechanical ventilation and an increased risk of developing BPD.[2–6] As the survival of the tiniest babies increases, it is important to determine if a better modality of invasive mechanical ventilation exists to minimize these exposures and prevent BPD. High-frequency ventilation does not reduce the incidence of BPD in the smallest, high-risk babies.[7] Volume-targeted ventilation still remains promising, but randomized trials remain small and unconvincing.[8] Newer approaches, including neurally adjusted ventilator assist, have not yet been adequately studied.[9] These data may point to the reality that the developing human lung at 22 to 26 weeks' gestation is uniquely susceptible to injury caused by invasive mechanical ventilation. If this is true, reducing the burden of BPD will come only with limiting the exposure to invasive mechanical ventilation.

Data from randomized controlled trials (RCTs) demonstrate that routine use of continuous positive airway pressure (CPAP) significantly reduces the combined outcome of BPD (assessed at 36 weeks' gestation) or death in at-risk preterm infants, with an number needed to treat of 17.7.[10] Two other similar meta-analyses have been performed, each including slightly different combinations of trials whose comparison groups go beyond strictly CPAP versus prophylactic surfactant.[11,12] In all of these meta-analyses, the signal for benefit always points toward CPAP. Unfortunately, the routine use of CPAP does not provide a larger treatment effect; the numbers needed to treat determined across these three analyses were 17.7,[10] 25,[11] and 35.[12] It is reasonable to ask why the treatment effect is not larger, and can more be done to enhance the benefit of CPAP.

If CPAP prevents BPD by limiting the exposure to mechanical ventilation, efforts to prevent CPAP failure would likely lead to increased protective effects. In the preterm infant at highest risk for developing BPD, CPAP failure is common. Data from three large RCTs evaluating routine CPAP versus routine intubation show that 45% to 50% of high-risk babies fail CPAP within the first week of life (**Table 1**). Data from

Table 1
Incidence of CPAP failure in large RCTs evaluating CPAP alone as primary mode of respiratory support

Trial	Year	Subjects Enrolled	GA	ACS, % (Any)	CPAP Failure, % (5–7 d)
COIN[13]	2008	610	25 0/7–28 6/7	94	46
SUPPORT[19]	2010	1316	24 0/7–27 6/7	>95	51.2
CURPAP[20]	2010	208	25 0/7–28 6/7	>95	33
Dunn[18]	2011	648	26 0/7–29 6/7	>98	45.1

Abbreviations: ACS, antenatal corticosteroids; GA, gestational age.

observational studies and RCT demonstrate that rates of CPAP failure are highest for the smallest babies, approaching 60% at 25 to 26 weeks' GA.[13–16] These data inform practice in one of two ways: either efforts to minimize CPAP failure in this group of infants will result in less BPD and improved outcomes; or, despite best efforts, CPAP failure in this group of patients will remain unacceptably high and the ability to detect who will fail must be improved to provided supportive therapy (eg, mechanical ventilation and/or surfactant) as soon as possible.

HOW TO PREVENT CONTINUOUS POSITIVE AIRWAY PRESSURE FAILURE: EVIDENCE-BASED INTERVENTIONS, FROM THE DELIVERY ROOM TO THE NEONATAL INTENSIVE CARE UNIT

Does Receipt of Antenatal Corticosteroids Decrease the Risk of Continuous Positive Airway Pressure Failure?

Antenatal corticosteroids (ACS) are considered "one of the most important antenatal therapies available to improve newborn outcomes," and are now recommended for threatened delivery at 24 0/7 weeks to 33 6/7.[17] It is reasonable to hypothesize that rates of CPAP failure would be higher among neonates that did not receive ACS. Among neonates enrolled in RCTs evaluating CPAP versus routine intubation, receipt of ACS was high (>90%, see **Table 1**).[13,18–20] These data suggest that even with the benefit of ACS, rates of CPAP failure remain high (~60%). So, the question remains: in the unfortunate circumstance that a baby at high risk of developing BPD (23–28 weeks) did not receive the benefit of ACS, should there be a lower threshold to intervene and provide exogenous surfactant?

Randomized studies performed in the 1980s and 1990s demonstrated that in large (>28 weeks' GA) intubated infants with respiratory distress syndrome (RDS), who often had not received ACS, early and even prophylactic surfactant treatment decreased mortality and air leak.[21,22] It is likely that a protective signal exists for earlier treatment of RDS in more immature infants 24 to 28 weeks' GA who did not receive ACS, but an RCT will never likely provide these answers.

Therefore, we recommend that a trial of CPAP should be attempted for all neonates born at less than 28 weeks' GA, but the threshold for intervention (ie, intubation and exogenous surfactant) should be considered early in the course of RDS if ACS were not administered. Quality of evidence: low, based on the lack of data in patient population of interest (24–28 weeks' GA). Strength of recommendation: weak, based on the lack of clear data guiding practice.

Does Routine Use of Sustained Lung Inflation Prevent Continuous Positive Airway Pressure Failure?

At delivery, term infants provide a sustained pressure (30–35 cm H_2O) over a long inspiratory time (4–5 seconds) to clear lung fluid and establish functional residual capacity (FRC).[23] Assisting preterm infants in the delivery room by providing positive pressure at 20 to 25 cm H_2O for 5 to 20 seconds via a nasopharyngeal tube or face-mask has been proposed as a method to establish FRC.[23] Smaller RCTs demonstrate that use of sustained lung inflation (SLI) decreases the need for mechanical ventilation at 72 hours, without increasing the risk of air leak.[24–27] A much larger trial powered to determine if use of SLI is safe and decreases the incidence of BPD or death in neonates born at 23 to 26 weeks' GA is ongoing.[28]

Therefore, we recommend SLI should be considered for all neonates born at less than 28 weeks' GA. Quality of evidence: moderate, based on consistent findings across multiple smaller RCTs. Strength of recommendation: strong recommendation, based on potential benefit and lack of data demonstrating harm.

Does the Modality of Assisted Ventilation Used in the Delivery (Resuscitation) Room Affect Continuous Positive Airway Pressure Failure?

Assisted ventilation in the delivery room is provided using one of three devices: (1) self-inflating bag, (2) flow-inflating bag, and (3) T-piece resuscitator. The theoretic advantages of the T-piece resuscitator include delivering a consistent end expiratory pressure while precisely delivering the desired peak inspiratory pressure. Whether use of the T-piece in the resuscitation suite prevents CPAP failure in the babies at highest risk of CPAP failure (<26 weeks' GA) is unknown. However, in babies greater than or equal to 26 weeks' GA, use of a T-piece resulted in less intubation in the delivery room when compared with use of a self-inflating bag. Importantly, use of the T-piece did not increase the need for chest compressions or air leak.[29]

Therefore, we recommend that when available, a T-piece resuscitator should be used to resuscitate neonates born at less than 28 weeks' GA. Quality of evidence: low, based on the lack of data in the population of interest (24–28 weeks' GA). Strength of recommendation: weak, based on the lack of clear data guiding practice balanced by the absence of evidence of harm.

Does Intubation, Surfactant, Extubation Improve Continuous Positive Airway Pressure Success?

Isayama and colleagues[30] recently published a systematic analysis comparing the intubation, surfactant, extubation (INSURE) approach with nasal CPAP. There were no statistically significant differences between the nasal CPAP and INSURE groups. However, the relative risks seemed to favor the INSURE group with a nonsignificant (12%) reduction in chronic lung disease and/or death (moderate-quality evidence), a 14% decrease in chronic lung disease (moderate-quality evidence), and a 50% decrease in air-leak (very-low-quality evidence).

We recommend that nasal CPAP should be offered to all preterm neonates with RDS; however, there is no benefit to routine surfactant administration followed by rapid extubation (INSURE) unless the likelihood of CPAP failure is very high. When the likelihood of CPAP failure is greatly increased, surfactant should be administered followed by rapid extubation. Quality of evidence: moderate. Strength of recommendation for using CPAP without prophylactic surfactant: strong.

Recently, there has been renewed interest in the INSURE approach using surfactant administration through a thin plastic catheter (minimally [or less] invasive surfactant therapy and less invasive surfactant administration [LISA]) (**Table 2**). Isayama and colleagues[31] recently published a meta-analysis comparing seven ventilation strategies (including LISA and INSURE). The primary outcome was death or BPD at 36 weeks' postmenstrual age. Compared with all other ventilatory strategies, LISA had the lowest risk of the primary outcome. However, this outcome was not robust for death when

Table 2
Need for CMV and incidence of BPD in preterm infants with RDS treated with INSURE approach using surfactant administration through a thin plastic catheter versus ETT

Study	N (Gestation, wk)	Need for CMV, % Catheter vs ETT	Incidence of BPD Catheter vs ETT, %	Entry Criteria for Catheter
Gopel et al,[80] 2015	2206 (26–28)	41 vs 62 (P<.001)	12 vs 18 (P = .001)	Cohort study not specified
Kanmaz et al,[81] 2013	200 (<32)	40 vs 49 (P = NS)	10.3 vs 20.2 Moderate-severe (P = .009)	F_{IO_2} >0.4 and CPAP
Gopel et al,[82] 2011	220 (26–28)	33 vs 73 (P<.0001)	8 vs 13 (P = .268)	F_{IO_2} >0.3 and CPAP
Kribs et al,[83] 2015	211 (23–26.8)	74.8 vs 99 (P<.001)	67.3 vs 58.7 Survival without BPD (P = NS)	F_{IO_2} >0.3 and CPAP in first 2 h
Mohammadizadeh et al,[84] 2015	38 (<34)	15.8 vs 10.5 (P = NS)	P = NS	CPAP and need for surfactant
Bao et al,[85] 2015	90 (27–32)	17.0 vs 23.3 (P = NS)	P = NS	F_{IO_2} = 0.30–0.35 and CPAP
Mirnia et al,[86] 2013	136 (27–32)	19 vs 22 (P = NS)	7.5 vs 7.1 (P = NS)	F_{IO_2} >0.3 and CPAP

Abbreviations: CMV, conventional mechanical ventilation; ETT, endotracheal tube; F_{IO_2}, fraction of inspired oxygen; NS, nonsignificant.

limited to higher quality studies. Rigo and colleagues[32] recently published a systematic analysis of four trials comparing surfactant administration through a thin plastic catheter versus INSURE. Compared with INSURE, less invasive surfactant therapy decreased of death/BPD or CPAP failure.

We do not recommend administration of surfactant using a thin plastic catheter (LISA). Quality of evidence for LISA: low, given the small number of patients randomized to this intervention. Strength of recommendation: strong, based on lack of large RCTs comparing LISA with other modes of surfactant administration.

Does Bubble Continuous Positive Airway Pressure Improve Rates of Continuous Positive Airway Pressure Success?

CPAP delivery devices are broadly grouped into continuous-flow and variable-flow systems. With continuous-flow devices this is achieved by using water-seal bubble CPAP (Fisher and Paykel Healthcare, Auckland, New Zealand; Babi-Plus, A Plus Medical, Hollister, CA; home-made) systems or via flow opposition, where the patient's expiratory flow opposes a constant flow from nasal prongs (conventional ventilator provided neonatal CPAP). Variable-flow devices that include the infant flow driver (IFD; infant flow nasal CPAP system, Care Fusion, Yorba Linda, CA), Benveniste gas jet valve CPAP (Dameca, Copenhagen, Denmark), Aladdin, and Arabella systems (Hamilton Medical AG, Reno, NV) use flow opposition with fluidic flow reversal during expiration, where gas is entrained during inspiration to maintain stable pressure and expiratory flow is diverted via a separate fluidic flip-flop.

Randomized Trials Comparing Continuous Positive Airway Pressure Devices

Randomized controlled trials performed at birth
Mazzella and colleagues[33] compared IFD CPAP with bi-nasal prongs and bubble CPAP through a single nasopharyngeal tube in preterm infants with RDS at less

than 12 hours of age. They reported a significant beneficial effect on oxygen requirement and respiratory rate with IFD CPAP, compared with bubble CPAP, and a trend toward a decreased need for mechanical ventilation. Tagare and colleagues[34] compared the efficacy and safety of bubble CPAP with ventilator-derived CPAP in preterm neonates with RDS. A higher percentage of infants was successfully treated with bubble CPAP (83% vs 63%; P = .03), suggesting superiority of bubble CPAP. Mazmanyan and colleagues[35] randomized preterm infants to bubble CPAP or IFD CPAP after stabilization at birth in a resource-poor setting. They reported bubble CPAP equivalent to IFD CPAP in the total number of days CPAP was required.

Randomized trials of continuous positive airway pressure after extubation

Stefanescu and colleagues[36] examined extremely low birth weight infants and compared IFD CPAP with ventilator-derived CPAP using INCA prongs and found no difference in the extubation success rate between the two groups. In a subsequent trial, Gupta and colleagues[37] randomized preterm infants 24 to 29 weeks' gestation or 600 to 1500 g at birth to receive bubble CPAP or IFD CPAP following the first attempt at extubation. Infants were stratified according to duration of initial ventilation ($\leq$14 days or >14 days). Although there was no statistically significant difference in the extubation failure rate (16.9% on bubble CPAP, 27.5% on IFD CPAP) for the entire study group, the median duration of CPAP support was 50% shorter in the infants on bubble CPAP, median 2 days (95% confidence interval, 1–3 days) on bubble CPAP versus 4 days (95% confidence interval, 2–6 days) on IFD CPAP (P = 0 .03). In infants ventilated for less than or equal to 14 days, the extubation failure rate was significantly lower with bubble CPAP (14.1%; 9 of 64) compared with IFD CPAP (28.6%; 18 of 63) (P = .046). This well-designed clinical trial suggests the superiority of postextubation bubble CPAP over IFD CPAP in preterm babies less than 30 weeks, who are initially ventilated for less than 14 days.

Therefore, we recommend the use of bubble CPAP over variable-flow CPAP devices for postextubation respiratory support, especially in infants ventilated for less than or equal to 2 weeks. Quality of evidence: low, for device preference when used to treat RDS after birth; moderate, for use of bubble CPAP following postextubation. Strength of recommendation: weak, based on only a slight difference between continuous- or variable-flow CPAP devices when used after birth but a trend in favor of bubble CPAP for postextubation support, especially in infants ventilated for less than 2 weeks.

Does the Interface Used to Deliver Continuous Positive Airway Pressure Affect Continuous Positive Airway Pressure Failure?

The ideal interface would reliably deliver consistent distending pressure while being comfortable to the infant and easy to use. Several options are available, including short binasal prongs, nasopharyngeal prongs, masks, and the RAM cannula. No adequately powered trial has directly compared all interfaces. Several have examined nasal mask versus nasal prongs to prevent CPAP failure, with one demonstrating less CPAP failure in infants less than 31 weeks with the use of nasal mask.[38] However, another found no difference in CPAP failure between mask and binasal prongs.[39] The variability in these results may be caused by different definitions of CPAP failure and difference in maximum noninvasive support provided (CPAP level, noninvasive positive-pressure ventilation).

RAM cannula has been used to deliver CPAP in neonates.[40] It provides positive distending pressure through longer nasal cannula prongs made from softer material.[41] Unfortunately, there are no clinical studies directly comparing RAM with other nasal interfaces for preventing CPAP failure. However, there are several preclinical studies using lung model systems that attempt to determine whether RAM cannula can reliably deliver mean airway pressure or peak inspiratory pressures. One demonstrated that when used as recommended with a 60% to 80% nasal occlusion, even with a closed mouth, the RAM cannula delivered on average 60% less mean airway pressure to the lungs than the set pressure.[42] Another showed RAM cannula resulted in significantly higher resistance and dramatically lower peak inspiratory pressures to the lungs than short binasal prongs.[43] The direct clinical relevance of these findings is unknown and deserves further study.

Therefore, we recommend use of either nasal mask or short binasal prongs for early CPAP administration. We recommend against the use of RAM cannula during the critical period determining CPAP success. Quality of evidence: low, based on the small number of patients studied. Strength of recommendation: strong, based on lack of clinical data directly comparing RAM cannula with CPAP.

Does Prone or Lateral Body Positioning Improve Continuous Positive Airway Pressure Success?

Prone positioning improves oxygenation in mechanically ventilated neonates,[44] infants, and children with acute respiratory distress.[45] Results in neonates on CPAP are conflicting, with several demonstrating improvements in oxygenation, respiratory rate, and end-expiratory lung volume with prone and lateral positioning.[46–48] However, another found no difference in vital signs or oxygen saturations regardless of position.[49] None of the studies found evidence of harm or adverse effect associated with prone or lateral positioning.

We recommend the prone and lateral positions for infants with the goal of increasing CPAP success. Quality of evidence: low, based on lack of trials evaluating position to prevent initial CPAP failure. Strength of recommendation: moderate, based on potential benefit and lack of demonstrated harm.

Does Timing of Caffeine Administration Affect Continuous Positive Airway Pressure Failure?

Importantly, the Caffeine for Apnea of Prematurity trial demonstrated that caffeine use was associated with a significant reduction in the duration of mechanical ventilation.[50] An enhanced protective effect on BPD and the duration of mechanical ventilation is observed when caffeine therapy is initiated early (before 2–3 days of life vs later than 2–3 days of life).[51–54] It is possible that these observations may be explained by later initiation of caffeine in infants with greater illness severity.[55] Additional prospective studies are needed to identify ideal timing of caffeine dosing.

Therefore, we recommend that caffeine should be administered to neonates both at and less than 28 weeks' GA, and there may be additional benefit of administering caffeine early in the first 24 to 72 hours of life. Quality of evidence: high, based on data from RCTs and large observational studies. Strength of recommendation: strong, based the consistent finding of benefit and the absence of evidence of harm.

WHEN NO EVIDENCE EXISTS, CAN ONE SUPPORT "BEST PRACTICE"?
Does Aggressive Airway Clearance Prevent Continuous Positive Airway Pressure Failure?

Effective delivery of noninvasive positive distending pressure cannot occur in the presence of obstructed nasal passages or oropharynx. Little evidence guides practice regarding how frequently one should preform nasal and oral suctioning. Although maintaining airway patency is paramount, aggressive suctioning can lead to edema, trauma, and bleeding, thus exacerbating plugging. In addition to the loss of positive distending pressure during suctioning, other more serious complications can occur including bradycardia, laryngospasm, and arrhythmias. In practice, indications and frequency of suctioning is variable.[56] Instructions on nontraumatic suctioning have been published.[57] Units with long experience in successful application of CPAP in the most premature infants recommend suctioning every 3 to 4 hours.[58]

Therefore, we recommend that nasal and oropharyngeal suctioning should be performed every 3 to 4 hours, and more frequently with signs of obstruction (apnea, desaturation, acute increase in work of breathing). Attention must be paid to avoiding excessive suctioning and causing trauma. Quality of evidence: low. Strength of recommendation: strong, based on physiologic benefit and the low likelihood of harm.

Can Quality Improvement Projects Improve Continuous Positive Airway Pressure Success Rates?

Multiple obstacles stand in the way of implementing early, aggressive, and successful CPAP in high-risk neonates. It takes time to technically train the multidisciplinary team (eg, nursing, respiratory therapist, neonatal nurse practitioner.) in correct CPAP application, administration, and maintenance. It requires education and consensus of the attending physicians, trainees at multiple levels, and nurse practitioners who are making decisions regarding what defines CPAP failure, and when invasive mechanical ventilation should be used. Not surprisingly, time and experience with CPAP has been shown to increase CPAP success and decrease rates of BPD.[59]

Several groups have implemented quality improvement studies demonstrating short-term success increasing CPAP use and decreasing rates of intubation.[60–63] Some,[60,61] but not all,[62,63] have decreased unit BPD rates during the study period. Importantly, sustained practice improvement and decreased rates of BPD have been demonstrated.[64] These findings support that targeted multidisciplinary quality improvement efforts can help improve CPAP success.

We recommend that any institution dedicated to adopting a strategy of early CPAP develop a multidisciplinary team to champion this cause, whether it is through a formal quality improvement project or as an annual unit goal. Quality of evidence: low, based on small number of studies. Strength of recommendation: strong, based on potential benefit.

IF BABIES MUST FAIL, CAN ONE PREDICT WHO WILL FAIL, AND INTERVENE EARLY?
Are There Antenatal Characteristics that Reliably Predict Continuous Positive Airway Pressure Failure?

Studies of antenatal identifiers of CPAP failure report discordant results. Many establish early GA and lower birth weight as predictive as CPAP failure.[16,65,66] Lack of ACS and male sex have correlated with CPAP failure in some studies.[66–68] However, others have shown aspects of medical history, including GA and birth weight, are not predictive of CPAP failure.[15,69]

None of these studies identified factors with adequate sensitivity or positive pressure ventilation in predicting CPAP failure. Thus, we recommend against using antenatal characteristics to exclude infants from a trial of CPAP. Quality of evidence: moderate, based on lack of convincing evidence. Strength of recommendation: strong, based on potential benefit of CPAP success.

Are There any Clinical Variables or Diagnostic Tests that Predict Continuous Positive Airway Pressure Failure?

Multiple studies have attempted to define clinical features of a neonate's initial NICU course that predict CPAP failure. Several groups have shown early higher fraction of inspired oxygen (F_{IO_2}) correlates with CPAP failure.[15,65,69] However, this relationship is confounded by including F_{IO_2} requirement in the definition of CPAP failure. The same can be said for the relationship between higher levels of CPAP and ultimate CPAP failure.[69] Importantly, one trial identified that infants who succeeded CPAP were started earlier (4.3 minutes vs 29 minutes), emphasizing the importance of early FRC establishment.[61] Multiple studies have performed sophisticated analyses to identify early clinical findings that predict CPAP failure (**Table 3**). Although no clinical variable is foolproof, thematic links begin to emerge. These studies would suggest that CPAP failure is more common in the most premature neonates, those with severe RDS on initial chest radiograph (CXR), and those requiring high levels of supplemental oxygen. Although none of these associations is surprising, these factors must be in the clinician's mind when attempting to determine if a neonate is "failing" CPAP. Other groups have recommended composite scoring and combining variables to help predict CPAP failure, such as birth weight less than 800 g, male sex, and F_{IO_2} greater than 0.25 at 1 or 2 hours,[14] the product of F_{IO_2} and CPAP level being greater than or equal to 1.28,[68] or creating a clinical score with features including GA, lack of antenatal corticosteroids, prolonged premature rupture of membranes, and the product of F_{IO_2} and CPAP level,[68] has also been considered.

Surfactant activity and/or production tests

A screening test able to identify surfactant deficiency would allow clinicians to target surfactant administrations to select patients at high risk of CPAP failure secondary to RDS. Surfactant activity level has been evaluated to predict CPAP failure using the surfactant adsorption test. The surfactant adsorption test is done on amniotic fluid and has demonstrated correlation with lamellar body counts and lung ultrasound scores. In a pilot study, infants failing CPAP have lower surfactant adsorption test levels than those who succeeded.[70]

The rapid bedside stable microbubble test evaluates if surfactant is present in tracheal, gastric, and amniotic fluid samples. This test has been used to stratify infants into high or low risk for CPAP failure.[71–74] Other tests of surfactant production include

Table 3
Clinical predictors of CPAP failure

Study	Infants Studied	Clinical Characteristics as Predictors of CPAP Failure	Odds Ratio (95% CI)
Ammari et al,[16] 2005	261 infants ≤1250 g	Severe RDS on initial CXR PPV at delivery A-a DO_2 >180 mm Hg	6.42 (2.75–15.0) 2.37 (1.02–5.52) 6.42 (2.75–15.0)
Pillai et al,[68] 2011	62 infants ≤1500 g	Product of CPAP and F_{IO_2} ≥1.28 PPROM GA <28 wk	3.9 (1.0–15.5) 5.3 (1.2–24.5) 6.5 (1.5–28.3)
Dargaville et al,[14] 2013	66 infants 25–28 wk GA	F_{IO_2} by 2 h Caesarean delivery	1.19 (1.06–1.33) 14.77 (1.47–148.55)
Tagliaferro et al,[66] 2015	235 infants ≤1000 g	GA ≤26 wk A-a DO_2 >180 mm Hg pH ≤7.27 Severe RDS on initial radiograph	6.19 (2.79–13.73) 2.18 (1.06–4.47) 2.69 (1.27–5.69) 10.81 (3.5–33.3)

Abbreviations: A-a DO_2, alveolar-arterial oxygen difference; CI, confidence interval; CXR, chest radiograph; F_{IO_2}, fraction of inspired oxygen; PPROM, prolonged premature rupture of membranes; PPV, positive pressure ventilation.

the click test, the shake test, and lamellar body counts, but have not been evaluating ability to predict CPAP failure.[75–78]

Chest radiographs

Severe RDS on a CXR obtained in the first hours of life has been identified as a predictive variable for CPAP failure in multiple studies.[14,16] A repeat study corroborated this finding in extremely low birth weight infants, finding that early radiologic evidence of severe RDS was a strong predictor of CPAP failure with a positive predictive value of 0.81. However, its utility as a screening tool is somewhat limited because the sensitivity of severe RDS on a CXR to predict CPAP failure was only 32%.[66] Because obtaining CXR is already a common part of clinical practice for these infants, incorporating a thoughtful interpretation of this modality to clinical decision making seems feasible and prudent to use it in decision making.

Lung ultrasound

Furthermore, a lung ultrasound score obtained in the first hours of life evaluating the patterns of aeration in different lung quadrants correlated well with CPAP level and oxygenation indices, such as alveolar-arterial gradient, oxygenation index, and arterial to alveolar ratio in infants 27 to 41 weeks.[79] Whether this information can be used to predict CPAP failure is unknown. Several of these diagnostic tools require further study before recommendation could be made for broad implementation.

We recommend against using a single antenatal risk factor or clinical finding to predict CPAP failure and implement surfactant treatment. At this point and pending further study, predicting CPAP failure depends on an individual's unique clinical characteristics. Quality of evidence: weak, based on lack of large studies and standardized criteria for defining CPAP failure. Strength of recommendation: strong, based on current available information. We also recommend that if an extremely premature neonate (<26 weeks GA) has a CXR with evidence of severe RDS, they be monitored closely and considered for early intubation and surfactant administration. Quality of evidence: moderate, based on support from multiple retrospective trials. Strength of recommendation: strong, based on ease of practice.

SUMMARY

Multiple studies support using CPAP as first-line therapy for many preterm infants requiring respiratory support. However, rates of CPAP failure remain high among neonates at highest risk for developing lung injury. Multiple interventions, from the delivery room to the NICU, stand to minimize the risk of CPAP failure. Future studies will determine whether SLI will decrease CPAP failure, and criteria used to predict CPAP failure require further refinement.

REFERENCES

1. Stoll BJ, Hansen NI, Bell EF, et al. Trends in care practices, morbidity, and mortality of extremely preterm neonates, 1993-2012. JAMA 2015;314: 1039–51.

2. May C, Patel S, Kennedy C, et al. Prediction of bronchopulmonary dysplasia. Arch Dis Child Fetal Neonatal Ed 2011;96:F410–6.

3. Ambalavanan N, Walsh M, Bobashev G, et al. Intercenter differences in bronchopulmonary dysplasia or death among very low birth weight infants. Pediatrics 2011;127:e106–16.

4. Laughon M, Bose C, Allred EN, et al. Antecedents of chronic lung disease following three patterns of early respiratory disease in preterm infants. Arch Dis Child Fetal Neonatal Ed 2011;96:F114–20.

5. Gagliardi L, Bellu R, Lista G, et al. Do differences in delivery room intubation explain different rates of bronchopulmonary dysplasia between hospitals? Arch Dis Child Fetal Neonatal Ed 2011;96:F30–5.

6. Ambalavanan N, Van Meurs KP, Perritt R, et al. Predictors of death or bronchopulmonary dysplasia in preterm infants with respiratory failure. J Perinatol 2008;28: 420–6.

7. Cools F, Offringa M, Askie LM. Elective high frequency oscillatory ventilation versus conventional ventilation for acute pulmonary dysfunction in preterm infants. Cochrane Database Syst Rev 2015;(3):CD000104.

8. Wheeler KI, Klingenberg C, Morley CJ, et al. Volume-targeted versus pressure-limited ventilation for preterm infants: a systematic review and meta-analysis. Neonatology 2011;100:219–27.

9. Stein H, Firestone K. Application of neurally adjusted ventilatory assist in neonates. Semin Fetal Neonatal Med 2014;19:60–9.

10. Wright CJ, Polin RA, Kirpalani H. Continuous positive airway pressure to prevent neonatal lung injury: how did we get here, and how do we improve? J Pediatr 2016;173:17–24.e2.

11. Schmolzer GM, Kumar M, Pichler G, et al. Non-invasive versus invasive respiratory support in preterm infants at birth: systematic review and meta-analysis. BMJ 2013;347:f5980.

12. Fischer HS, Buhrer C. Avoiding endotracheal ventilation to prevent bronchopulmonary dysplasia: a meta-analysis. Pediatrics 2013;132:e1351–60.

13. Morley CJ, Davis PG, Doyle LW, et al. Nasal CPAP or intubation at birth for very preterm infants. N Engl J Med 2008;358:700–8.

14. Dargaville PA, Aiyappan A, De Paoli AG, et al. Continuous positive airway pressure failure in preterm infants: incidence, predictors and consequences. Neonatology 2013;104:8–14.

15. Fuchs H, Lindner W, Leiprecht A, et al. Predictors of early nasal CPAP failure and effects of various intubation criteria on the rate of mechanical ventilation in preterm infants of <29 weeks gestational age. Arch Dis Child Fetal Neonatal Ed 2011;96:F343–7.

16. Ammari A, Suri M, Milisavljevic V, et al. Variables associated with the early failure of nasal CPAP in very low birth weight infants. J Pediatr 2005;147:341–7.

17. Committee opinion No. 677 summary: antenatal corticosteroid therapy for fetal maturation. Obstet Gynecol 2016;128:940–1.

18. Dunn MS, Kaempf J, de Klerk A, et al. Randomized trial comparing 3 approaches to the initial respiratory management of preterm neonates. Pediatrics 2011;128: e1069–76.

19. Finer NN, Carlo WA, Walsh MC, et al. Early CPAP versus surfactant in extremely preterm infants. N Engl J Med 2010;362:1970–9.

20. Sandri F, Plavka R, Ancora G, et al. Prophylactic or early selective surfactant combined with nCPAP in very preterm infants. Pediatrics 2010;125:e1402–9.

21. Seger N, Soll R. Animal derived surfactant extract for treatment of respiratory distress syndrome. Cochrane Database Syst Rev 2009;(2):CD007836.

22. Rojas-Reyes MX, Morley CJ, Soll R. Prophylactic versus selective use of surfactant in preventing morbidity and mortality in preterm infants. Cochrane Database Syst Rev 2012;(3):CD000510.

23. Lista G, Castoldi F, Cavigioli F, et al. Alveolar recruitment in the delivery room. J Matern Fetal Neonatal Med 2012;25(Suppl 1):39–40.

24. Lista G, Boni L, Scopesi F, et al. Sustained lung inflation at birth for preterm infants: a randomized clinical trial. Pediatrics 2015;135:e457–64.

25. te Pas AB, Walther FJ. A randomized, controlled trial of delivery-room respiratory management in very preterm infants. Pediatrics 2007;120:322–9.

26. Lindner W, Hogel J, Pohlandt F. Sustained pressure-controlled inflation or intermittent mandatory ventilation in preterm infants in the delivery room? A randomized, controlled trial on initial respiratory support via nasopharyngeal tube. Acta Paediatr 2005;94:303–9.

27. El-Chimi MS, Awad HA, El-Gammasy TM, et al. Sustained versus intermittent lung inflation for resuscitation of preterm infants: a randomized controlled trial. J Matern Fetal Neonatal Med 2017;30(11):1273–8.

28. Foglia EE, Owen LS, Thio M, et al. Sustained Aeration of Infant Lungs (SAIL) trial: study protocol for a randomized controlled trial. Trials 2015;16:95.

29. Szyld E, Aguilar A, Musante GA, et al. Comparison of devices for newborn ventilation in the delivery room. J Pediatr 2014;165:234–9.e3.

30. Isayama T, Chai-Adisaksopha C, McDonald SD. Noninvasive ventilation with vs without early surfactant to prevent chronic lung disease in preterm infants: a systematic review and meta-analysis. JAMA Pediatr 2015;169:731–9.

31. Isayama T, Iwami H, McDonald S, et al. Association of noninvasive ventilation strategies with mortality and bronchopulmonary dysplasia among preterm infants: a systematic review and meta-analysis. JAMA 2016;316:611–24.

32. Rigo V, Lefebvre C, Broux I. Surfactant instillation in spontaneously breathing preterm infants: a systematic review and meta-analysis. Eur J Pediatr 2016;175: 1933–42.

33. Mazzella M, Bellini C, Calevo MG, et al. A randomised control study comparing the infant flow driver with nasal continuous positive airway pressure in preterm infants. Arch Dis Child Fetal Neonatal Ed 2001;85:F86–90.

34. Tagare A, Kadam S, Vaidya U, et al. Bubble CPAP versus ventilator CPAP in preterm neonates with early onset respiratory distress: a randomized controlled trial. J Trop Pediatr 2013;59:113–9.

35. Mazmanyan P, Mellor K, Dore CJ, et al. A randomised controlled trial of flow driver and bubble continuous positive airway pressure in preterm infants in a resource-limited setting. Arch Dis Child Fetal Neonatal Ed 2016;101:F16–20.

36. Stefanescu BM, Murphy WP, Hansell BJ, et al. A randomized, controlled trial comparing two different continuous positive airway pressure systems for the successful extubation of extremely low birth weight infants. Pediatrics 2003;112: 1031–8.

37. Gupta S, Sinha SK, Tin W, et al. A randomized controlled trial of post-extubation bubble continuous positive airway pressure versus infant flow driver continuous positive airway pressure in preterm infants with respiratory distress syndrome. J Pediatr 2009;154:645–50.

38. Kieran EA, Twomey AR, Molloy EJ, et al. Randomized trial of prongs or mask for nasal continuous positive airway pressure in preterm infants. Pediatrics 2012; 130:e1170–6.

39. Goel S, Mondkar J, Panchal H, et al. Nasal mask versus nasal prongs for delivering nasal continuous positive airway pressure in preterm infants with respiratory distress: a randomized controlled trial. Indian Pediatr 2015;52:1035–40.

40. Nzegwu NI, Mack T, DellaVentura R, et al. Systematic use of the RAM nasal cannula in the Yale-New Haven Children's Hospital neonatal intensive care unit: a quality improvement project. J Matern Fetal Neonatal Med 2015;28:718–21.

41. Neotech Ram Cannula Sell Sheet. Valencia (CA): Neotech Products LLC; 2017. Available at: https://www.neotechproducts.com/n17/wp-content/uploads/2017/07/M555_RevC_RAM_Sell_Sheet.pdf. Accessed May 18, 2017.

42. Gerdes JS, Sivieri EM, Abbasi S. Factors influencing delivered mean airway pressure during nasal CPAP with the RAM cannula. Pediatr Pulmonol 2016;51:60–9.

43. Mukerji A, Belik J. Neonatal nasal intermittent positive pressure ventilation efficacy and lung pressure transmission. J Perinatol 2015;35:716–9.

44. Rivas-Fernandez M, Roque IFM, Diez-Izquierdo A, et al. Infant position in neonates receiving mechanical ventilation. Cochrane Database Syst Rev 2016;(11):CD003668.

45. Gillies D, Wells D, Bhandari AP. Positioning for acute respiratory distress in hospitalised infants and children. Cochrane Database Syst Rev 2012;(7):CD003645.

46. Gouna G, Rakza T, Kuissi E, et al. Positioning effects on lung function and breathing pattern in premature newborns. J Pediatr 2013;162:1133–7, 1137.e1.

47. Maynard V, Bignall S, Kitchen S. Effect of positioning on respiratory synchrony in non-ventilated pre-term infants. Physiother Res Int 2000;5:96–110.

48. Montgomery K, Choy NL, Steele M, et al. The effectiveness of quarter turn from prone in maintaining respiratory function in premature infants. J Paediatr Child Health 2014;50:972–7.

49. Brunherotti MA, Martinez EZ, Martinez FE. Effect of body position on preterm newborns receiving continuous positive airway pressure. Acta Paediatr 2014;103:e101–5.

50. Schmidt B, Roberts RS, Davis P, et al. Caffeine therapy for apnea of prematurity. N Engl J Med 2006;354:2112–21.

51. Lodha A, Seshia M, McMillan DD, et al. Association of early caffeine administration and neonatal outcomes in very preterm neonates. JAMA Pediatr 2015;169:33–8.

52. Taha D, Kirkby S, Nawab U, et al. Early caffeine therapy for prevention of bronchopulmonary dysplasia in preterm infants. J Matern Fetal Neonatal Med 2014;27:1698–702.

53. Patel RM, Leong T, Carlton DP, et al. Early caffeine therapy and clinical outcomes in extremely preterm infants. J Perinatol 2013;33:134–40.

54. Dobson NR, Patel RM, Smith PB, et al. Trends in caffeine use and association between clinical outcomes and timing of therapy in very low birth weight infants. J Pediatr 2014;164:992–8.e3.

55. Jensen EA, Foglia EE, Schmidt B. Evidence-based pharmacologic therapies for prevention of bronchopulmonary dysplasia: application of the grading of recommendations assessment, development, and evaluation methodology. Clin Perinatol 2015;42:755–79.

56. Mann B, Sweet M, Knupp AM, et al. Nasal continuous positive airway pressure: a multisite study of suctioning practices within NICUs. Adv Neonatal Care 2013;13:E1–9.

57. Waisman D. Non-traumatic nasopharyngeal suction in premature newborn infants with upper airway obstruction from secretions following nasal CPAP. J Pediatr 2006;149:279.

58. Sahni R, Schiaratura M, Polin RA. Strategies for the prevention of continuous positive airway pressure failure. Semin Fetal Neonatal Med 2016;21:196–203.

59. Aly H, Milner JD, Patel K, et al. Does the experience with the use of nasal continuous positive airway pressure improve over time in extremely low birth weight infants? Pediatrics 2004;114:697–702.

60. Birenbaum HJ, Dentry A, Cirelli J, et al. Reduction in the incidence of chronic lung disease in very low birth weight infants: results of a quality improvement process in a tertiary level neonatal intensive care unit. Pediatrics 2009;123:44–50.

61. Levesque BM, Kalish LA, LaPierre J, et al. Impact of implementing 5 potentially better respiratory practices on neonatal outcomes and costs. Pediatrics 2011; 128:e218–26.

62. Payne NR, Finkelstein MJ, Liu M, et al. NICU practices and outcomes associated with 9 years of quality improvement collaboratives. Pediatrics 2010;125:437–46.

63. Walsh M, Laptook A, Kazzi SN, et al. A cluster-randomized trial of benchmarking and multimodal quality improvement to improve rates of survival free of bronchopulmonary dysplasia for infants with birth weights of less than 1250 grams. Pediatrics 2007;119:876–90.

64. Birenbaum HJ, Pfoh ER, Helou S, et al. Chronic lung disease in very low birth weight infants: persistence and improvement of a quality improvement process in a tertiary level neonatal intensive care unit. J Neonatal Perinatal Med 2016;9: 187–94.

65. De Jaegere AP, van der Lee JH, Cante C, et al. Early prediction of nasal continuous positive airway pressure failure in preterm infants less than 30 weeks gestation. Acta Paediatr 2012;101:374–9.

66. Tagliaferro T, Bateman D, Ruzal-Shapiro C, et al. Early radiologic evidence of severe respiratory distress syndrome as a predictor of nasal continuous positive airway pressure failure in extremely low birth weight newborns. J Perinatol 2015;35:99–103.

67. Dargaville PA, Aiyappan A, De Paoli AG, et al. Minimally-invasive surfactant therapy in preterm infants on continuous positive airway pressure. Arch Dis Child Fetal Neonatal Ed 2013;98:F122–6.

68. Pillai MS, Sankar MJ, Mani K, et al. Clinical prediction score for nasal CPAP failure in pre-term VLBW neonates with early onset respiratory distress. J Trop Pediatr 2011;57:274–9.

69. Rocha G, Flor-de-Lima F, Proenca E, et al. Failure of early nasal continuous positive airway pressure in preterm infants of 26 to 30 weeks gestation. J Perinatol 2013;33:297–301.

70. Autilio C, Echaide M, Benachi A, et al. A noninvasive surfactant adsorption test predicting the need for surfactant therapy in preterm infants treated with continuous positive airway pressure. J Pediatr 2017;182:66–73.e61.

71. Chida S, Fujiwara T. Stable microbubble test for predicting the risk of respiratory distress syndrome: I. Comparisons with other predictors of fetal lung maturity in amniotic fluid. Eur J Pediatr 1993;152:148–51.

72. Bhatia R, Morley CJ, Argus B, et al. The stable microbubble test for determining continuous positive airway pressure (CPAP) success in very preterm infants receiving nasal CPAP from birth. Neonatology 2013;104:188–93.

73. Daniel IW, Fiori HH, Piva JP, et al. Lamellar body count and stable microbubble test on gastric aspirates from preterm infants for the diagnosis of respiratory distress syndrome. Neonatology 2010;98:150–5.

74. Fiori HH, Fritscher CC, Fiori RM. Selective surfactant prophylaxis in preterm infants born at < or =31 weeks' gestation using the stable microbubble test in gastric aspirates. J Perinat Med 2006;34:66–70.

75. Bhuta T, Kent-Biggs J, Jeffery HE. Prediction of surfactant dysfunction in term infants by the click test. Pediatr Pulmonol 1997;23:287–91.
76. Fiori HH, Varela I, Justo AL, et al. Stable microbubble test and click test to predict respiratory distress syndrome in preterm infants not requiring ventilation at birth. J Perinat Med 2003;31:509–14.
77. Mehrpisheh S, Mosayebi Z, Memarian A, et al. Evaluation of specificity and sensitivity of gastric aspirate shake test to predict surfactant deficiency in Iranian premature infants. Pregnancy Hypertens 2015;5:182–6.
78. Verder H, Ebbesen F, Brandt J, et al. Lamellar body counts on gastric aspirates for prediction of respiratory distress syndrome. Acta Paediatr 2011;100:175–80.
79. Brat R, Yousef N, Klifa R, et al. Lung ultrasonography score to evaluate oxygenation and surfactant need in neonates treated with continuous positive airway pressure. JAMA Pediatr 2015;169. e151797.
80. Gopel W, Kribs A, Hartel C, et al. Less invasive surfactant administration is associated with improved pulmonary outcomes in spontaneously breathing preterm infants. Acta Paediatr 2015;104:241–6.
81. Kanmaz HG, Erdeve O, Canpolat FE, et al. Surfactant administration via thin catheter during spontaneous breathing: randomized controlled trial. Pediatrics 2013; 131:e502–9.
82. Gopel W, Kribs A, Ziegler A, et al. Avoidance of mechanical ventilation by surfactant treatment of spontaneously breathing preterm infants (AMV): an open-label, randomised, controlled trial. Lancet 2011;378:1627–34.
83. Kribs A, Roll C, Gopel W, et al. Nonintubated surfactant application vs conventional therapy in extremely preterm infants: a randomized clinical trial. JAMA Pediatr 2015;169:723–30.
84. Mohammadizadeh M, Ardestani AG, Sadeghnia AR. Early administration of surfactant via a thin intratracheal catheter in preterm infants with respiratory distress syndrome: feasibility and outcome. J Res Pharm Pract 2015;4:31–6.
85. Bao Y, Zhang G, Wu M, et al. A pilot study of less invasive surfactant administration in very preterm infants in a Chinese tertiary center. BMC Pediatr 2015;15:21.
86. Mirnia K, Heidarzadeh M, Hosseini M, et al. Comparison outcome of surfactant administration via tracheal catheterization during spontaneous breathing with INSURE. Medical Journal of Islamic World Academy of Sciences 2013;21:143–8.

Optimizing Caffeine Use and Risk of Bronchopulmonary Dysplasia in Preterm Infants

A Systematic Review, Meta-analysis, and Application of Grading of Recommendations Assessment, Development, and Evaluation Methodology

Mitali Atul Pakvasa, MD, Vivek Saroha, MD, PhD, Ravi Mangal Patel, MD, MSc*

KEYWORDS

- Infant • Neonate • Preterm • Caffeine • Methylxanthine • Dose • Timing • Duration

KEY POINTS

- Earlier initiation of caffeine, compared to later initiation, is associated with a decreased risk of bronchopulmonary dysplasia.
- High-dose caffeine, compared to standard-dose caffeine, may reduce the risk of bronchopulmonary dysplasia.
- The overall quality of evidence of studies on the dose and timing of caffeine and risk of bronchopulmonary dysplasia is low.
- Higher-quality evidence is needed to understand the risks and benefits of early initiation and high-dose caffeine to decrease the risk of bronchopulmonary dysplasia.

Conflicts of Interest: None of the authors report any relationship with a commercial company that has a direct financial interest in subject matter or materials discussed in the article or with a company making a competing product.

The review was supported, in part, by the National Institutes of Health under awards KL2 TR000455, UL1 TR000454, and K23 HL128942 (R.M. Patel), which had no role in the content of this review.

Division of Neonatal-Perinatal Medicine, Department of Pediatrics, Emory University School of Medicine, 2015 Uppergate Drive Northeast, 3rd Floor, Atlanta, GA 30322, USA

* Corresponding author.

E-mail address: rmpatel@emory.edu

Clin Perinatol 45 (2018) 273–291
https://doi.org/10.1016/j.clp.2018.01.012
0095-5108/18/© 2018 Elsevier Inc. All rights reserved.

INTRODUCTION
Rationale

From the first described use in the 1970s as a treatment of apnea of prematurity,[1,2] caffeine is now one of the most commonly administered medications in neonatal intensive care units worldwide.[3,4] The Caffeine for Apnea of Prematurity (CAP) trial demonstrated several beneficial effects of caffeine in extremely preterm infants, including a lower risk of bronchopulmonary dysplasia (BPD)[5] and death or disability at 18 to 21 months[6] with benefits persisting into middle childhood.[7] A post hoc subgroup analysis of this trial reported a greater reduction in the duration of respiratory support among infants who initiated caffeine early (before day 3) compared with later (3–10 days) in life.[8] Multiple observational studies have also evaluated the timing of caffeine initiation and neonatal outcomes,[9,10] and the optimal timing of caffeine administration for maximal beneficial effect remains the subject of more recent investigation.[11] The standard dosing for caffeine citrate used in the CAP trial was 20 mg/kg loading followed by 5 to 10 mg/kg/d as maintenance.[5] Although some studies have shown respiratory benefits with a higher dose of caffeine,[12] another study raised concerns regarding the potential harms.[13] Additionally, clinicians have used a variety of dosing regimens to balance the optimal benefit of caffeine with the potential for adverse effects in routine practice.[14] Variation also exists in the age at cessation of caffeine therapy.[14,15] The authors' rationale for this review was that given the common use of caffeine in preterm infants, optimizing its use may enhance the known benefits of caffeine therapy.

Objective

The objective of this systematic review was to evaluate the following question: Among preterm infants, does the timing of caffeine initiation, the dose of caffeine, or the duration of caffeine therapy influence clinical outcomes, including BPD?

METHODS
Protocol/Registration

The authors used the Preferred Reporting Items for Systematic Reviews and Meta-Analyses (PRISMA) guidelines to report the systematic review and meta-analysis[16] and registered the protocol with PROSPERO (https://www.crd.york.ac.uk/PROSPERO/) on August 31, 2017 (No. 75841).

Eligibility Criteria

Studies: All meta-analyses, randomized controlled trials (RCT), and observational studies were considered for qualitative inclusion. Only individual RCTs and observational studies were quantitatively synthesized. The authors excluded case reports, editorials, and reviews without meta-analyses and resolved discrepancies by consensus of all investigators.

Participants: The participants were infants of less than 37 weeks' gestation.

Interventions: (1) For the timing of initiation, intervention is early initiation of caffeine as defined by the study. (2) For the dose of caffeine, intervention is a high dose as defined by the study or the higher dose for 2 or more comparison groups. (3) For the duration of treatment, intervention is the longer duration of caffeine for 2 or more comparison groups.

Comparators: (1) For the timing of initiation, comparator is the later initiation of caffeine as defined by the study. (2) For the dose of caffeine, comparator is the standard dose or lower dose as defined by the study. (3) For the duration of treatment, comparator is the shorter duration of caffeine for 2 or more comparison groups.

Outcomes: The primary outcome of the review was BPD. Secondary outcomes included BPD or death, death, intraventricular hemorrhage (IVH), periventricular leukomalacia (PVL), patent ductus arteriosus (PDA), necrotizing enterocolitis (NEC), retinopathy of prematurity (ROP), duration of mechanical ventilation, and neurodevelopmental impairment. Additional adverse neonatal outcomes were summarized if reported by the study.

Outcome definitions

Study-specific definitions were used to define BPD and other outcomes. For studies reporting multiple definitions for BPD, the authors used the need for oxygen at 36 weeks' postmenstrual age as the definition of BPD.

Information Sources and Search

The authors conducted a systematic search of PubMed using the MeSH terms *INFANT* and *CAFFEINE* with exclusion of non-English articles without restriction of publication date or type of study. Additional studies were identified through review of study reference lists. The authors initially performed the search in January 2017 and updated the search in July 2017.

Study Selection

Three researchers conducted this review. Two reviewers independently conducted the search (M.A.P. and V.S.) using the same search strategy to identify studies. Both reviewers decided on the selection of studies for the review and included meta-analyses, RCTs, and observational studies that assessed one of the following aspects of caffeine use: the timing of initiation, dose, or duration of treatment. The authors resolved discrepancies by consensus of all authors.

Data Collection Process and Data Items

One reviewer independently extracted data on studies on the timing of caffeine (V.S.), and another reviewer independently extracted data on studies on the dose and duration of caffeine (M.A.P.). All the authors reviewed extracted data for accuracy.

Risk of Bias Within and Across Studies

The authors applied the Grading of Recommendations Assessment, Development, and Evaluation (GRADE) framework to assess the overall quality of the evidence for the primary study outcome of BPD.[17,18] They used GRADEpro GDT: GRADEpro Guideline Development Tool Software, McMaster University, 2015 (developed by Evidence Prime, Inc and available from gradepro.org) to apply an overall GRADE. All eligible studies, regardless of the quality of evidence, were synthesized. No interrater assessment of quality was performed. Evidence from RCTs start with a high rating but can be downgraded for study limitations, indirectness of evidence, imprecision of estimate, inconsistency of the evidence, or publication bias (http://gdt.guidelinedevelopment.org/app/handbook/handbook.html). Observational studies start with a low rating and can be downgraded for the aforementioned reasons or upgraded for a large magnitude of effect, evidence of dose-response relationship, or the effect of plausible residual confounding.

Summary Measures and Synthesis of Results

Data reported in the individual studies were included. No additional data were sought from study investigators. All selected studies and outcomes underwent a descriptive synthesis. A quantitative synthesis was performed for studies reporting on the primary outcome of BPD. Random-effects meta-analyses generating pooled odds ratios (ORs) were used for the effect measure for all analyses, given the decision to search for both observational studies and randomized trials and the authors' goal to have the same effect measure for all meta-analyses. Random effects, rather than fixed effects, was used for primary reporting given the anticipated differences in intervention and comparison groups and populations across studies. The I^2 statistical was used to report measures of statistical heterogeneity. Randomized trials and observational studies were evaluated separately. For randomized trials, an intention-to-treat approach was used and all randomized infants were included in the denominator. For observational studies, the study-reported denominator was used. For randomized trials reporting on BPD with similar intervention and comparator groups, events and randomized infants were pooled in a meta-analysis using the Mantel-Haenszel (M-H) approach. For observational studies reporting on BPD, a similar approach was used to generate unadjusted pooled estimates and the inverse variance (IV) approach used to generate adjusted pooled estimates. Publication bias was visually assessed using funnel plots. Review Manager (RevMan) Version 5.3 was used for meta-analysis (Source: The Nordic Cochrane Centre, Copenhagen; The Cochrane Collaboration, 2014).

RESULTS
Study Selection

Of the 548 records screened, the authors identified 21 studies for inclusion (**Fig. 1**).

Study Characteristics

Timing of caffeine initiation

Five studies compared early versus late caffeine initiation and reported on the risk of BPD (**Table 1**). A reduction in the risk of BPD with earlier initiation of caffeine (<day of life 3), compared with later initiation (≥day of life 3), has been reported in 2 separate meta-analyses,[19,20] one post hoc subgroup analysis of a large RCT[8] and 4 observational studies,[9,21–23] whereas one study reported no difference[24] (**Table 2**). Two small randomized trials studied the timing of caffeine.[11,25] One of these 2 trials reported on oxygen at 36 weeks post-menstrual age and found no difference among early caffeine (mean age of initiation 1 hour after birth) vs. later caffeine (mean age of initiation 12 hours after birth) groups.[11] One observational study reported an association of early caffeine initiation and death,[21] and this weighed substantially on the overall pooled higher odds for death associated with earlier initiation in a meta-analysis of observational studies,[20] although the absolute risk difference was small and the interpretation was limited by survival bias. Two meta-analyses of observational studies reported associations between early caffeine and a decreased risk for ROP, IVH, and PVL. Several observational studies reported associations between early caffeine use and a decreased risk for a PDA. Several of the observational studies had large sample sizes, a multicenter design and used propensity matching or covariate adjustment.[9,21]

High- versus low-dose caffeine

Three studies evaluated the effect of high- versus low-dose caffeine on the risk of BPD (see **Table 1**). One follow-up study of a randomized trial also reported on BPD[26], but was not included as short-term outcomes were previously published in a separate study.[12] Of 3 studies evaluating caffeine dose and extubation, all 3 found that high-dose caffeine, compared with standard or lower dose, was associated with a reduction in extubation failure[12,27,28] (**Table 3**). Three of the 4 studies evaluating apnea of prematurity were RCTs and showed an increased efficacy of high-dose caffeine, compared

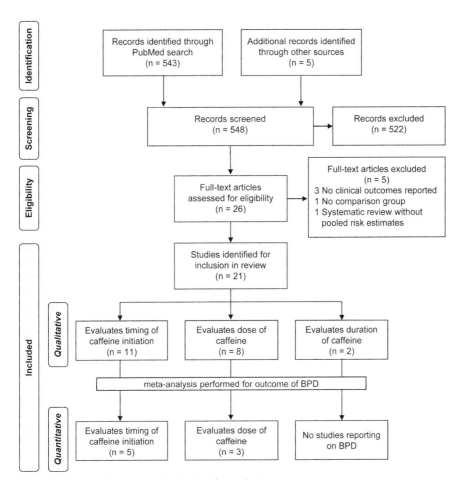

Fig. 1. Study identification and selection for inclusion.

with standard or lower dose, in the prevention of apnea.[12,27–29] Five studies evaluated the total number of ventilator days, 2 evaluated the number of continuous-positive-airway-pressure days, and one evaluated days of oxygen therapy; no study found a difference in duration of therapy among those receiving high- versus standard or lower-dose caffeine.[12,27,28,30] Among the 4 studies that evaluated the risk of BPD or death, as a composite outcome, before hospital discharge, there was no difference found among either group of infants.[12,13,27,30]

Four studies assessed ROP, and 5 studies assessed NEC. None found a difference among either outcome between infants receiving high-dose versus standard or lower-dose caffeine.[12,13,27,28,30] One study reported an association between the cumulative dose of caffeine and the risk of ROP.[31] One study evaluated seizures and reported that there was a higher seizure burden in infants who received high dose caffeine, although this was not statistically significant.[30] Overall, there was no difference in the risk of any IVH between high- and standard or lower-dose caffeine[12,13,27,28,30]; however, one study reported a high frequency of cerebellar hemorrhage among infants receiving high-dose compared with standard or lower-dose caffeine.[13] One trial comparing higher vs. lower dose caffeine followed infants up to 1 year of corrected age and found no

Table 1
Grading of Recommendations Assessment, Development, and Evaluation summary of evidence

No. of Studies	Study Design	Risk of Bias	Inconsistency	Indirectness	Imprecision	Other Considerations	Early Initiation/High Dose of Caffeine	Late Initiation/Standard Dose of Caffeine	Relative (95% CI)	Absolute (95% CI)	Certainty	Importance
Certainty Assessment							**No. of Patients**		**Effect**			
BPD (early vs late initiation of caffeine)												
5	Observational studies	Not serious (adjusted estimates)	Not serious	Not serious	Not serious	None	20,495	16,871	OR 0.69 (0.64–0.75)	Unable to calculate	⊕⊕◯◯ Low	Critical
5	Observational studies	Very serious[a] (unadjusted estimates)	Serious[b]	Not serious	Not serious	None	7578 of 36,851 (20.6%)	8909 of 26,198 (34.0%)	OR 0.59 (0.39–0.90)	107 fewer per 1000 (from 23 fewer to 173 fewer)	⊕◯◯◯ Very low	Critical
BPD (high vs standard dose of caffeine)												
3	Randomized trials	Not serious	Not serious	Serious[c]	Serious[d]	None	65 of 213 (30.5%)	88 of 219 (40.2%)	OR 0.65 (0.43–0.97)	98 fewer per 1000 (from 7 fewer to 178 fewer)	⊕⊕◯◯ Low	Critical

Abbreviation: CI, confidence interval.
[a] Confounding was not addressed (for unadjusted analyses).
[b] Wide variance in estimates without overlapping confidence intervals; high statistical heterogeneity ($I^2 = 97\%$).
[c] Differences in interventions: caffeine initiated at different postnatal ages and doses.
[d] Optimal information size not met: total number of events less than 200.

Table 2
Summary of studies evaluating timing of caffeine initiation

Author, Year, Outcome	Study Type	Population, Intervention, and Comparison[a]	Results[b]
BPD			
Davis et al,[8] 2010	RCT, subgroup analysis, multicenter	BW <1250 g (n = 1917) (caffeine vs placebo across 2 subgroups: early 0–2 d; late: 3–10 d)	Early: 28% vs 45% (OR 0.48; 95% CI 0.36–0.65); late: 42% vs 49% (OR 0.77; 0.61–0.98); interaction P = .02
Dobson et al,[21] 2014	OBS (retrospective), multicenter	BW <1500 g (n = 29,070; matched)	23% vs 31% (OR 0.68; 99% CI 0.63–0.73; P<.001)
Hand et al,[24] 2016	OBS (retrospective), single center	GA <29 wk (n = 150) (early: 0–2 d; late/very late: ≥3 d; early vs very late for multivariable analysis)	27% vs 35% (OR 0.39; 0.13–1.22; P = .16)
Kua & Lee,[19] 2017	Meta-analysis of OBS studies	Preterm infants, 5 cohort studies (n = 37,383)	26% vs 31% (RR 0.80; 0.66–0.96; P = .02)
Kua & Lee,[19] 2017	Meta-analysis of RCT	Preterm infants, 2 RCTs (n = 999)	28% vs 42% (RR 0.67; 56–0.81; P<.001)
Lodha et al,[9] 2015	OBS (retrospective), multicenter	GA <31 wk (n = 5101)	28% vs 28% (OR 0.79; 0.64–0.96)
Park et al,[20] 2015	Meta-analysis	BW <1500 g; 1 RCT and 3 OBS (retrospective) (n = 58,761)	20% vs 34% (OR 0.51; 0.39–0.65; P<.001)
Patel et al,[22] 2013	OBS (retrospective), single center	BW <1250 g (n = 140)	24% vs 51% (OR 0.33; 0.14–0.98; P = .04)
Taha et al,[23] 2014	OBS (retrospective), multicenter	BW <1250 g (n = 2951)c	36% vs 47% (OR 0.69; 0.58–0.83; P<.001)
Katheria et al,[11] 2015	RCT, single center	GA <29 wk (n = 20) [early: mean initiation age 1 h; Routine: mean age 12 h]	9% vs 20% (P = .59)
BPD or death			
Dobson et al,[21] 2014	OBS (retrospective), multicenter	BW <1500 g (n = 29,070; matched)	27% vs 34% (OR 0.74; 99% CI 0.69–0.80; P<.001)
Kua & Lee,[19] 2017	Meta-analysis of OBS studies	Preterm infants, 4 cohort studies (n = 37,262)	28% vs 33% (RR 0.84; 0.73–0.95)
Park et al,[20] 2015	Meta-analysis	Infants <1500 g at birth, 3 OBS (retrospective) (n = 57,798)	24% vs 38% (OR 0.53; 0.38–0.72; P<.001)
Patel et al,[22] 2013	OBS (retrospective), single center	BW <1250 g (n = 140)	25% vs 53% (OR 0.32; 0.15–0.63; P<.01)

(continued on next page)

Table 2
(continued)

Author, Year, Outcome	Study Type	Population, Intervention, and Comparison[a]	Results[b]
Taha et al,[23] 2014	OBS (retrospective), multicenter	BW <1250 g (n = 2951)[c]	46% vs 55% (OR 0.77; 0.63–0.94; P = .01)
Death before hospital discharge			
Dobson et al,[21] 2014	OBS (retrospective), multicenter	BW <1500 g (n = 29,070, matched), excluded death on DOL 0–3	4.5% vs 3.7% (OR 1.23; 99% CI 1.05–1.43; P<.001)
Kua & Lee,[19] 2017	Meta-analysis of OBS studies	Preterm infants, 3 studies (n = 34,311)	4.8% vs 3.9% (RR 1.16; 1.02–1.32)
Kua & Lee,[19] 2017	Meta-analysis of RCT	Preterm infants, 2 RCTs (n = 973)	40% vs 40% (RR 1.00; 0.86–1.17; P = .95)
Lodha et al,[9] 2015	OBS (retrospective), multicenter	GA <31 wk (n = 5101)	6% vs 6% (OR 0.98; 0.70–1.37)
Park et al,[20] 2015	Meta-analysis	BW <1500 g, 2 OBS (retrospective) (n = 54,852)	3.8% vs 4.2% (OR 0.90; 0.83–0.98; P = .02)
Patel et al,[22] 2013	OBS (retrospective), single center	BW <1250 g (n = 140)	6% vs 5% (OR 1.47; 0.30–7.26; P = .64)
IVH			
Dekker et al,[25] 2017	RCT, single center	GA <30 wk (n = 23) (Early: <7 min of birth; late: after NICU admission)	23% vs 30% (P = NS)
Dobson et al,[21] 2014	OBS (retrospective), multicenter	BW <1500 g (n = 29,070; matched)	Any IVH: 29% vs 33% (P<.001) Severe IVH: 5% vs 8% (P<.001)
Gupte et al,[10] 2016	OBS (retrospective), single center	BW <1500 g & GA <32 wk (n = 160) (early: 0–2 d; late: ≥3 d; no caffeine)	26% vs 30% vs 21%; NS
Kua & Lee,[19] 2017	Meta-analysis of OBS studies	Preterm infants, 4 cohort studies (n = 32,282)	5% vs 8% (RR 0.68; 0.63–0.75)
Lodha et al,[9] 2015	OBS (retrospective), multicenter	GA <31 wk (n = 5101)	12% vs 14% (OR 0.80; 0.63–1.01)
Park et al,[20] 2015	Meta-analysis	4 OBS (retrospective) (n = not specified)	OR 0.54; 0.36–0.80; P = .002
Patel et al,[22] 2013	OBS (retrospective), single center	BW <1250 g (n = 140)	Severe IVH: 14% vs 14% (P = .94)
Taha et al,[23] 2014	OBS (retrospective), multicenter	BW <1250 g (n = 2951)[c]	Severe IVH: OR 0.72; 0.52–0.99; P = .05
Katheria et al,[11] 2015	RCT, single center	GA <29 wk (n = 20) [early: mean initiation age 1 h; Routine: mean age 12 h)	0% vs 10% (P = .48)
PVL			
Dobson et al,[21] 2014	OBS (retrospective), multicenter	BW <1500 g (n = 29,070; matched)	1.6% vs 2.1% (P = .001)
Hand et al,[24] 2016	OBS (retrospective), single center	GA <29 wk (n = 150)	4.7% vs 3.1% (P = .27)

Kua & Lee,[19] 2017	Meta-analysis of OBS studies	Preterm infants, 2 studies (n = 29,210)	1.6% vs 2.1% (RR 0.76; 0.65–0.71)
Park et al,[20] 2015	Meta-analysis	2 OBS (retrospective) (n = not specified)	1.4% vs 2.4% (OR 0.56; 0.49–0.63; $P<.001$)
Patel et al,[22] 2013	OBS (retrospective), single center	BW <1250 g (n = 140)	8% vs 7% ($P = 1.0$)
PDA			
Davis et al,[8] 2010	Subgroup analysis of RCT	BW <1250 g (n = 2000) (caffeine vs placebo across 2 subgroups: early 0–2 d; late: 3–10 d)	Early: 2.7% vs 12.0% (OR 0.20; 0.10–0.38); late 6% vs 14% (OR 0.40; 0.26–0.61); interaction $P = .08$
Dobson et al,[21] 2014	OBS (retrospective), multicenter	BW <1500 g (n = 29,070; matched)	12% vs 19% (OR 0.60; 99% CI 0.55–0.65; $P<.001$)
Hand et al,[24] 2016	OBS (retrospective), single center	GA <29 wk (n = 150)	PDA: 48% vs 57% ($P = .61$) PDA surgery: 4.7% vs 6.2% ($P = .32$)
Kua & Lee,[19] 2017	Meta-analysis of OBS studies	Preterm infants, 4 studies (n = 37,262) for PDA, 2 (n = 5241) for PDA surgery	PDA: RR 0.71; 0.60–0.84 PDA surgery: RR 0.41; 0.18–0.90
Kua & Lee,[19] 2017	Meta-analysis of RCT	Preterm infants, 2 RCTs (n = 1037)	PDA: RR 0.77; 0.23–2.61
Lodha et al,[9] 2015	OBS (retrospective), multicenter	GA <31 wk (n = 5101)	13% vs 25% (OR 0.58; 0.42–0.80)
Park et al,[20] 2015	Meta-analysis	1 RCT & 2 OBS (n = not specified)	9% vs 19% (OR 0.40; 0.38–0.42; $P<.001$)
Patel et al,[22] 2013	OBS (retrospective), single center	BW <1250 g (n = 140)	10% vs 36% (OR 0.28; 0.10–0.73; $P = .01$)
Katheria et al,[11] 2015	RCT, single center	GA <29 wk (n = 20) [early: mean initiation age 1 h; Routine: mean age 12 h]	18% vs 40% ($P = .36$)
NEC			
Dobson et al,[21] 2014	OBS (retrospective), multicenter	BW <1500 g (n = 29,070; matched)	8% vs 8% ($P = .50$)
Hand et al,[24] 2016	OBS (retrospective), single center	GA <29 wk (n = 150)	9% vs 12% ($P = 1.0$)
Kua & Lee,[19] 2017	Meta-analysis of OBS studies	Preterm infants, 5 studies (n = 37,383)	8% vs 8% (RR 1.03; 0.90–1.18)
Lodha et al,[9] 2015	OBS (retrospective), multicenter	GA <31 wk (n = 5101)	6% vs 6% (OR 0.88; 0.65–1.20)
Park et al,[20] 2015	Meta-analysis	2 OBS (retrospective) (n = not specified)	2.6% vs 2.4% (OR 0.98; 0.71–1.33); $P = .89$
Patel et al,[22] 2013	OBS (retrospective), single center	BW <1250 g (n = 140)	10% vs 18% ($P = .15$); surgery: 1% vs 5% ($P = .30$)
Taha et al,[23] 2014	OBS (retrospective), multicenter	BW <1250 g (n = 2951)c	7.3% vs 5.9% (OR 1.41; 1.04–1.91; $P = .03$)

(continued on next page)

Table 2
(continued)

Author, Year, Outcome	Study Type	Population, Intervention, and Comparison[a]	Results[b]
Neurodevelopmental impairment			
Davis et al,[8] 2010	Subgroup analysis of RCT	BW <1250 g (n = 1725) (caffeine vs placebo across 2 subgroups: early 0–2 d; late: 3–10 d)	Cognitive delay: early: 35% vs 41% (OR 0.80; 0.59–1.08); late: 33% vs 35% (OR 0.84; 0.65–1.09) Interaction P = .80; cerebral palsy: early: 4.1% vs 8.6% (OR 0.54; 0.24–0.85); late: 4.6% vs 6.3% (OR 0.72; 0.42–1.23); interaction P = .27
Gupte et al,[10] 2016	OBS (retrospective), single center	BW <1500 g & GA <32 wk (n = 160) (early: 0–2 d; late: ≥3 d vs no caffeine)	43% vs 16% vs 23% (P<.001)
ROP			
Dobson et al,[21] 2014	OBS (retrospective), multicenter	BW <1500 g (n = 29,070; matched)	ROP: 31% vs 36% (P<.001) ROP treatment: 2.8% vs 5.0%. (P<.001)
Hand et al,[24] 2016	OBS (retrospective), single center	GA <29 wk (n = 150)	8.0% vs 3.1% (P = .10)
Kua & Lee,[19] 2017	Meta-analysis of OBS studies	Preterm infants, 5 studies (n = 37,383)	24% vs 32% (RR 0.85; 0.83–0.88)
Lodha et al,[9] 2015	OBS (retrospective), multicenter	GA <31 wk (n = 5101)	10% vs13% (OR 0.78; 0.56–1.10)
Park et al,[20] 2015	Meta-analysis	3 OBS (retrospective) (n = not specified)	ROP laser surgery: OR 0.45; 0.22–0.90; P = .02
Patel et al,[22] 2013	OBS (retrospective), single center	BW <1250 g (n = 140)	ROP > stage 1: 30% vs 41% (P = .20) ROP laser surgery: 3% vs 10% (P = .24)
Taha et al,[23] 2014	OBS (retrospective), multicenter	BW <1250 g (n = 2951)[c]	ROP laser surgery: OR 0.74; 0.52–1.06; P = .10

Duration of mechanical ventilation			
Davis et al,[8] 2010	Subgroup analysis of RCT	BW <1250 g (n = 2004) (caffeine vs placebo across 2 subgroups: early 0–2 d; late: 3–10 d)	Early: 29 vs 31 mean wk PMA (weighted mean difference −1.08; −1.51, −0.6); late 31 vs 31 wk (0.37; −0.79 to −0.05); interaction $P = .04$
Dobson et al,[21] 2014	OBS (retrospective), multicenter	BW <1500 g (n = 29,070; matched)	Median (IQR) 3 (1–12) vs 6 (0–25) d ($P<.001$)
Park et al,[20] 2015	Meta-analysis	2 OBS (retrospective) (n = not specified)	Standard mean difference 0.17 d (−0.45, 0.11; $P = .24$)
Patel et al,[22] 2013	OBS (retrospective), single center	BW <1250 g (n = 140)	Median 6 d vs 22 d ($P<.01$)
Lodha et al,[9] 2015	OBS (retrospective), multicenter	GA <31 wk (n = 5101)	Median (IQR) 2 (1–9) vs 4 (1–23) d ($P<.01$)
Taha et al,[23] 2014	OBS (retrospective), multicenter	BW <1250 g (n = 2951)[c]	Mean (SD) 16.7 (21.7) vs 23.7 (23.7) d ($P<.001$)
Katheria et al,[11] 2015	RCT, single center	GA <29 wk (n = 20) [early: mean initiation age 1 h; Routine: mean age 12 h]	Mean [SD] 6 [9] vs 3 [5] d ($P = .40$)
Discharge home on oxygen			
Kua & Lee,[19] 2017	Meta-analysis of OBS studies	Preterm infants, 2 studies (n = 8052)	22% vs 25% (RR 0.87; 0.67–1.12)
Lodha et al,[9] 2015	OBS (retrospective), multicenter	GA <31 wk (n = 1501)	25% vs 25% ($P = .73$)
Taha et al,[23] 2014	OBS (retrospective), multicenter	BW <1250 g (n = 2951)[c]	18% vs 24% (OR 0.73; 0.55–0.96; $P = .025$)

Abbreviations: BW, birth weight; GA, gestational age; HOL, hour of life; IQR, interquartile range; NICU, neonatal intensive care unit; NS, not significant; OBS, observational study; PMA, postmenstrual age; RR, relative risk.

[a] Unless otherwise noted in DOL, the intervention group (early) initiated caffeine on DOL 0 to 2 and the comparison group (late) on DOL 3 or greater.

[b] Estimates provided compare the intervention group (early caffeine) with the comparison group (late caffeine) unless otherwise noted, and adjusted or matched estimates (if unadjusted or unmatched estimates were also reported) with 95% confidence interval are noted in parenthesis unless otherwise stated.

[c] Comparison group was DOL 3 to 10.

Table 3
Summary of studies evaluating high- versus standard-dose caffeine

Author, Year, Outcome	Study Type	Population	Intervention: Higher-Dose Caffeine[a]	Comparison – Standard/Lower-Dose Caffeine[a]	Results[b]
BPD					
McPherson et al,[13] 2015[c]	RCT, single center	GA ≤30 wk (n = 74)	L: 40, 20 (12 h); 10 (24 h); 10 (36 h); M: 10	L: 20 within <24 HOL; M: 10	51% vs 49% (P = .82)
Mohammed et al,[27] 2015	RCT, single center	GA <32 wk; apnea <10 DOL (n = 120)	L: 40; M: 20	L: 20; M: 10	22% vs 32% (RR 0.59; 0.26–1.35; P = .31)
Steer et al,[12] 2004[d]	RCT, multicenter	GA <30 wk; ventilation ≥48 h (n = 234)	L: 80; M: 20	L: 20; M: 5	34% vs 48% (RR 0.72; 0.51–1.01; P = .06)
BPD or death					
Mohammed et al,[27] 2015	RCT, single center	GA <32 wk; apnea <10 DOL (n = 120)	L: 40; M: 20	L: 20; M: 10	33% vs 43% (RR 0.65; 0.31–1.37; P = .26)
Death before hospital discharge					
McPherson et al,[13] 2015[c]	RCT, single center	GA ≤30 wk (n = 74)	L: 40, 20 (12 h); 10 (24 h); 10 (36 h); M:10	L: 20 within <24 HOL; M: 10	19% vs 14% (P = .53)
Mohammed et al,[27] 2015	RCT, single center	GA <32 wk; apnea <10 DOL (n = 120)	L: 40; M: 20	L: 20; M: 10	12% vs 15% (RR 0.74; 0.25–2.16; P = .78)
Steer et al,[12] 2004[d]	RCT, multicenter	GA <30 wk; ventilation ≥48 h (n = 234)	L: 80; M: 20	L: 20; M: 5	4% vs 6% (RR 0.77; 0.25–2.34; P = .64)
IVH or PVL					
Mohammed et al,[27] 2015	RCT, single center	GA <32 wk; apnea <10 DOL (n = 120)	L: 40; M: 20	L: 20; M: 10	Severe IVH: 12% vs 8% (RR 1.22; 0.61–2.44; P = .76). PVL: 8% vs 7% (RR 1.27; 0.32–4.99; P = .99)
Steer et al,[12] 2004[d]	RCT, multicenter	GA <30 wk; ventilation ≥48 h (n = 234)	L: 80; M: 20	L: 20; M: 5	IVH: 30% vs 28% (RR 1.04; 0.68–1.58; P = .86) Severe IVH: 4.0% vs 0.8% (P = .11)

Study	Design	Population	Dosing (high)	Dosing (low/moderate)	Outcome
Steer et al,[28] 2003	RCT, single center	GA <32 wk; ventilated ≥48 h (n = 127)	Very high: L: 30; M: 1 High: L: 15; M: 1 (peri-extubation)	L: 3; M: 1	Severe IVH: 4% vs 0% vs 0% (P not reported)
McPherson et al,[13] 2015c	RCT, single center	GA ≤30 wk (n = 74)	L: 40, 20 (12 h); 10 (24 h); 10 (36 h); M:10	L: 20 within <24 HOL; M: 10	IVH: 27% vs 32% (P = .61). Severe IVH: 11% vs 11% (P>.99). Cerebellar hemorrhage: 36% vs 10% (OR 5.0; 1.2–20.17; P = .03). PVL: 8% vs 5% (P = .78)
Patent ductus arteriosus					
McPherson et al,[13] 2015c	RCT, single center	GA ≤30 wk (n = 74)	L: 40, 20 (12 h); 10 (24 h); M: 10 (36 h); M: 10	L: 20 within <24 HOL; M: 10	54% vs 54% (P>.99)
Steer et al,[28] 2003	RCT, single center	GA <32 wk; ventilated ≥48 h (n = 127)	Very high: L: 30; M: 1 High: L: 15; M: 1 (peri-extubation)	L: 3; M: 1	20% vs 7% vs 21% (P not reported)
NEC					
McPherson et al,[13] 2015	RCT, single center	GA ≤30 wk (n = 74)	L: 40, 20 (12 h); 10 (24 h); M: 10 (36 h); M: 10	L: 20 within <24 HOL; M: 10	16% vs 14% (P = .74)
Mohammed et al,[27] 2015	RCT, single center	GA <32 wk; apnea <10 DOL (n = 120)	L: 40; M: 20	L: 20; M: 10	7% vs 10% (RR 0.64; 0.17–2.40; P = .74)
Steer et al,[12] 2004	RCT, multicenter	GA <30 wk; ventilation ≥48 h (n = 234)	L: 80; M: 20	L: 20; M: 5	0% vs 4% (P not reported)
Steer et al,[28] 2003	RCT, single center	GA <32 wk; ventilated ≥48 h (n = 127)	Very high: L: 30; M: 1 High: L: 15; M: 1 (peri-extubation)	L: 3; M: 1	0% vs 5% vs 0% (P = not reported)
ROP					
Hussein et al,[31] 2014	OBS, single center	BW <1500 g or GA <32 wk; selected infants with BW 1500–2000 g or GA >32 wk (n = 350; 338 treated)	Total cumulative caffeine dose given throughout NICU stay	No comparison group	Cumulative caffeine dose associated with any ROP (RR 1.03; 1.01–1.06; P = .003); and ROP receiving treatment (RR 1.07; 1.02–1.12; P = .006)

(continued on next page)

Table 3
(continued)

Author, Year, Outcome	Study Type	Population	Intervention: Higher-Dose Caffeine[a]	Comparison – Standard/Lower-Dose Caffeine[a]	Results[b]
McPherson et al,[13] 2015[c]	RCT, single center	GA ≤30 wk (n = 74)	L: 40, 20 (12 h); 10 (24 h); 10 (36 h); M: 10	L: 20 within <24 HOL; M: 10	5% vs 11% (P = .68)
Mohammed et al,[27] 2015	RCT, single center	GA <32 wk; apnea <10 DOL (n = 120)	L: 40; M: 20	L: 20; M: 10	8% vs 8% (RR 1.0; 0.27–3.65; P = 1.0)
Steer et al,[12] 2004[d]	RCT, multicenter	GA <30 wk; ventilation ≥48 h (n = 234)	L: 80; M: 20	L: 20; M: 5	Any ROP: 23% vs 33% (RR 0.68; 0.43–1.09; P = .11) ROP stage 3 and 4: 3% vs 8% (RR 0.42; 0.11–1.52; P = .22)
Duration of mechanical ventilation (d)					
Mohammed et al,[27] 2015	RCT, single center	GA <32 wk; apnea <10 DOL (n = 120)	L: 40; M: 20	L: 20; M: 10	Median (IQR): 3.5 (1–10) vs 5 (2–13) (P = .61)
Steer et al,[12] 2004[d]	RCT, multicenter	GA <30 wk; ventilation ≥48 h (n = 234)	L: 80; M: 20	L: 20; M: 5	Median (IQR]: 7.4 (3.3–16.5) vs 9 (0.5–77) (P = .38)
Steer et al,[28] 2003	RCT, single center	GA <32 wk; ventilated ≥48 h (n = 127)	Very high: L: 30; M: 1 High: L: 15; M: 1 (peri-extubation)	L: 3; M: 1	Mean (SD): 3.9 (2.7) vs 3.1 (2.2) vs 3.5 (2.3)
McPherson et al,[13] 2015[c]	RCT, single center	GA ≤30 wk (n = 74)	L: 40, 20 (12 h); 10 (24 h); 10 (36 h); M: 10	L: 20 within <24 HOL; M: 10	Median (IQR): 4 (1–22) vs 3 (1–22) (P = .95)
Extubation failure					
Mohammed et al,[27] 2015	RCT, single center	GA <32 wk; apnea <10 DOL (n = 120)	L: 40; M: 20	L: 20; M: 10	22% vs 47% (P = .02)
Steer et al,[12] 2004	RCT, multicenter	GA <30 wk; ventilation ≥48 h (n = 234)	L: 80; M: 20	L: 20; M: 5	15.0% vs 29.8% (RR 0.51; 0.31–0.85; P<.01)

Study	Design	Population	Intervention dose	Comparison dose	Outcome
Steer et al,[28] 2003	RCT, single center	GA <32 wk; ventilated ≥48 h (n = 127)	Very high: L: 30; M: 1 High: L: 15; M: 1 (peri-extubation)	L: 3; M: 1	24% vs 25% vs 45% (P = .06)
Apnea of prematurity					
Mohammed et al,[27] 2015	RCT, single center	GA <32 wk; apnea <10 DOL (n = 120)	L: 40; M: 20	L: 20; M: 10	Frequency, median (IQR): 9 (6–16) vs 16 (14–17) (P<.001); Days: 2.5 (1–4) vs 5 (4–6) (P<.001)
Romagnoli et al,[29] 1992	OBS, single center	GA <32 wk (n = 37)	L: 10; M: 5	L: 10; M: 2.5	Significant decrease in apnea, although numeric data not provided (P<.01)
Steer et al,[12] 2004[d]	RCT, multicenter	GA <30 wk; ventilation ≥48 h (n = 234)	L: 80; M: 20	L: 20; M: 5	Episodes, median (IQR): 4 (1–12) vs 7 (2–22) (P<.01), days: 0.6 (0.1–2.1) vs 1.3 (0.3–4.3) (P = .02)
Steer et al,[28] 2003	RCT, single center	GA <32 wk; ventilated ≥48 h (n = 127)	Very high: L: 30; M: 1 High: L: 15; M: 1 (peri-extubation)	L: 3; M: 1	Apnea/day, median (range): 0.2(0–13) vs 0.4 (0–11) vs 1.3 (0–14) (P = .01)
Neurodevelopmental impairment					
Gray et al,[26] 2011	RCT, multicenter	GA <30 wk; ventilation ≥48 hr (n = 287 with 1 y follow-up on n = 190). Excluded infants receiving caffeine ≤7 d	L: 80; M: 20	L: 20; M: 5	Major disability 9% vs 16% (RR 0.73; 95% CI 0.43–1.25; P = .28) Mean [SD] cognitive score at 1 y corrected age: 98.0 [13.8] vs 93.6 [16.5] (P = .048)
Seizure activity					
Vesoulis et al,[30] 2016	RCT, single center	GA <30 wk (n = 74)	L: 40, 20 (12 h); 10 (24 h); 10 (36 h); M: 10	L: 20 within <24 HOL; M: 10	58% vs 40% (P = .19); duration: 170.9 s vs 48.9 s (P = .10)

Abbreviations: BW, birth weight; GA, gestational age; HOL, hour of life; IQR, interquartile range; L, loading dose; M, maintenance dose; NICU, neonatal intensive care unit; OBS, observational study; RR, relative risk.

a Loading dose and maintenance dose in milligrams per kilogram of caffeine citrate.

b Estimates compare the intervention group with the comparison group, and 95% confidence intervals provided with corresponding RR estimates.

c Also reported by Vesoulis 2016[30].

d Also reported by Gray et al, 2011[26] and not reported again given overlap in study populations.

difference in major disability but a higher general quotient on cognitive testing on the Griffiths Mental Development Scales among infants receiving high-dose caffeine.[27]

Duration of caffeine therapy

The authors identified 2 studies that investigated outcomes associated with the duration of caffeine treatment.[32,33] No studies reported on the outcome of BPD and, therefore, studies were not quantitatively synthesized. Rhein and colleagues[32] conducted a randomized trial (n = 95) comparing extended use of caffeine beyond 34 weeks' postmenstrual age (PMA) versus cessation of caffeine and found extended use resulted in less intermittent hypoxia episodes at 35 and 36 weeks' PMA. Tabacaru and colleagues[33] compared the PMA at last caffeine use in a single-center observational study of 302 infants 32 or less weeks' gestation and found no association between the last PMA at cessation of caffeine (mean 33 weeks) and central apnea, bradycardia, or desaturation events.

Synthesis of Results

Five observational studies evaluating the timing of caffeine and the risk of BPD were included for meta-analysis. Earlier initiation of caffeine before day of life 3, compared with later initiation, was associated with a decreased risk of BPD in both unadjusted and adjusted analyses (unadjusted OR 0.59; 95% confidence interval [CI] [random] 0.39 to 0.90 [n = 63,049]; adjusted OR 0.69; 95% CI [random] 0.64–0.75; **Fig. 2**). There was low statistical heterogeneity (I^2 = 10% for adjusted estimates). The overall quality of evidence was low for studies reporting adjusted estimates (see **Table 1**). Visual assessment of funnel plots of early versus late caffeine and estimates of BPD suggested asymmetry for adjusted but not unadjusted estimates. Most studies had similar estimates, so no downgrade for publication bias was given. One randomized trial comparing early caffeine to routine caffeine with reporting on oxygen at 36 weeks postmenstrual age was identified[14] and, therefore, no meta-analysis could be performed and the study was not included in GRADE assessment. Three randomized trials comparing high-dose caffeine with standard-dose caffeine were included for meta-analysis. High-dose caffeine, compared with standard dose, resulted in a decreased risk of BPD

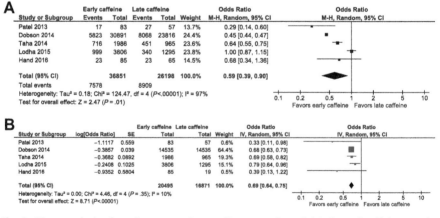

Fig. 2. Meta-analysis of studies comparing earlier versus later initiation of caffeine on the risk of BPD. Forest plot of unadjusted (A) and adjusted (B) individual and pooled estimates from observational studies. All studies defined early caffeine as initiation before day of life 3, but late caffeine was defined differently among studies. See **Table 2** for details.

Study or Subgroup	High-dose Events	High-dose Total	Standard dose Events	Standard dose Total	Weight	Odds Ratio M-H, Random, 95% CI
McPherson 2015	19	37	18	37	19.7%	1.11 [0.45, 2.77]
Mohammed 2015	13	60	19	60	24.3%	0.60 [0.26, 1.36]
Steer 2004	33	116	51	122	56.0%	0.55 [0.32, 0.95]
Total (95% CI)		**213**		**219**	**100.0%**	**0.65 [0.43, 0.97]**
Total events	65		88			

Heterogeneity: $Tau^2 = 0.00$; $Chi^2 = 1.72$, df = 2 ($P = .42$); $I^2 = 0\%$

Test for overall effect: Z = 2.11 ($P = .03$)

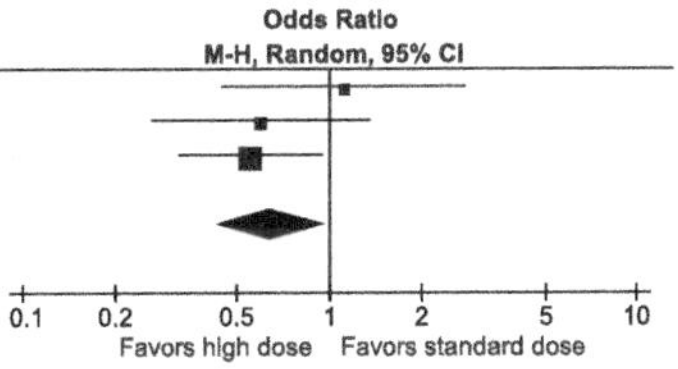

Fig. 3. Meta-analysis of randomized trials comparing the effect of a high versus standard dose of caffeine on the risk of BPD.

(OR 0.65; 95% CI [random] 0.43 to 0.97 [n = 432]; **Fig. 3**). There was low statistical heterogeneity ($I^2 = 0\%$). The pooled risk difference in BPD between high and standard caffeine groups was -0.10 (95% CI [random] -0.19, -0.01). The overall quality of evidence was low (see **Table 1**). There was no evidence of publication bias by visual assessment of funnel plots.

Discussion

Results from the authors' review on optimal timing of caffeine initiation suggests a significant treatment benefit of earlier initiation of caffeine, compared with later initiation of caffeine, in decreasing the risk of BPD. However, these results are based only on observational studies and, therefore, could be influenced by confounding by indication for early caffeine treatment. One post hoc subgroup analysis of the CAP trial also supports the beneficial effect of earlier initiation of caffeine on the risk of BPD.[8] However, one study reported an increased risk of death associated with early caffeine, which may be the result of survivor treatment selection bias.[21] As the data regarding optimal timing of caffeine are based on observational studies and the overall GRADE quality of evidence is low, additional randomized trials are necessary to provide higher quality evidence to determine the efficacy and safety of early caffeine. The authors' goal was to summarize the existing literature but not provide guideline recommendations; therefore, they used the GRADE framework to assess the quality of evidence across all evaluated studies but not provide strong or weak recommendations. Of note, the 2016 European consensus guidelines on the management of respiratory distress syndrome note that "early caffeine should be considered for all babies at high risk of needing [mechanical ventilation], such as those less than 1250 g birth weight, who are managed on non-invasive respiratory support"[34] and assign this a strong recommendation based on low-quality evidence.

The authors' analysis indicates that high-dose caffeine, compared with standard-dose caffeine, may decrease the risk of BPD. However, the overall GRADE quality of evidence was low, largely owing to the small sample sizes of trials and imprecision in estimates. In addition, one study raised concerns regarding the risk of cerebellar hemorrhage with high-dose caffeine use.[13] Guidance from the American Academy of Pediatrics states that "Caffeine citrate is a safe and effective treatment of apnea of prematurity when administered at a 20-mg/kg loading dose and 5 to 10 mg/kg per day maintenance"[35]; no published guidelines, to the authors' knowledge, recommend high-dose caffeine. There are insufficient studies on the duration of caffeine to guide use, and additional studies are needed.

SUMMARY

Earlier initiation of caffeine and/or use of high-dose caffeine may reduce the risk of BPD, when compared with later initiation or the standard dose of caffeine, respectively. However, the overall quality of evidence is low; higher-quality evidence is necessary to guide caffeine use to optimize outcomes.

REFERENCES

1. Aranda JV, Gorman W, Bergsteinsson H, et al. Efficacy of caffeine in treatment of apnea in the low-birth-weight infant. J Pediatr 1977;90(3):467–72.
2. Kuzemko JA, Paala J. Apnoeic attacks in the newborn treated with aminophylline. Arch Dis Child 1973;48(5):404–6.
3. Hsieh EM, Hornik CP, Clark RH, et al. Medication use in the neonatal intensive care unit. Am J Perinatol 2014;31(9):811–21.
4. Krzyzaniak N, Pawlowska I, Bajorek B. Review of drug utilization patterns in NICUs worldwide. J Clin Pharm Ther 2016;41(6):612–20.
5. Schmidt B, Roberts RS, Davis P, et al. Caffeine therapy for apnea of prematurity. N Engl J Med 2006;354(20):2112–21.
6. Schmidt B, Roberts RS, Davis P, et al. Long-term effects of caffeine therapy for apnea of prematurity. N Engl J Med 2007;357(19):1893–902.
7. Schmidt B, Roberts RS, Anderson PJ, et al. Academic performance, motor function, and behavior 11 years after neonatal caffeine citrate therapy for apnea of prematurity: an 11-year follow-up of the CAP randomized clinical trial. JAMA Pediatr 2017;171(6):564–72.
8. Davis PG, Schmidt B, Roberts RS, et al. Caffeine for apnea of prematurity trial: benefits may vary in subgroups. J Pediatr 2010;156(3):382–7.
9. Lodha A, Seshia M, McMillan DD, et al. Association of early caffeine administration and neonatal outcomes in very preterm neonates. JAMA Pediatr 2015;169(1):33–8.
10. Gupte AS, Gupta D, Ravichandran S, et al. Effect of early caffeine on neurodevelopmental outcome of very low-birth weight newborns. J Matern Fetal Neonatal Med 2016;29(8):1233–7.
11. Katheria AC, Sauberan JB, Akotia D, et al. A pilot randomized controlled trial of early versus routine caffeine in extremely premature infants. Am J Perinatol 2015;32(9):879–86.
12. Steer P, Flenady V, Shearman A, et al. High dose caffeine citrate for extubation of preterm infants: a randomised controlled trial. Arch Dis Child Fetal Neonatal Ed 2004;89(6):F499–503.
13. McPherson C, Neil JJ, Tjoeng TH, et al. A pilot randomized trial of high-dose caffeine therapy in preterm infants. Pediatr Res 2015;78(2):198–204.
14. Abu Jawdeh EG, O'Riordan M, Limrungsikul A, et al. Methylxanthine use for apnea of prematurity among an international cohort of neonatologists. J Neonatal Perinatal Med 2013;6(3):251–6.
15. Eichenwald EC, Blackwell M, Lloyd JS, et al. Inter-neonatal intensive care unit variation in discharge timing: influence of apnea and feeding management. Pediatrics 2001;108(4):928–33.
16. Moher D, Liberati A, Tetzlaff J, et al. Preferred reporting items for systematic reviews and meta-analyses: the PRISMA statement. BMJ 2009;339:b2535.
17. Guyatt GH, Oxman AD, Vist GE, et al. GRADE: an emerging consensus on rating quality of evidence and strength of recommendations. BMJ 2008;336(7650):924–6.
18. Schunemann HJ, Jaeschke R, Cook DJ, et al. An official ATS statement: grading the quality of evidence and strength of recommendations in ATS guidelines and recommendations. Am J Respir Crit Care Med 2006;174(5):605–14.

19. Kua KP, Lee SW. Systematic review and meta-analysis of clinical outcomes of early caffeine therapy in preterm neonates. Br J Clin Pharmacol 2017;83(1):180–91.
20. Park HW, Lim G, Chung SH, et al. Early caffeine use in very low birth weight infants and neonatal outcomes: a systematic review and meta-analysis. J Korean Med Sci 2015;30(12):1828–35.
21. Dobson NR, Patel RM, Smith PB, et al. Trends in caffeine use and association between clinical outcomes and timing of therapy in very low birth weight infants. J Pediatr 2014;164(5):992–8.e3.
22. Patel RM, Leong T, Carlton DP, et al. Early caffeine therapy and clinical outcomes in extremely preterm infants. J Perinatol 2013;33(2):134–40.
23. Taha D, Kirkby S, Nawab U, et al. Early caffeine therapy for prevention of bronchopulmonary dysplasia in preterm infants. J Matern Fetal Neonatal Med 2014;27(16):1698–702.
24. Hand I, Zaghloul N, Barash L, et al. Timing of caffeine therapy and neonatal outcomes in preterm infants: a retrospective study. Int J Pediatr 2016;2016:9478204.
25. Dekker J, Hooper SB, van Vonderen JJ, et al. Caffeine to improve breathing effort of preterm infants at birth: a randomized controlled trial. Pediatr Res 2017;82(2):290–6.
26. Gray PH, Flenady VJ, Charles BG, et al. Caffeine Collaborative Study Group. Caffeine citrate for very preterm infants: Effects on development, temperament and behaviour. J Paediatr Child Health 2011;47(4):167–72.
27. Mohammed S, Nour I, Shabaan AE, et al. High versus low-dose caffeine for apnea of prematurity: a randomized controlled trial. Eur J Pediatr 2015;174(7):949–56.
28. Steer PA, Flenady VJ, Shearman A, et al. Periextubation caffeine in preterm neonates: a randomized dose response trial. J Paediatr Child Health 2003;39(7):511–5.
29. Romagnoli C, De Carolis MP, Muzii U, et al. Effectiveness and side effects of two different doses of caffeine in preventing apnea in premature infants. Ther Drug Monit 1992;14(1):14–9.
30. Vesoulis ZA, McPherson C, Neil JJ, et al. Early high-dose caffeine increases seizure burden in extremely preterm neonates: a preliminary study. J Caffeine Res 2016;6(3):101–7.
31. Hussein MA, Coats DK, Khan H, et al. Evaluating the association of autonomic drug use to the development and severity of retinopathy of prematurity. J AAPOS 2014;18(4):332–7.
32. Rhein LM, Dobson NR, Darnall RA, et al. Effects of caffeine on intermittent hypoxia in infants born prematurely: a randomized clinical trial. JAMA Pediatr 2014;168(3):250–7.
33. Tabacaru CR, Jang SY, Patel M, et al. Impact of caffeine boluses and caffeine discontinuation on apnea and hypoxemia in preterm infants. J Caffeine Res 2017;7(3):103–10.
34. Sweet DG, Carnielli V, Greisen G, et al. European consensus guidelines on the management of respiratory distress syndrome - 2016 update. Neonatology 2017;111(2):107–25.
35. Eichenwald EC, American Academy of Pediatrics Committee on Fetus and Newborn. Apnea of prematurity. Pediatrics 2016;137(1).

Oxygen Therapy in the Delivery Room

What Is the Right Dose?

Vishal Kapadia, MD, MSCS*, Myra H. Wyckoff, MD

KEYWORDS

- Oxygen • Oxygen saturation • Newborn • Resuscitation • Delivery room

KEY POINTS

- Oxygen delivery depends on multiple factors, including fraction of inspired oxygen, ventilation, pulmonary blood flow, cardiac output, hemoglobin type and content, and local tissue factors.
- The goal of oxygen therapy is normoxia and is achieved by avoiding oxygen toxicity owing to excess oxygen exposure while delivering sufficient oxygen to prevent hypoxia.
- Initiate resuscitation with 21% oxygen in infants 35 weeks gestational age or older and 21% to 30% oxygen in preterm infants less than 35 weeks gestational age.
- Titrate oxygen to maintain oxygen saturations that are an approximation of the interquartile range of oxygen saturations of healthy term newborns delivered vaginally at sea level.
- Further research is urgently needed as the current recommendations are based on a low to moderate quality of evidence.

INTRODUCTION

Oxygen is the single most commonly used medication during resuscitation of the newborn in the delivery room (DR). The goal of oxygen therapy is to prevent hypoxemia and hyperoxemia, because both can have detrimental effects on the health of the newborn.[1,2] To achieve this goal, DR care providers must accurately recognize the need for oxygen in the newborn after birth and adjust the fraction of inspired oxygen (Fio2) as needed while simultaneously ensuring adequate ventilation. This article reviews the unique physiology of fetal and newborn oxygenation, oxygen transport,

Disclosure Statement: The authors do not have any relationship with a commercial company that has a direct financial interest in the subject matter or materials discussed in article or with a company making a competing product. Neither author has any relationship with a commercial company.
Department of Pediatrics, Division of Neonatal-Perinatal Medicine, University of Texas Southwestern Medical Center, 5323 Harry Hines Boulevard, Dallas, TX 75390-9063, USA
* Corresponding author.
E-mail address: Vishal.kapadia@utsouthwestern.edu

Clin Perinatol 45 (2018) 293–306
https://doi.org/10.1016/j.clp.2018.01.014
0095-5108/18/© 2018 Elsevier Inc. All rights reserved.

perinatology.theclinics.com

and delivery; different techniques to measure adequacy of oxygen therapy in the DR; the importance of appropriate oxygen therapy during this critical transition period; and the current recommendations for oxygen therapy and its limitations.

OXYGEN FROM A PHYSIOLOGIC PERSPECTIVE

To understand optimal oxygen therapy in the DR, understanding oxygen physiology during fetal transition from the low-oxygen intrauterine environment to the high-oxygen extrauterine environment is essential. Oxygen is a critical fuel source for aerobic metabolism and is required in numerous crucial oxidative metabolic reactions.[3] A constant and adequate supply of oxygen at the cellular level is vital. Oxygen physiology can be conceptualized in 3 steps: oxygenation, oxygen delivery, and oxygen consumption. Oxygenation is the process by which oxygen diffuses passively from the alveolus to the pulmonary capillary. High altitude, hypoventilation, ventilation–perfusion mismatch, and limited diffusion owing to lung disease or right-to-left shunts owing to congenital cardiac anomalies can affect oxygenation.[3] Most of the oxygen is bound to hemoglobin, but some dissolves in plasma. Oxygen delivery is the rate of oxygen transport from the lungs to the peripheral tissues. Oxygen delivery depends on the oxygen content of the blood and cardiac output.[3] The oxygen content of the blood depends on hemoglobin and oxygen saturation. The rate at which peripheral tissues remove oxygen from the blood is called oxygen consumption. Hypoxia arises when the oxygen supply is inadequate to meet the demands of the peripheral tissues. Hypoxia can occur owing to inadequate oxygenation, inadequate oxygen delivery, or very high oxygen consumption. Hypoxemia is defined as an abnormally low level of oxygen in the blood. Hyperoxemia, or excess oxygen in the blood, can lead to oxidative stress and cause tissue damage. The goal of oxygen therapy is to achieve normoxia, which is discussed in additional detail elsewhere in this article.

FETAL OXYGEN DELIVERY

The fetus thrives in the low-oxygen intrauterine environment where the partial pressure of oxygen in the descending aorta is close to 18 mm Hg.[4–7] The highest partial pressure of oxygen in the umbilical vein is close to 30 mm Hg.[8] The fetus is able to maintain normoxia in this low oxygen environment owing to

- Fetal hemoglobin (HbF): HbF shifts the oxygen–hemoglobin dissociation curve to the left (**Fig. 1**). This increases the affinity of hemoglobin for oxygen and allows efficient loading of oxygen in the low-oxygen environment of the placenta. HbF allows efficient unloading of oxygen from the blood to peripheral tissues owing to the steepness of the oxygen–hemoglobin dissociation curve.[3]
- Elevated hemoglobin levels: The higher hematocrit of the fetus compared with adults increases the oxygen content of the blood.[3]
- High cardiac output: Fetal cardiac output is 4 times higher than that of adults.[3,9,10] This improves oxygen delivery even at such low oxygen saturations.[3]

TRANSITION FROM THE INTRAUTERINE TO EXTRAUTERINE ENVIRONMENT

On average, the HbF saturation is around 50% during labor.[11–13] It takes approximately 10 minutes after birth to achieve oxygen saturation close to 90% in spontaneously breathing healthy term and late preterm newborns.[14,15] The transition from fetus to newborn is a complex process.[3,8,16,17] After birth, fluid in the alveoli is absorbed and replaced by air.[18] As a result of gaseous distension and possibly increased oxygen in the alveoli, pulmonary vascular resistance decreases.[19] The decrease in the

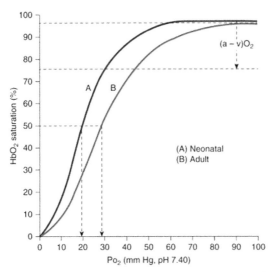

Fig. 1. Oxyhemoglobin dissociation curve. (*From* McNamara PJ, El-Khuffash A. Oxygen transport and delivery. In: Abman SH, Rowitch DH, Benitz WE, et al, editors. Fetal and neonatal physiology. 5th edition. Philadelphia: Elsevier; 2016;728; with permission.)

pulmonary vascular resistance, along with increased systemic blood pressure, increases pulmonary blood flow. Spontaneously breathing preterm neonates on continuous positive airway pressure achieve higher oxygen saturations compared with those who require positive pressure ventilation.[20] Many early or moderate preterm newborns have difficulty with oxygenation owing to the high prevalence of surfactant deficiency contributing to difficulty with transition. This condition makes it challenging to define normoxia in the DR for preterm neonates.

MEASUREMENT OF OXYGENATION IN THE DELIVERY ROOM

Studies indicate that visual assessment of cyanosis, peripheral or central, is not reliable to assess oxygenation in the newly born.[21] Pulse oximetry during neonatal resuscitation and stabilization is the standard used to guide oxygen therapy in the DR.[1,2] A pulse oximeter should be used when resuscitation is anticipated, when positive pressure ventilation is needed for more than few breaths, when cyanosis is persistent, or whenever supplementary oxygen is administered.[22] Oxygen saturation is the percentage of hemoglobin bound with oxygen. Oxygenated and deoxygenated hemoglobin absorb light differently. Oxyhemoglobin absorbs light maximally in the infrared spectrum and deoxyhemoglobin absorbs light maximally in the red spectrum.[23] Pulse oximeters calculate the ratio of tissue absorption of red and infrared light to derive the oxygen saturation of hemoglobin.[23] The pulse oximeter should be set to a shorter averaging time (2 s) to allow rapid detection of changes in oxygen saturation[24] and set to high sensitivity to allow measurement during low perfusion states.[23] To avoid a delay in obtaining accurate measurements, turn the oximeter on with the oximeter cable connected. Next, apply the probe to the baby and connect it to the oximeter cable.[25–27] Although a recent study suggested that application of the probe to the newborn first achieved a signal faster, reliable signals were obtained in a similar time by either method.[28] Preductal saturations during transition are 5% to 8% higher than postductal saturations.[15] Because preductal saturations reflect the saturation of blood perfusing the brain, and the nomograms used by the International Liaison Committee on Resuscitation (ILCOR) and Neonatal Resuscitation Program (NRP) are based on preductal saturations measured mostly at the wrist, it is recommended to apply the probe on the right hand or wrist.[1] Although manufacturers recommend that the pulse oximeter probe be applied to the hand, application to the right wrist is also acceptable.[29] It is important to assess the quality of the signal based on the manufacturer's recommendations and to compare it with the heart rate obtained by auscultation or with a cardiac monitor.[23] Most studies show that, by 1 to 2 minutes of life, the pulse oximeter is able to achieve a reliable signal.[22,30] If ambient light is excessive, the pulse oximeter probe should be shielded by an opaque wrap to achieve accurate readings.

It is important to assess for factors affecting oxygen delivery along with measuring oxygenation. Bradycardia will impair oxygen uptake and delivery. An increasing heart rate is the most important indicator of adequacy of resuscitation in neonates with initial bradycardia. Adequate ventilation and normal heart rate are important for good oxygenation of peripheral tissues. In rare situations, excessive fetal blood loss may impair oxygenation of peripheral tissues.

THE IMPORTANCE OF APPROPRIATE OXYGENATION IN THE DELIVERY ROOM

Optimal oxygen therapy should follow the "Goldilocks principle"[31] and avoid both extremes of hypoxemia as well as hyperoxemia. The goal of oxygen therapy is to restore normoxia quickly. However, normoxia in infants undergoing transition remains poorly defined. The interquartile ranges of oxygen saturations of healthy term newborns delivered vaginally at sea level can be used as a guide. The pros and cons of such approach are discussed in additional detail herein.

Birth is an oxidative challenge to the newborn.[32] The sharp postnatal transition from the relatively low oxygen intrauterine environment to a significantly higher oxygen extrauterine environment can result in formation of reactive O_2 species.[32] The use of high O_2 concentrations during DR resuscitation further exacerbates the generation of reactive O_2 and nitrogen species, which can overwhelm newborn antioxidant capacity and damage cell components such as lipids, proteins, RNA, and DNA.[32] Even a few minutes of excess O_2 exposure immediately after birth increases oxidative stress and reduces antioxidant capacity.[33,34] In animal experiments, O_2 causes DNA damage in a dose-dependent manner.[4,35–39] Preterm infants are more vulnerable to oxidative stress owing to reduced antioxidant defenses and frequent exposure to oxygen in the DR.[40] Several animal studies demonstrate that hyperoxemic resuscitation results in worse brain injury.[41–45] Exposure to early hyperoxemia is also associated with the development of hypoxic ischemic encephalopathy in term neonates with severe perinatal acidosis.[32] Animal studies demonstrate clear links between excessive O_2 exposure, resultant oxidative stress, and lung injury.[46–48] Three clinical studies have shown an increased incidence of bronchopulmonary dysplasia with hyperoxemic resuscitation.[33,39,49] However, a recent metaanalysis of randomized, controlled trials did not shown any adverse impact on clinical outcomes in preterm neonates when resuscitation was initiated with 30% or less initial Fio_2 versus 60% or greater Fio_2.[50] Interestingly, in the same metaanalysis, masked studies showed lower mortality with 30% or less initial Fio_2 where unmasked studies showed lower mortality with 60% or greater Fio_2. Hyperoxemic resuscitation has also been associated with increased cardiac and renal damage[51] and with childhood cancer in large cohort studies.[52,53] A metaanalysis of multiple clinical trials shows higher mortality with 100% O_2 DR resuscitation in term neonates.[54]

In contrast, hypoxemia, especially for prolonged periods, can result in inadequate oxygen delivery to vital organs and anaerobic metabolism, and may result in adverse clinical outcomes, including increased mortality.[55] Excess oxygen exposure after hypoxemia, the now well-recognized "oxygen paradox," may exacerbate free radical damage and reperfusion injury.[32,56]

CURRENT RECOMMENDATION REGARDING THE ADMINISTRATION OF SUPPLEMENTAL OXYGEN IN TERM INFANTS AND PRETERM INFANTS GREATER THAN 35 WEEKS GESTATIONAL AGE

Based on the most recent ILCOR consensus of science,[2] current NRP guidelines recommend that resuscitation of term infants and preterm infants 35 weeks gestational age or greater be initiated with room air and oxygen subsequently titrated to achieve a preductal oxygen saturation approximating the interquartile range of healthy term infants after vaginal delivery at sea level.[1] If the heart rate of the newborn is less than 60 bpm after 90 seconds of resuscitation with a lower concentration of oxygen, the Fio_2 should be increased to 100% until recovery of a normal heart rate. Once the heart rate is recovered, the oxygen should be weaned to maintain goal saturations and avoid hyperoxia.

Initial Fraction of Inspired Oxygen

Before 2010, pure oxygen was routinely used to resuscitate term neonates in the majority of the medical centers in the United States. Pulse oximetry was not used routinely to guide oxygen therapy. Evidence gradually accumulated regarding the superiority of room air as the initial gas for resuscitation in term infants. Multiple animal studies showed that exposure to high levels of oxygen does not improve response to resuscitative efforts and causes harm by the creation of reactive oxygen species.[57] Clinical studies showed that resuscitation with room air as the initial ventilation gas was feasible and resulted in no harm compared with 100% oxygen resuscitation.[57] Clinical studies demonstrated that neonates resuscitated with room air as the initial gas for resuscitation had a shorter time to first breath, higher Apgar scores, and less oxidative stress at 28 days.[37,38,58] A metaanalysis of such trials suggested lower mortality at 1 week and 1 month of age.[59] There was no difference in rates of hypoxic ischemic encephalopathy or neurodevelopmental impairment between the room air and the 100% oxygen groups. Clinical studies included in these metaanalyses had several limitations. Some were quasirandomized and not blinded. Large numbers of neonates crossed over from room air to 100% oxygen owing to a poor response after 90 seconds of resuscitation. Some of these studies were done in developing countries and the applicability of such results (especially for the outcome of mortality) to patients in higher resourced countries may be limited. Neurodevelopmental assessment did not use strict objective criteria and a significant percentage (>25%) of all neonates were lost to follow-up.[60]

Initially, there was a concern that, if pure oxygen was not used for DR resuscitation, the desired decrease in pulmonary vascular resistance would be hampered because oxygen is a potent vasodilator. Animal studies done by Lakshminrusimha and colleagues[61] showed that, although the use of pure oxygen during neonatal resuscitation initially enhances the speed and degree of relaxation of the pulmonary vascular bed, there are consequences later in the neonatal course from less pulmonary vascular relaxation owing to excess free radicals.

Given the limitations of the existing evidence while giving high priority to avoidance of harm from exposure to excess oxygen, the current recommendation of initiating resuscitation of term neonates with room air is reasonable, although supplemental oxygen should be available if needed. Because the majority of studies examined the effect of room air versus 100% oxygen, the effect of initiating resuscitation with an intermediate oxygen concentration remains unknown.[62] Because this recommendation is weak, with a low quality of evidence, further studies on this subject are needed. The tracking of the outcomes in large population databases over time will be also be important to look for impact of a low oxygen strategy on neonatal morbidity and mortality.

Oxygen Saturation Targets During Resuscitation of the Term Newborn

DR medical providers must balance 2 objectives: the need to prevent the toxic effects of excess oxygen and the need to give enough oxygen to prevent hypoxia. The question remains: if we start at room air, how to best titrate the oxygen to meet these 2 objectives? The fetus in labor has an oxygen saturation of around 50%, which can decrease to as low as 30% without adversely affecting the fetus.[11,13,63] Multiple studies have demonstrated that a term newborn takes about 10 minutes after birth to reach an oxygen saturation of greater than 90%.[14,15] Based on preductal saturations obtained by Mariani and colleagues[15] (**Fig. 2**) for healthy term newborns who were breathing spontaneously and born vaginally at sea level, an approximated interquartile range was recommended as the target goal saturations during the first 10 minutes after birth by the NRP.[1,14] This finding was based on expert consensus as a reasonable compromise to avoid too much or too little oxygen administration. Dawson and colleagues[14] published a large cohort study that included reference ranges for oxygen saturations for the first 10 minutes after birth in term infants. No randomized controlled trial has compared different goal saturations during the first 10 minutes of life. Clinicians should use their best judgment on how frequently and how fast to titrate the oxygen up or down to meet the transitional goal saturations. Delayed cord clamping results in slightly higher oxygen saturations during the first 10 minutes after birth.[64] Curves for normal saturation ranges for newborns with delayed cord clamping are lacking. In animal studies, initiating ventilation before cord clamping in preterm lambs results in higher oxygen saturations and higher heart rates after birth, and it also

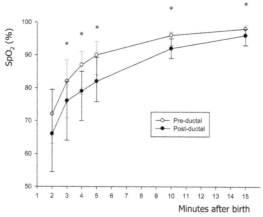

Fig. 2. Preductal saturations by Mariani. (*From* Mariani G, Dik PB, Ezquer A, et al. Pre-ductal and post-ductal O_2 saturation in healthy term neonates after birth. J Pediatr 2007;150(4):420; with permission.)

results in a smoother transition.[65] Studies are underway to examine the effects of establishing ventilation before clamping of the umbilical cord. Such changes in umbilical cord management may impact what are considered the optimal goal saturations.

Use of 100% Oxygen During Neonatal Cardiopulmonary Resuscitation

The NRP recommends to increase the oxygen concentration to 100% whenever cardiac compressions are needed.[1] This guideline is a best practice because there is no evidence from any human study to support or refute such a practice. Multiple animal studies have shown that there is no difference in the return of spontaneous circulation and survival when air of 100% oxygen is used during cardiopulmonary resuscitation, at least when the asphyxial insult is brief.[2,66] Evidence is conflicting when it comes to oxidative injury and neurologic outcome.[2,66] The optimal oxygen concentration for neonatal cardiopulmonary resuscitation remains a significant knowledge gap. Until new evidence is available, it is reasonable to use 100% Fio_2 when the need for chest compressions is recognized. Forgetting to turn the Fio_2 to 100% during neonatal cardiopulmonary resuscitation is a common error recognized during neonatal simulation training as well as during DR resuscitations. It is also important that, as soon as the HR is greater than 100 bpm, the oxygen should be weaned if oxygen saturations are above the goal saturation of peripheral oxygen (SpO_2) to limit hyperoxia and reperfusion injury.[32]

CURRENT RECOMMENDATIONS ABOUT THE ADMINISTRATION OF SUPPLEMENTAL OXYGEN IN PRETERM INFANTS

Based on the ILCOR consensus of science, current NRP guidelines recommend that resuscitation of preterm infants less than 35 weeks gestational age should be initiated with 21% to 30% oxygen and oxygen should be adjusted to maintain oxygen saturation within the same target range as defined for full term newborns.[1,2,66]

Initial Fraction of Inspired Oxygen

Before 2010, the majority of centers in North America started preterm resuscitation with 100% oxygen. Multiple animal studies showed increasing oxidative stress even with brief exposure to oxygen and worsening organ damage with hyperoxic resuscitation.[4,34,35,44] Initial studies showed that resuscitation of preterm infants was feasible with a low Fio_2.[33,67,68] Multiple studies demonstrate that preterm neonates need some supplemental oxygen to achieve target saturations but, irrespective of starting Fio_2, most infants needed approximately 30% oxygen by the time of stabilization.[33,39,67–70] When compared with static 100% oxygen and static goal saturations of 85% to 95% since birth, it is clear that low Fio_2 resuscitation decreases oxygen load in the DR and decreases oxidative stress in preterm neonates.[33,49] Three studies found less bronchopulmonary dysplasia with initiating resuscitation with low Fio_2,[33,39,49] but a recent metaanalysis of all available trials found no difference in bronchopulmonary dysplasia with low versus high Fio_2.[50] A recent study by Oei and colleagues,[71] the largest study so far comparing 21% versus 100% oxygen as initial Fio_2 during resuscitation of preterm infants, was powered for death or neurodevelopmental impairment at 2 years of age, but was stopped early owing to failure to reach target recruitment (292 enrolled of the needed 1976 preterm neonates). Room air infants had lower oxygen load in the DR, lower respiratory support, and lower incidence of patent ductus arteriosus ligation. There was no difference in bronchopulmonary dysplasia, intraventricular hemorrhage, or mortality. On subgroup analysis of 100 neonates less than 28 weeks of gestational age, mortality was higher in the room air versus the oxygen group (22% vs 6%). When included in a recent metaanalysis, there still was no difference in bronchopulmonary dysplasia, intraventricular hemorrhage, retinopathy of prematurity, or mortality between the low Fio_2 and high Fio_2 groups.[50] It is important to acknowledge that this trial was limited by premature termination and the subgroup of less than 28 weeks gestational age infants is significantly underpowered because 1 more death in the 100% oxygen group would have changed the conclusion. The heart rate was lower in the room air group in this trial for the first 3 minutes after birth compared with the 100% oxygen group. There was no difference in heart rate between the 2 groups in other trials comparing 21% versus 100% oxygen.[33,39,50,67–71] Studies show conflicting evidence regarding neurodevelopment outcomes. A randomized trial by Boronat and colleagues[72] compared initial oxygen of 30% versus 60% and found no difference in neurodevelopmental outcomes in preterm neonates. Two retrospective cohort studies from the Canadian Neonatal Network show conflicting results. Rabi and colleagues[73] found an increased incidence of death or severe intraventricular hemorrhage/periventricular leukomalacia after a change in the Canadian neonatal resuscitation policy to titrate oxygen starting at 21% compared with the previous policy of starting at 100% in preterm infants less than 28 weeks' gestational age Another study by the same group showed that in a more recent cohort of preterm neonates less than 29 weeks' gestational age, 100% oxygen use was associated with increased odds of severe neurodevelopmental impairment among survivors compared with room air.[74] There was no difference in the composite outcome of death or neurodevelopmental impairment in preterm infants who received room air, intermediate oxygen, or 100% oxygen at the initiation of resuscitation.

Based on the currently available literature, it is reasonable to start resuscitation of preterm neonates less than 35 weeks' gestation with 21% to 30% oxygen. In making this recommendation (a strong recommendation with a moderate quality of evidence), ILCOR placed higher value on not exposing preterm newborns to additional oxygen without proven benefit for important clinical outcomes.[2,66] Given the conflicting evidence and small size of the available studies, large randomized controlled trials adequately powered for long-term outcomes are necessary to answer this question. Fortunately, such trials are underway.[75,76]

Oxygen Target Saturation for Preterm Resuscitation

Multiple studies have shown that the majority of preterm neonates need supplemental oxygen for the first few minutes after birth because they are not able to achieve the target oxygen saturations recommended by the NRP.[30,77,78] The likelihood of not being able to achieve NRP-recommended oxygen saturations is higher if resuscitation is initiated with 21% to 30% Fio_2 and if the preterm infant requires positive pressure ventilation.[20] The likelihood of overshooting the target saturations is higher if resuscitation is initiated with and Fio_2 of 60% or greater.[33,67–69,77,79] Given the difficulty in keeping the newborns in target saturations, additional aids such as Transitioning Oxygen Target System have been developed. Transitioning Oxygen Target System gives a graphic display of prespecified high and low SpO_2 limits, as well as a real-time display of SpO_2 and administered supplemental oxygen values. This system allows resuscitation teams a visual target in the DR. The use of such aids slightly improves achievement of the NRP-recommended goal saturations. However, it remains difficult to maintain the NRP-recommended target oxygen saturations.[30]

It remains uncertain if the NRP-recommended goal saturations are optimal goals for preterm infants during the first 10 minutes after birth, because recommendations these are based on the saturations of healthy term newborns. It is possible that preterm neonates, who may have surfactant deficiency and poor antioxidant defenses, require different target oxygen saturations. No randomized controlled trial to date has examined the effects of different target oxygen saturations during preterm resuscitation. It is also important to remember that the trials included in the most recent metaanalysis followed different titration strategies, which have the potential to change the oxygen load in the DR irrespective of the initial Fio_2.[50] This makes it a challenge to speculate as to the optimal oxygen strategy from results of metaanalysis of small randomized trials. Future large randomized controlled trials are underway that may fill some of these knowledge gaps. Until more evidence is available, it is reasonable to titrate oxygen to maintain the NRP-recommended goal saturations with vigilance to avoid excess oxygen administration and to avoid low oxygen saturations.

THE ROLE OF VENTILATION AND PERFUSION IN OXYGEN UPTAKE AND DELIVERY

To achieve adequate oxygenation after birth, apart from oxygen administration, it is equally important, if not more, to adequately ventilate the lungs. Normal transition may not occur in many term and preterm neonates who do not breathe immediately after birth and/or require resuscitation at birth.[8,19,80] Bradycardia further decreases oxygen delivery to tissues by decreasing cardiac output. In a neonate who requires resuscitation, clinicians should consider achieving adequate ventilation as the primary step in preventing hypoxia in addition to increasing the Fio_2 in response to low oxygen saturations.

MEASURING CEREBRAL OXYGEN STATUS USING NEAR INFRARED SPECTROSCOPY

Near infrared spectroscopy (NIRS) has been used in multiple studies as an adjunct tool to evaluate oxygen delivery to the brain during the first few minutes after birth in newborn.[16] It measures cerebral skeletal muscle tissue oxygenation (StO_2), which is mixed oxygen saturation in a multicompartment system. It is noninvasive and available within 1 to 2 minutes of application in most cases and provides continuous measurement. SpO_2, hemoglobin content, cardiac output, local blood flow blood volume, and oxygen extraction of the organ affect StO_2 values. The NIRS device and sensor type must be taken into account when NIRS monitoring of cerebral oxygenation is applied in clinical care.[81] Studies have shown that cerebral tissue oxygenation reaches a plateau earlier compared with oxygen saturation. This finding may indicate preferential oxygen delivery to the brain in the first few minutes after birth.[16] There are cerebral StO_2 reference ranges available for transitioning term and preterm infants.[16] Caution should be used when using these reference ranges because the optimal cerebral StO_2 values during transition in term and preterm neonates remain unknown. A small randomized controlled trial has shown that by using NIRS in the DR, StO_2 values of less than the 10th percentile can be minimized, which possibly represents a decrease in cerebral hypoxia.[82] Larger studies are underway to define role of this additional tool in the search for optimizing oxygen therapy in the DR.

SUMMARY

Oxygen therapy in the DR for resuscitation of the newly born should be titrated to avoid excess oxygen exposure and to give sufficient oxygen to ensure adequate oxygen delivery. Such an approach will avoid oxygen toxicity and hypoxia. Both hyperoxemia and hypoxia during transition are associated with adverse neonatal outcomes. The current recommendations are based on limited evidence but seem reasonable while we await results of ongoing studies. Close attention should be paid to oxygen titration to achieve the recommended goal saturations. The avoidance of bradycardia and adequate ventilation are equally important for oxygen delivery as Fio_2.

Best Practices

Major recommendations

- Initiate resuscitation with 21% oxygen in term and preterm infants 35 weeks' gestational age or older and 21% to 30% oxygen in preterm infants less than 35 weeks' gestational age.

- Titrate oxygen to maintain oxygen saturations, which are an approximation of the interquartile range of oxygen saturations of healthy term newborns delivered vaginally at sea level.

- When heart rate remains less than 60 bpm even after all the efforts to provide adequate ventilation, chest compressions are indicated. Increase the oxygen concentration to 100% whenever chest compressions are provided. Once the heart rate is recovered, the oxygen should be weaned to maintain goal saturations and avoid hyperoxia.

Rating for the strength of the evidence

- Further research is urgently needed as the current recommendations are based on a low to moderate quality of evidence.

REFERENCES

1. Wyckoff MH, Aziz K, Escobedo MB, et al. Part 13: neonatal resuscitation: 2015 American Heart Association guidelines update for cardiopulmonary resuscitation and emergency cardiovascular care. Circulation 2015;132(18 suppl 2):S543–60.

2. Perlman JM, Wyllie J, Kattwinkel J, et al. Part 7: neonatal resuscitation: 2015 International Consensus on Cardiopulmonary Resuscitation and Emergency Cardiovascular Care Science with treatment recommendations. Circulation 2015; 132(16 suppl 1):S204–41.

3. McNamara PJ, El-Khuffash A. Oxygen transport and delivery. In: Abman SH, Rowitch DH, Benitz WE, et al, editors. Fetal and neonatal physiology. 5th edition. Philadelphia: Elsevier; 2016. p. 724–37.e72.

4. Torres-Cuevas I, Parra-Llorca A, Sánchez-Illana A, et al. Oxygen and oxidative stress in the perinatal period. Redox Biol 2017;12:674–81.

5. Battaglia FC, Meschia G. Review of studies in human pregnancy of uterine and umbilical blood flows. Med Wieku Rozwoj 2013;17(4):287–92.

6. Mukai M, Uchida T, Itoh H, et al. Tissue oxygen saturation levels from fetus to neonate. J Obstet Gynaecol Res 2017;43(5):855–9.

7. East CE, Begg L, Colditz PB, et al. Fetal pulse oximetry for fetal assessment in labour. Cochrane Database Syst Rev 2014;10:CD004075.

8. Berger TM. Neonatal resuscitation: foetal physiology and pathophysiological aspects. Eur J Anaesthesiol 2012;29(8):362–70.

9. Kiserud T, Ebbing C, Kessler J, et al. Fetal cardiac output, distribution to the placenta and impact of placental compromise. Ultrasound Obstet Gynecol 2006;28(2):126–36.

10. Mielke G, Benda N. Cardiac output and central distribution of blood flow in the human fetus. Circulation 2001;103(12):1662–8.

11. Dildy GA, van den Berg PP, Katz M, et al. Intrapartum fetal pulse oximetry: fetal oxygen saturation trends during labor and relation to delivery outcome. Am J Obstet Gynecol 1994;171(3):679–84.

12. Vayssiere C, Haberstich R, Sebahoun V, et al. Fetal electrocardiogram ST-segment analysis and prediction of neonatal acidosis. Int J Gynecol Obstet 2007;97(2):110–4.

13. Dildy GA. Fetal pulse oximetry. Clin Obstet Gynecol 2011;54(1):66–73.
14. Dawson JA, Kamlin CO, Vento M, et al. Defining the reference range for oxygen saturation for infants after birth. Pediatrics 2010;125(6):e1340–7.
15. Mariani G, Dik PB, Ezquer A, et al. Pre-ductal and post-ductal O2 saturation in healthy term neonates after birth. J Pediatr 2007;150(4):418–21.
16. Pichler G, Schmölzer GM, Urlesberger B. Cerebral tissue oxygenation during immediate neonatal transition and resuscitation. Front Pediatr 2017;5:29.
17. Hooper SB, te Pas AB, Lewis RA, et al. Establishing functional residual capacity at birth. NeoReviews 2010;11(9):e474–83.
18. Hooper SB, te Pas AB, Kitchen MJ. Respiratory transition in the newborn: a three-phase process. Arch Dis Child Fetal Neonatal Ed 2016;101(3):F266–71.
19. Lang JAR, Pearson JT, Binder-Heschl C, et al. Increase in pulmonary blood flow at birth: role of oxygen and lung aeration. J Physiol 2016;594(5):1389–98.
20. Phillipos E, Solevåg AL, Aziz K, et al. Oxygen saturation and heart rate ranges in very preterm infants requiring respiratory support at birth. J Pediatr 2017;182: 41–6.e2.
21. O'Donnell CPF, Kamlin COF, Davis PG, et al. Clinical assessment of infant colour at delivery. Arch Dis Child Fetal Neonatal Ed 2007;92(6):F465–7.
22. Kattwinkel J, Perlman JM, Aziz K, et al. Neonatal resuscitation: 2010 American Heart Association guidelines for cardiopulmonary resuscitation and emergency cardiovascular care. Pediatrics 2010;126(5):e1400–13.
23. Rabi Y, Dawson JA. Oxygen therapy and oximetry in the delivery room. Semin Fetal Neonatal Med 2013;18(6):330–5.
24. Ahmed SJM, Rich W, Finer NN. The effect of averaging time on oximetry values in the premature infant. Pediatrics 2010;125(1):e115–21.
25. O'Donnell CPF, Kamlin COF, Davis PG, et al. Feasibility of and delay in obtaining pulse oximetry during neonatal resuscitation. J Pediatr 2005;147(5):698–9.
26. O'Donnell CPF, Kamlin COF, Davis PG, et al. Obtaining pulse oximetry data in neonates: a randomised crossover study of sensor application techniques. Arch Dis Child - Fetal Neonatal Ed 2005;90(1):F84–5.
27. Saraswat A, Simionato L, Dawson JA, et al. Determining the best method of Nellcor pulse oximeter sensor application in neonates. Acta Paediatr 2012;101(5): 484–7.
28. Louis D, Sundaram V, Kumar P. Pulse oximeter sensor application during neonatal resuscitation: a randomized controlled trial. Pediatrics 2014;133(3): 476–82.
29. Phattraprayoon N, Sardesai S, Durand M, et al. Accuracy of pulse oximeter readings from probe placement on newborn wrist and ankle. J Perinatol 2012;32(4): 276–80.
30. Gandhi B, Rich W, Finer N. Achieving targeted pulse oximetry values in preterm infants in the delivery room. J Pediatr 2013;163(2):412–5.
31. Southey R. The story of the three bears. In: Warter JW, editor. The doctor. London: Longman, Brown, Green and Longmans; 1848. p. 327–9.
32. Kapadia VS, Chalak LF, DuPont TL, et al. Perinatal asphyxia with hyperoxemia within the first hour of life is associated with moderate to severe hypoxic-ischemic encephalopathy. J Pediatr 2013;163(4):949–54.
33. Kapadia VS, Chalak LF, Sparks JE, et al. Resuscitation of preterm neonates with limited versus high oxygen strategy. Pediatrics 2013;132(6):e1488–96.
34. Perez-de-Sa V, Cunha-Goncalves D, Nordh A, et al. High brain tissue oxygen tension during ventilation with 100% oxygen after fetal asphyxia in newborn sheep. Pediatr Res 2009;65(1):57–61.

35. Solberg R, Andresen JH, Escrig R, et al. Resuscitation of hypoxic newborn piglets with oxygen induces a dose-dependent increase in markers of oxidation. Pediatr Res 2007;62(5):559–63.
36. Trindade CEP, Rugolo LMSS. Free radicals and neonatal diseases. NeoReviews 2007;8(12):e522–32.
37. Vento M, Asensi M, Sastre J, et al. Resuscitation with room air instead of 100% oxygen prevents oxidative stress in moderately asphyxiated term neonates. Pediatrics 2001;107(4):642–7.
38. Vento M, Asensi M, Sastre J, et al. Oxidative stress in asphyxiated term infants resuscitated with 100% oxygen. J Pediatr 2003;142(3):240–6.
39. Vento M, Moro M, Escrig R, et al. Preterm resuscitation with low oxygen causes less oxidative stress, inflammation, and chronic lung disease. Pediatrics 2009; 124(3):e439–49.
40. O'Donovan DJ, Fernandes CJ. Free radicals and diseases in premature infants. Antioxid Redox Signal 2004;6(1):169–76.
41. Dalen ML, Liu X, Elstad M, et al. Resuscitation with 100% oxygen increases injury and counteracts the neuroprotective effect of therapeutic hypothermia in the neonatal rat. Pediatr Res 2012;71(3):247–52.
42. Koch JD, Miles DK, Gilley JA, et al. Brief exposure to hyperoxia depletes the glial progenitor pool and impairs functional recovery after hypoxic-ischemic brain injury. J Cereb Blood Flow Metab 2008;28(7):1294–306.
43. Markus T, Hansson S, Amer-Wahlin I, et al. Cerebral inflammatory response after fetal asphyxia and hyperoxic resuscitation in newborn sheep. Pediatr Res 2007; 62(1):71–7.
44. Munkeby BH, Borke WB, Bjornland K, et al. Resuscitation with 100% O2 increases cerebral injury in hypoxemic piglets. Pediatr Res 2004;56(5):783–90.
45. Vereczki V, Martin E, Rosenthal RE, et al. Normoxic resuscitation after cardiac arrest protects against hippocampal oxidative stress, metabolic dysfunction, and neuronal death. J Cereb Blood Flow Metab 2005;26(6):821–35.
46. Buczynski BW, Maduekwe ET, O'Reilly MA. The role of hyperoxia in the pathogenesis of experimental BPD. Semin Perinatol 2013;37(2):69–78.
47. Gien J, Kinsella JP. Pathogenesis and treatment of bronchopulmonary dysplasia. Curr Opin Pediatr 2011;23(3):305–13.
48. Jobe AH, Bancalari E. Bronchopulmonary dysplasia. Am J Respir Crit Care Med 2001;163(7):1723–9.
49. Kapadia VS, Lal CV, Kakkilaya V, et al. Impact of the neonatal resuscitation program–recommended low oxygen strategy on outcomes of infants born preterm. J Pediatr 2017;191:35–41.
50. Oei JL, Vento M, Rabi Y, et al. Higher or lower oxygen for delivery room resuscitation of preterm infants below 28 completed weeks gestation: a meta-analysis. Arch Dis Child - Fetal Neonatal Ed 2017;102(1):F24–30.
51. Vento M, Sastre J, Asensi MA, et al. Room-air resuscitation causes less damage to heart and kidney than 100% oxygen. Am J Respir Crit Care Med 2005;172(11): 1393–8.
52. Naumburg E, Bellocco R, Cnattingius S, et al. Supplementary oxygen and risk of childhood lymphatic leukaemia. Acta Paediatr 2002;91(12):1328–33.
53. Spector LG, Klebanoff MA, Feusner JH, et al. Childhood cancer following neonatal oxygen supplementation. J Pediatr 2005;147(1):27–31.
54. Saugstad OD, Ramji S, Soll RF, et al. Resuscitation of newborn infants with 21% or 100% oxygen: an updated systematic review and meta-analysis. Neonatology 2008;94(3):176–82.

55. Goldsmith JP, Kattwinkel J. The role of oxygen in the delivery room. Clin Perinatol 2012;39(4):803–15.

56. Saugstad OD. The oxygen paradox in the newborn: keep oxygen at normal levels. J Pediatr 2013;163(4):934–5.

57. Tan A, Schulze AA, O'Donnell CPF, et al. Air versus oxygen for resuscitation of infants at birth. Cochrane Database Syst Rev 2005;(2):CD002273.

58. Saugstad OD. Resuscitation of newborn infants: from oxygen to room air. Lancet 2010;376(9757):1970–1.

59. Rabi Y, Rabi D, Yee W. Room air resuscitation of the depressed newborn: a systematic review and meta-analysis. Resuscitation 2007;72(3):353–63.

60. Shah PS. Meta-analysis of neurodevelopmental outcome after room air versus 100% oxygen resuscitation: generating more questions than answers? Neonatology 2012;102(2):104–6.

61. Lakshminrusimha S, Steinhorn RH, Wedgwood S, et al. Pulmonary hemodynamics and vascular reactivity in asphyxiated term lambs resuscitated with 21 and 100% oxygen. J Appl Physiol (1985) 2011;111(5):1441–7.

62. Hellström-Westas L, Forsblad K, Sjörs G, et al. Earlier Apgar score increase in severely depressed term infants cared for in Swedish level III units with 40% oxygen versus 100% oxygen resuscitation strategies: a population-based register study. Pediatrics 2006;118(6):e1798–804.

63. Garite TJ, Dildy GA, McNamara H, et al. A multicenter controlled trial of fetal pulse oximetry in the intrapartum management of nonreassuring fetal heart rate patterns. Am J Obstet Gynecol 2000;183(5):1049–58.

64. Smit M, Dawson JA, Ganzeboom A, et al. Pulse oximetry in newborns with delayed cord clamping and immediate skin-to-skin contact. Arch Dis Child Fetal Neonatal Ed 2014;99(4):F309–14.

65. Polglase GR, Dawson JA, Kluckow M, et al. Ventilation onset prior to umbilical cord clamping (physiological-based cord clamping) improves systemic and cerebral oxygenation in preterm lambs. PLoS One 2015;10(2):e0117504.

66. Perlman JM, Wyllie J, Kattwinkel J, et al. Part 7: neonatal resuscitation: 2015 international consensus on cardiopulmonary resuscitation and emergency cardiovascular care science with treatment recommendations (reprint). Pediatrics 2015; 136(Suppl 2):S120–66.

67. Escrig R, Arruza L, Izquierdo I, et al. Achievement of targeted saturation values in extremely low gestational age neonates resuscitated with low or high oxygen concentrations: a prospective, randomized trial. Pediatrics 2008;121(5):875–81.

68. Wang CL, Anderson C, Leone TA, et al. Resuscitation of preterm neonates by using room air or 100% oxygen. Pediatrics 2008;121(6):1083–9.

69. Rabi Y, Singhal N, Nettel-Aguirre A. Room-air versus oxygen administration for resuscitation of preterm infants: the ROAR study. Pediatrics 2011;128(2): e374–81.

70. Rook D, Schierbeek H, Vento M, et al. Resuscitation of preterm infants with different inspired oxygen fractions. J Pediatr 2014;164(6):1322–6.e3.

71. Oei JL, Saugstad OD, Lui K, et al. Targeted oxygen in the resuscitation of preterm infants, a randomized clinical trial. Pediatrics 2017;139(0031) [pii:e20161452].

72. Boronat N, Aguar M, Rook D, et al. Survival and neurodevelopmental outcomes of preterms resuscitated with different oxygen fractions. Pediatrics 2016;138(6) [pii: e20161405].

73. Rabi Y, Lodha A, Soraisham A, et al. Outcomes of preterm infants following the introduction of room air resuscitation. Resuscitation 2015;96:252–9.

74. Soraisham AS, Rabi Y, Shah PS, et al. Neurodevelopmental outcomes of preterm infants resuscitated with different oxygen concentration at birth. J Perinatol 2017; 37(10):1141–7.

75. ClinicalTrials.gov. Study of room air versus 60% oxygen for resuscitation of premature infants (PRESOX). 2013-; Identifier: NCT01773746. Available at: https://clinicaltrials.gov/ct2/show/NCT01773746. Accessed September 19, 2017.

76. Australian New Zealand Clinical Trials Registry. Trial ID: ACTRN12615000115538. 2015-; The Torpido2 Study: Targeted Oxygenation in the Respiratory care of Premature Infants at Delivery: Effects on developmental Outcome. Available at: https://www.anzctr.org.au/Trial/Registration/TrialReview.aspx?id=367725. Accessed September 19, 2017.

77. White LN, Thio M, Owen LS, et al. Achievement of saturation targets in preterm infants <32 weeks' gestational age in the delivery room. Arch Dis Child Fetal Neonatal Ed 2017;102(5):F423–7.

78. Goos TG, Rook D, van der Eijk AC, et al. Observing the resuscitation of very preterm infants: are we able to follow the oxygen saturation targets? Resuscitation 2013;84(8):1108–13.

79. Ezaki S, Suzuki K, Kurishima C, et al. Resuscitation of preterm infants with reduced oxygen results in less oxidative stress than resuscitation with 100% oxygen. J Clin Biochem Nutr 2009;44(1):111–8.

80. Saugstad OD. Physiology of resuscitation. In: Abman SH, Rowitch DH, Benitz WE, et al, editors. Fetal and neonatal physiology. 5th edition. Philadelphia: Elsevier; 2016. p. 619–26.e611.

81. Dix LML, van Bel F, Lemmers PMA. Monitoring cerebral oxygenation in neonates: an update. Front Pediatr 2017;5:160.

82. Pichler G, Urlesberger B, Baik N, et al. Cerebral oxygen saturation to guide oxygen delivery in preterm neonates for the immediate transition after birth: a 2-center randomized controlled pilot feasibility trial. J Pediatr 2016;170:73–8.e1–4.

Detection and Prevention of Perinatal Infection

Cytomegalovirus and Zika Virus

Amber M. Wood, MD*, Brenna L. Hughes, MD

KEYWORDS

- Congenital cytomegalovirus infection • Congenital Zika virus syndrome
- Perinatal infections • Ultrasound diagnosis

KEY POINTS

- Cytomegalovirus is the most common viral congenital infection and can lead to significant neonatal sequelae, including sensineuronal hearing loss, seizures, and death.
- Diagnosis of cytomegalovirus infection is based on maternal serologic testing, with amniocentesis available for confirmatory fetal diagnosis.
- There are no current therapies for congenital cytomegalovirus; therefore, prevention and education efforts are vital to decrease the risk of congenital cytomegalovirus.
- Zika virus is a mosquito-borne flavivirus transmitted via mosquitoes or bodily, and has been found to cause congenital Zika syndrome in the setting of transplacental infection.
- Diagnosis in pregnancy is complicated by limitations to screening and diagnostic testing; prevention is focused on education of risk factors and avoidance of endemic areas.

Viral infections in pregnancy may affect both mother and fetus. Maternal illness may be mild; however, transplacental transmission of the virus can lead to neonatal infection and sequelae. Identification and diagnosis of fetal viral infection can be challenging, because maternal symptoms may be mild or absent, and there are variable prenatal and postnatal findings. In this review, we present the epidemiology, diagnosis, and prevention strategies for cytomegalovirus, which is the most common congenital infection, as well as Zika virus (ZIKV), which is an emerging virus that has been associated with multiple perinatal complications.

CYTOMEGALOVIRUS
Epidemiology

Cytomegalovirus (CMV) is a double-stranded DNA herpes virus. It is transmitted via body fluids, such as blood, saliva, and urine. Although CMV infection in pregnancy

Disclosure Statement: The authors report no conflict of interest.
Division of Maternal Fetal Medicine, Department of Obstetrics and Gynecology, Duke University Medical Center, Durham, NC 27710, USA
* Corresponding author. Duke University, DUMC 3967, Durham, NC 27710.
E-mail address: amber.wood@duke.edu

Clin Perinatol 45 (2018) 307–323
https://doi.org/10.1016/j.clp.2018.01.005
0095-5108/18/© 2018 Elsevier Inc. All rights reserved.
perinatology.theclinics.com

normally causes only minimal maternal symptoms, CMV infection can be transmitted vertically during pregnancy and can have significant effects if fetal infection occurs, leading to congenital CMV. Congenital CMV is the most common viral congenital infection, and affects between 0.2% and 2.2% of all neonates.[1–3] There are an estimated 27,000 to 40,000 new cases in the United States annually.[4,5]

The prevalence of exposure before pregnancy varies by location, socioeconomic status, and ethnicity, and ranges from 40% to 83%.[6,7] Previously seronegative women have up to a 1% to 4% risk of developing a primary infection during pregnancy,[4,6] and vertical transmission of CMV can occur via transplacental infection after primary or secondary infection, although it is much more likely to occur in primary infection (30%–50% in primary infection vs 0.15%–2% in secondary infection).[1,8,9] Secondary infection may occur after reactivation of the latent virus or by reinfection with a different strain of CMV.[10]

The risk of transmission to the fetus depends on the trimester in which CMV infection occurs. The greatest risk of transmission is in the third trimester; however, the most significant neonatal sequelae occur when transmission occurs in the first trimester.[6,11–13] **Table 1** details the transmission rates of CMV based on trimester in women diagnosed with CMV in pregnancy. Of note, CMV transmission has been described in the preconception period (1–10 weeks before the last menstrual period) and periconceptual period (1 week before the last menstrual period to 4 weeks 6 days gestational age).[11,12]

When fetal infection occurs after a primary CMV infection, up to 18% of neonates are symptomatic at birth.[14] Symptoms include jaundice, petechial rash, hepatosplenomegaly, or death. However, the absence of symptoms at birth does not exclude the possibility of sequelae developing later in life. Up to 25% of neonates who are asymptomatic at birth may develop later complications, including sensorineural hearing loss, cognitive deficits, chorioretinitis, seizures, and death.[14]

Diagnosis

Most women (75%) experiencing CMV infection are asymptomatic.[9] Even when symptomatic, most women have mild, nonspecific symptoms, such as a low-grade fever, fatigue, headache, myalgias, abnormal liver function tests, and lymphadenopathy.[7,10] Therefore, clinical symptoms are unreliable and insensitive for diagnosis.

Table 1
Risk of cytomegalovirus transmission during preconception, periconception, and each trimester

Trimester	Risk of Perinatal Transmission (%)
Preconceptional[a]	8.9–16.7
Periconceptual[b]	19–38.5
First trimester	30.1–31.8
Second trimester	35.9–38.2
Third trimester	42.9–72.2

[a] Defined as 1 to 10 weeks before the last menstrual period.
[b] Defined as 1 week before the last menstrual period to 4 weeks and 6 days of gestation.
Data from Enders G, Daiminger A, Bader U, et al. Intrauterine transmission and clinical outcome of 248 pregnancies with primary cytomegalovirus infection in relation to gestational age. J Clin Virol 2011;52:244–6; and Picone O, Vauloup-Fellous C, Cordier AG, et al. A series of 238 cytomegalovirus primary infections during pregnancy: description and outcome. Prenat Diagn 2013;33:751–8.

One of the most accurate methods to diagnose maternal CMV infection in pregnancy is documentation of seroconversion of a previously seronegative patient (the development of IgG antibodies to CMV in a patient who was previously negative for these antibodies).[9] However, routine screening for CMV in pregnancy is not recommended by either the Centers for Disease Control and Prevention (CDC) or the American College of Obstetricians and Gynecologists, because it is difficult to differentiate primary from recurrent infection by maternal IgM antibody screening. Further, there is risk that the reactivation of the virus may lead to neonatal infection, and there is no effective treatment or vaccine currently available.[15,16] Therefore, alternate methods may be required for diagnosis because maternal serologic status is typically unknown. The CDC recommends testing for CMV in pregnant women with symptoms similar to mononucleosis with negative Epstein-Barr virus testing, or signs of hepatitis but negative hepatitis A, B, and C.[16] Serologic testing may also be considered in addition to amniocentesis if there are characteristic findings on ultrasound examination (**Table 2**) or significant documented exposure.[15]

Maternal CMV infection may be diagnosed based on serologic testing of anti-CMV IgM, anti-CMV IgG, and low IgG avidity for CMV. IgM alone, although classically thought to indicate acute infection in disease processes, is an unreliable indicator for acute CMV infection. IgM may be produced in reactivation or reinfections, may persist for months after natural infection, and is frequently falsely positive (up to 90%) in patients with other viral infections or autoimmune diseases.[9,17–19] Consequently, the presence of CMV IgM alone is not sufficient for a diagnosis of acute or primary infection. The anti-CMV IgG avidity test should be performed in addition to CMV IgM and IgG to aid in diagnosis. Antibody avidity indicates the strength with which the antibody binds the antigen. Early in infection, IgG antibodies have a low avidity for the antigen. As the infection progresses, the avidity increases. Therefore, the earlier the infection, the lower the avidity of the anti-CMV IgG will be. Low to

Table 2
Ultrasound abnormalities in congenital cytomegalovirus infection

Ultrasound Finding	Frequency, %
Cerebral calcifications	0.6–17.4
Microcephaly	14.5
Echogenic bowel	4.5–13.0
Fetal growth restriction	1.9–13.0
Subependymal cysts	11.6
Cerebral ventriculomegaly	4.5–11.6
Ascites	8.7
Pericardial effusion	7.2
Hyperechogenic kidneys	4.3
Hepatomegaly	4.3
Placentomegaly or placental calcifications	4.3
Hepatic calcifications	1.4
Hydrops	0.6

Data from Picone O, Vauloup-Fellous C, Cordier AG, et al. A series of 238 cytomegalovirus primary infections during pregnancy: description and outcome. Prenat Diagn 2013;33:751–8; and Guerra B, Simonazzi G, Puccetti C, et al. Ultrasound prediction of symptomatic congenital cytomegalovirus infection. Am J Obstet Gynecol 2008;198:380.e1–7.

moderate avidity IgG are found only after acute infection and usually last for 16 to 18 weeks after infection.[9]

Therefore, the combination of a positive IgM antibody and a low to moderate avidity IgG indicates an infection within the past 3 to 4 months. Rates of congenital infection in women with positive IgM and low to moderate avidity have been shown to be similar to rates of congenital infection in women with documented seroconversion.[20] **Fig. 1** demonstrates the recommended testing strategy for maternal and fetal CMV infection.

Fetal Diagnosis

The diagnosis of fetal infection is possible by either amniocentesis or cordocentesis. Given the increased risk of complications and technical difficulty of the cordocentesis, amniocentesis is the most commonly used method for diagnosis, and the use of cordocentesis is not generally recommended.[15] In the setting of a primary maternal infection without confirmed fetal infection, the risk of sequelae is approximately 3% and any adverse outcome approximately 8%.[21] Diagnostic fetal testing with polymerase chain reaction (PCR) should be offered because it can add additional counseling benefit if fetal infection is definitively diagnosed. It is important to note that the presence of a positive PCR result does not indicate the severity of infection.[22–24]

In the setting of a serologic diagnosis of maternal primary CMV infection, amniocentesis for the diagnosis of fetal infection should ideally be performed at greater than 21 weeks of gestation and more than 6 weeks after maternal infection. PCR for CMV has improved sensitivity over culture and should be the test of choice for evaluation. When performed in this time frame, the sensitivity for PCR is 78% to 98%, with a specificity of 92% to 98%.[25–31] In those without fetal ultrasound findings, amniocentesis for CMV PCR should not be performed before 21 weeks of gestation, because

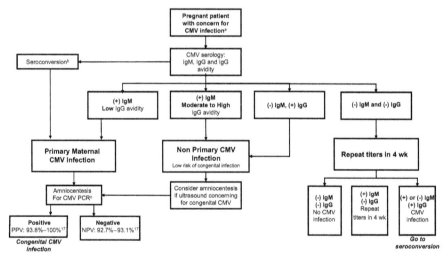

Fig. 1. Testing for CMV infection in pregnancy. [a] The Centers for Disease Control and Prevention recommend testing patients with symptoms similar to mononucleosis and negative Epstein-Barr virus, or signs of hepatitis with negative hepatitis testing.[15] Testing should also be considered if there are characteristic findings on ultrasound examination. [b] Seroconversion of previously negative immunoglobulins to positive, or a significant (>4-fold) increase in anti-CMV IgG titers.[14] [c] Amniocentesis should be performed after 21 weeks gestation. CMV, cytomegalovirus; IgM, immunoglobulin M; IgG, Immunoglobulin G; PCR, polymerase chain reaction; PPV, positive predictive value; NPV, negative predictive value.

the sensitivity is much lower at earlier gestational ages.[31] In a retrospective cohort of 52 women, Donner and colleagues[27] found that the sensitivity of amniocentesis before 21 weeks was as low as 45%, and several women had a initially negative PCR that was subsequently found to be positive when performed after 21 weeks.

Ultrasound examination may also aid in fetal diagnosis, because the characteristic ultrasound findings may be seen in fetuses with congenital CMV. It is important to note, however, that not all affected fetuses will have typical ultrasound findings. In a recent retrospective cohort evaluating the ultrasound examinations of 650 fetuses from mothers with primary CMV infection, Guerra and colleagues[32] found that ultrasound abnormalities were found in only 8.5% of cases of mothers with primary infection and 14.9% of congenitally infected fetuses. Symptomatic congenital infection occurred in 68 of 131 cases without abnormal ultrasonographic findings, with a positive predictive value of ultrasound findings of approximately 30%. Therefore, although ultrasound examination can be a useful adjunct in diagnosis, the absence of ultrasound findings does not exclude congenital CMV infection. When fetal infection is confirmed, abnormal ultrasound findings occur in approximately 15% to 52% of fetuses.[32,33] **Table 2** details the ultrasound findings seen in prenatal CMV infection.

Prevention

There is no vaccine for prevention of CMV currently available. A phase II trial, published in 2009, demonstrated that a vaccine consisting of recombinant CMV envelope glycoprotein B had an efficacy of 50%, but lacked long-term efficacy.[34] Part of the difficulty in development of an effective vaccine is that reinfection may occur with new strains of CMV, and a vaccine would need to cover multiple strains and may not protect against reinfection. Additionally, CMV is a large virus with multiple immunogenic proteins, making vaccine design challenging. Vaccine development remains a high priority in the Institute of Medicine vaccine prioritization reports.[35]

In the absence of an effective vaccine, the only available prevention strategies involve patient and provider education and prevention of exposure to the virus. Knowledge is a key component; in a recent survey of more than 4000 participants, Cannon and colleagues[36] demonstrated that only 7% of men and 13% of women had heard of congenital CMV. Provider counseling and knowledge is also limited. A survey of practicing obstetrician/gynecologists demonstrated that fewer than 50% routinely counseled patients on CMV.[37]

There is some evidence that education may decrease the risk of seroconversion. Revello and colleagues[38] conducted a mixed interventional and observational controlled study evaluating prevention of exposure to CMV in women at high risk for CMV infection. In the intervention group, seronegative women were given information about CMV as well as hygiene, and tested for CMV until delivery. Women were specifically counseled on washing hands after exposure to young children's bodily fluids, as well as surfaces touched by children. They were also counseled on avoidance of kissing on the mouth/cheeks and not to share utensils, food, drinks, washcloths, and such items. In the observation group, women were not educated on CMV or prevention. In the intervention group, there was a significant difference in the number of women who seroconverted during pregnancy (1.2% in the intervention group vs 6.7% in the comparison group; $P<.001$). This study was limited, however, by the intervention and control groups being in different geographic areas, which may indicate underlying differences in the rates of CMV infection in the different areas.

In a recent randomized, controlled trial by Hughes and colleagues,[39] pregnant women were randomized to a brief behavioral intervention composed of a video about congenital CMV, hygiene education, and a reminder calendar and weekly text messages, versus standard care (a CDC brochure). The primary outcome of the study was change in reported compliance with recommended hygiene measures between baseline and follow-up assessments, measured by a behavioral compliance score. The study demonstrated a higher than anticipated baseline compliance with desired hygiene measures and a modest statistically significant increase in the compliance score in the intervention arm ($P = .007$) as well as a slight increase in compliance in the control arm, who only received a brochure. This study was limited by the inability to detect whether education impacted seroconversion; such a study would likely be prohibitively large. Currently, the CDC recommends regular hand washing, particularly after contact with body fluids of young children, to potentially reduce exposure to CMV.[16]

Management of Perinatal Cytomegalovirus Infection

All current management options for congenital CMV infection are considered experimental. Present areas of research include the use of antiviral medications or CMV hyperimmune globulin (HIG). At this time, antiviral medications for CMV such as ganciclovir, valganciclovir, and foscarnet are only approved by the US Food and Drug Administration for the treatment of patients with acquired immunodeficiency syndrome or organ transplants.[10] A study evaluating the efficacy of valacyclovir for the in utero treatment of symptomatic CMV-infected fetuses found that treatment with valacyclovir until delivery seemed to improve hearing and neurodevelopmental measures at 6 months of age.[40] A subsequent open-label, nonrandomized, phase II study of 43 women with fetuses with symptomatic CMV treated with valacyclovir until delivery demonstrated that valacyclovir decreased fetal blood viral loads and increased platelet counts, and significantly increased the proportion of asymptomatic neonates (in comparison with a historical cohort). These neonates remained symptom free at 12 months.[41] Unfortunately, limited conclusions can be drawn from this study because it was not a randomized, controlled trial and the only comparison group was a historical cohort, which may introduce bias or other confounding factors. Further research is needed to determine whether valacyclovir is efficacious for treating neonatal CMV and preventing long-term sequelae.

CMV HIG has also been used in experimental settings to prevent congenital CMV. In 2005, Nigro and colleagues[42] published the results of a nonrandomized, prospective cohort study in women with primary CMV infection in pregnancy, which found that CMV HIG therapy was associated with a significantly lower risk of congenital CMV. However, a follow-up randomized, controlled trial of 124 women with primary CMV infection in pregnancy published by Revello and colleagues[43] in 2014 demonstrated no significant difference in congenital infection between women treated with CMV HIG and those who were not treated (30% vs 44%; $P = .13$). There was also a nonsignificantly higher risk of adverse obstetric events, including preterm delivery and intrauterine growth restriction, within the treatment group.

Currently, use of either antiviral medications or CMV HIG are not recommended for treatment of primary CMV infection in pregnancy outside of clinical trials. Presently, there is 1 ongoing randomized clinical trial evaluating CMV HIG in CMV in pregnancy (clinicaltrials.gov: NCT01376778). There is another trial in progress evaluating valacyclovir therapy in Israel (clinicaltrials.gov: NCT02351102).

ZIKA VIRUS
Epidemiology

ZIKV is a mosquito-borne flavivirus that is closely related to dengue virus, and is transmitted by the Aedes species mosquito. It was initially described in Uganda in

1947,[44] and previous historical outbreaks of ZIKV were limited and occurred primarily in Southeast Asia and Africa. Recently, in 2013 a ZIKV outbreak occurred in French Polynesia. Subsequently, in late 2014, ZIKV was found in Brazil when clusters of patients with rash, mild fevers, and arthralgias were noted.[44] Since that time, ZIKV has spread across the Americas and at least 50 countries or territories have been affected, including Puerto Rico, Florida, and Texas.[45] The ZIKV outbreak gained worldwide attention when concern for perinatal transmission of ZIKV was noted, primarily based on increased rates of microcephaly in Brazil that were coincident with the ZIKV outbreak.[46] Since that time, a causal link has been established between prenatal ZIKV and microcephaly, as well as other severe brain abnormalities,[47] and characteristic findings of the congenital Zika syndrome have been described (**Table 3**).[48–57] Because most of these findings are based on case reports and smaller series, the incidence of each of these findings in congenital Zika syndrome is unknown. Although several features of congenital ZIKV syndrome overlap with other congenital infections, other features that are either rarely seen in other infections or unique to ZIKV (**Box 1**).[56] The presence of ZIKV has also been demonstrated in brain and placental tissue from affected fetuses, providing direct evidence for its association with microcephaly and other brain anomalies.[58] Infection in pregnancy has also been associated with first trimester miscarriage and second and third trimester fetal loss.[50,51]

Table 3
Features associated with congenital Zika syndrome

Category	Clinical Features Associated with Congenital Zika Syndrome
Neurologic sequelae – imaging findings	• Congenital microcephaly • Intracranial calcifications (often subcortical) • Cerebral atrophy • Abnormal cortical formation • Cortical thinning • Cerebellar hypoplasia • Absence or hypoplasia of the corpus callosum • Hydranencephaly • Ventriculomegaly • Fetal brain disruption sequence (severe microcephaly, overlapping cranial sutures, prominent occipital bone, redundant scalp skin, neurologic impairment)
Neurologic sequelae – clinical findings	• Sensorineural hearing loss • Altered motor activity • Seizures • Hypertonia • Hyperreflexia • Irritability
Eye abnormalities	• Structural eye anomalies (microphthalmia and coloboma) • Cataracts • Intraocular calcifications • Chorioretinal atrophy • Optic nerve atrophy/anomalies • Focal pigmentary mottling of the retina
Musculoskeletal abnormalities	• Arthrogryposis • Clubfoot • Congenital hip dysplasia

Data from Refs.[51,54,56]

> **Box 1**
> **Unique features in congenital Zika infection**
>
> Features rarely seen in other congenital disorders or unique to ZIKV congenital infection
>
> - Severe microcephaly with partially collapsed skull.
> - Thin cerebral cortices with subcortical calcification.
> - Macular scarring and focal pigmentary retinal mottling.
> - Congenital contractures.
> - Marked early hypertonia and symptoms of extrapyramidal involvement.
>
> *Data from* Moore CA, Staples JE, Dobyns WB, et al. Characterizing the pattern of anomalies in congenital Zika syndrome for pediatric clinicians. JAMA Pediatr 2017;171:288–95.

ZIKV can be transmitted in several different ways: by the *Aedes* species mosquito, vertically from mother to child in pregnancy, through sexual contact, and through blood transfusion. ZIKV has been identified in human serum, saliva, semen, urine, and vaginal secretions.[49,50,59–62] Osuna and colleagues[63] demonstrated that, in a macaque monkey model, inoculation with ZIKV resulted in infection and viral RNA was found in saliva, urine, and cerebrospinal fluid, as well as transiently in vaginal secretions. Given the potential for ZIKV to be transmitted by body fluids as well as through the *Aedes* mosquito, there are multiple ways in which pregnant women may be exposed or acquire the virus during pregnancy, putting the fetus at risk for vertical transmission.

Diagnosis

Symptoms of ZIKV infection include fever, headache, arthralgia, myalgia, and a maculopapular rash. However, symptoms are not a reliable screening tool for ZIKV because only 1 out of every 4 to 5 people with infection will display characteristic symptoms.[64–67] Given that approximately 80% of women with ZIKV infection in pregnancy will remain asymptomatic, alternate methods for the identification and testing of at risk women must be used. Currently, it is recommended by the CDC that all pregnant women should be screened for ZIKV exposure by travel and sexual history. The most current information about affected areas may be found at https://www.cdc.gov/zika/geo/index.html. All pregnant women in the United States and in US territories should be assessed for ZIKV exposure at each prenatal visit by asking about the following[68]:

- Travel to or residence in any areas with risk for ZIKV transmission before and during the current pregnancy.
- Sexual exposure before and during the current pregnancy.
- A diagnosis of laboratory confirmed ZIKV infection before the current pregnancy.
- Symptoms of ZIKV disease (fever, rash, conjunctivitis, arthralgia).

Pregnant women should be tested if they have recent possible ZIKV exposure and symptoms of ZIKV disease (**Fig. 2**). Routine testing is no longer recommended in women who have recent possible ZIKV exposure but are asymptomatic and without ongoing exposure, although testing may be considered using a shared decision model in these cases. Testing is also indicated for the following[68]:

- Asymptomatic women with ongoing possible ZIKV exposure should be offered ZIKV nucleic acid testing (NAT) of serum and urine 3 times during pregnancy; IgM testing is not routinely recommended for these patients.

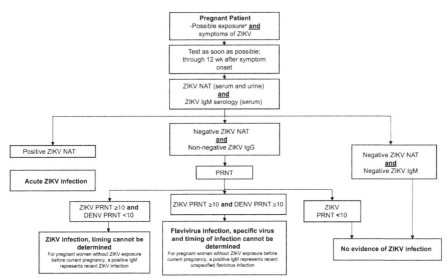

Fig. 2. Recommended strategy for ZIKV testing in symptomatic women. [a] Possible exposure to ZIKV includes travel or residence in areas with active ZIKV transmission, or sexual contact (oral, vaginal, or anal sex, or sharing of sex toys) without a barrier method with a partner who traveled to, or lives in an area with active ZIKV transmission. ZIKV, Zika virus; DENV, dengue virus; IgM, immunoglobulin M; PRNT, plaque reduction neutralization test; NAT, nucleic acid test. (*Adapted from* the Centers for Disease Control and Prevention Website. Available at: https://www.cdc.gov/zika/hc-providers/pregnant-women/testing-and-diagnosis.html. Accessed August 1, 2017.)

- Pregnant women who have recent possible ZIKV exposure and who have a fetus with prenatal ultrasound findings consistent with congenital ZIKV syndrome should receive ZIKV testing (NAT and IgM).

The CDC updates testing guidelines as knowledge regarding ZIKV evolves. The most recent interim guidance for health care providers was published on July 24, 2017.[68] It is important to note that these guidelines may change in the future, therefore providers are urged to check the CDC website at https://www.cdc.gov/zika/hc-providers/pregnant-women/testing-and-diagnosis.html for updates on testing and diagnosis of ZIKV in pregnancy.

Methods for testing include both serologic and molecular tests. Laboratory tests in the algorithm include ZIKV IgM, ZIKV NAT, and plaque reduction neutralization testing. These tests and their limitations are outlined herein.

ZIKV IgM is the only current immunoglobin test available for immunologic ZIKV testing. The ZIKV IgM is only temporally present in serum after a ZIKV infection, and the duration of IgM antibody persistence after ZIKV infection is unknown. IgM antibodies for West Nile virus (a closely related flavivirus) have been detected for at least 3 months after the viremic period in asymptomatic, infected blood donors, and for more than 1 year in patients with West Nile encephalitis.[69,70] These results have been extrapolated to ZIKV and used as potential testing window for patients with suspected infection. ZIKV IgM may also cross-react with related flaviviruses,[71] such as dengue, making positive IgM results more difficult to interpret. Therefore, a plaque reduction neutralization test should be performed in the case of a positive IgM antibody test to confirm diagnosis of ZIKV.[71] There is not currently a validated IgG antibody or avidity test available for ZIKV.

Molecular diagnostic testing for ZIKV is available in the form of NAT, which is used to identify viral RNA in clinical or pathologic specimens.[68] A positive result typically indicates infection, although false positives have been reported.[61,72] A negative test does not rule out infection,[71] because the duration and persistence of viremia are not known at this time. In a recent report of ZIKV in body fluids in a cohort of 150 participants with symptomatic and PCR positive ZIKV, the investigators found that the median and 95th percentiles for time until the loss of ZIKV RNA detection was 14 and 54 days, respectively, in serum, 8 and 39 days in urine, and 34 and 81 days in semen.[61] These findings indicate that the time frame in which ZIKV is present in bodily fluids is variable, and testing too late after symptom onset may result in a false-negative NAT result.

Amniocentesis for ZIKV NAT may also be performed in cases of concern for maternal infection based on positive laboratory results or abnormal fetal ultrasound results with known maternal exposure to ZIKV. However, the sensitivity, specificity, and predictive values of NAT on amniotic fluid are unknown. Schaub and colleagues[73] have demonstrated that detection of ZIKV RNA in amniotic fluid from fetuses with ZIKV associated birth defects indicates fetal infection. However, in several cases with initially positive results, subsequent amniocenteses were negative, indicating ZIKV presence in amniotic fluid may be transient and not always detectable. The optimal gestational age for amniocentesis is unknown. These limitations of amniotic fluid testing should be reviewed with the patient. Finally, any pregnant women with serologic or molecular evidence of recent ZIKV infection should be reported to the US Zika Pregnancy Registry or the Puerto Rico Zika Active Pregnancy Surveillance System in addition to being followed for possible adverse pregnancy outcomes.[71]

Fetal Diagnosis

The risk of microcephaly in ZIKV infection has been estimated to be from 1% to 13% based on models of outbreaks in Brazil and French Polynesia.[74,75] As more ZIKV infections are identified in pregnant women and more outcome data are obtained, it will become possible to estimate the frequency with which fetuses are affected during ZIKV infection in pregnancy; however, it is important to note that the majority of these data are preliminary and limited by smaller numbers.

In a prospective cohort of pregnant women in Rio De Janeiro[50] who presented with a rash and were tested for ZIKV with real-time reverse transcription PCR, the authors found that of 117 live infants born to 116 ZIKV positive women, 49 (42%) were found to have grossly abnormal clinical or brain imaging findings, or both. Of those infants, 4 (3.4%) were found to have microcephaly. In comparison, in the 61 pregnancies in women who were negative for ZIKV, only 3 infants (5%) had abnormalities in brain imaging or clinical examination. In a prospective cohort of women from the United States with laboratory evidence of possible recent ZIKV infection with 442 completed pregnancies, Honein and colleagues[51] found that birth defects potentially related to ZIKV were found in 26 (6%; 95% confidence interval, 4%–8%) of fetuses or infants. This wide range of incidence of findings related to ZIKV infection indicate that further research is needed into the congenital Zika syndrome.

There is evidence that vertical transmission to the fetus may occur in any trimester[50,56]; therefore, ZIKV infection at any point in pregnancy should lead to counseling on potential neonatal effects of ZIKV, as well as after the pregnancy for adverse outcomes. As more is learned about ZIKV, it is likely that a clearer picture regarding incidence of birth defects and risk of transmission in each trimester will develop. A currently enrolling observational cohort study, the Zika in Infants and Pregnancy (ZIP) study (clinicaltrials.gov number NCT02856984) is a multisite, multicountry prospective study that aims to assess the strength the association of ZIKV infection in pregnancy with adverse maternal and neonatal outcomes. These investigators will enroll women in the first trimester and follow patients through pregnancy to assess for ZIKV infection, as well as maternal and neonatal outcomes. The goal enrollment is 10,000 pregnant women from ZIKV-endemic regions.

Fetal ultrasound examination is a key component of evaluation in suspected or confirmed ZIKV infection in pregnancy. Currently, the CDC, American Congress of Obstetricians and Gynecologists,[76] the International Society of Ultrasound in Obstetrics and Gynecology,[77] and the Society for Maternal-Fetal Medicine[78] have all recommended ultrasound for evaluation of the fetus in cases of proven or suspected ZIKV infection in pregnancy. One of the characteristic findings on ultrasound examination is microcephaly. The Society for Maternal-Fetal Medicine defines isolated microcephaly as a head circumference (HC) or 3 or more standard deviations below the mean for gestational age,[78] although it is important to note this value may encompass some normal fetuses as well.[79] The diagnosis of pathologic microcephaly is considered to be certain when the HC is 5 or more standard deviations below the mean.[80]

The Society for Maternal-Fetal Medicine and the International Society of Ultrasound in Obstetrics and Gynecology recommend that if the HC 3 or more standard deviations below the mean, the intracranial anatomy should be carefully evaluated.[77,78] It is important to note that abnormalities may not be evident on initial ultrasound evaluation, but may develop over time; therefore, follow-up ultrasound examinations should be performed every 3 to 4 weeks when there is evidence of maternal infection.[78] In a retrospective evaluation of 19 cases of microcephaly in mothers with definite or a high probability of ZIKV infection, Carvalho and colleagues[81] report that all but one of the 19 fetuses had a normal ultrasound examination at 18 to 24 weeks of gestation, with the subsequent development of abnormal ultrasound findings. This finding underscores the importance of serial ultrasound examinations within this population. In addition to microcephaly, other ultrasound anomalies that have been described in fetuses found to have congenital Zika syndrome include the following[50,81–83]:

- Periventricular and intraparenchymal calcifications;
- Ventriculomegaly;
- Cerebellar hypoplasia;
- Cortical atrophy; and
- Corpus callosum abnormalities.

It is important to note that studies that have reported high rates of ultrasound-based abnormalities in the setting of ZIKV infection have included other abnormalities detected on ultrasound examination, such as fetal growth restriction, abnormal umbilical cord Doppler examinations, and amniotic fluid abnormalities,[50,81] so there may be a percentage of affected fetuses that do not have intracranial abnormalities on ultrasound examination.

Additionally, there have been highly concerning reports of neonatal anomalies that have been identified after delivery or during the infant period in cases of ZIKV in the absence of microcephaly. Van der Linden and colleagues[53] describe 13 infants born in Brazil with a normal HC at birth and laboratory evidence of ZIKV infection. These infants had brain abnormalities on postnatal neuroimaging, including decreased brain volume, ventriculomegaly, subcortical calcifications, and cortical malformations. Although born without microcephaly, head growth was noted to decelerate, and 11 infants developed microcephaly. Therefore, patients with a positive maternal or fetal ZIKV test should be counseled that the absence of prenatal ultrasound findings does not preclude the development of congenital Zika syndrome, and infant development should be carefully monitored.

Prevention

Current CDC recommendations[68,84] for prevention of ZIKV include the following:

- Avoidance of travel to ZIKV endemic areas during pregnancy.
- The use of N,N-Diethyl-meta-toluamide, which has been recommended in pregnancy to prevent ZIKV infection,[85] long sleeves and pants or permethrin-treated clothing, and use of mosquito nets and window screens if living in or traveling to an endemic area.
- If living in an endemic area, areas of standing water (such as tires, buckets, planters, etc) should be eliminated because they are a breeding area for mosquitoes.
- All pregnant women and their partners should receive counseling on prevention measures including avoidance of mosquito bites and sexual transmission.
- If a couple has a male partner and he travels to an area with ZIKV, they should use condoms or abstain from sexual activity for 6 months (even in the absence of symptoms).
- If a female travels to an area with risk of ZIKV, condoms or abstinence from sexual activity for 8 weeks (even in the absence of symptoms) is recommended.
- If a pregnant patient and her partner travel to or live in an area with ZIKV, condoms should be used each time the couple has sex for the remainder of pregnancy, or they should abstain from sexual activity.

There is no current vaccine therapy for ZIKV. A search of clinicaltrials.gov reveals that there are currently 9 active vaccine trials evaluating ZIKV; this number will likely increase over time. These trials include several phase I trials led by the National Institute of Allergy and Infectious Diseases (clinicaltrial.gov numbers NCT02996461, NCT03008122, and NCT02963909). Although research into a ZIKV vaccine is moving forward quickly, there remain multiple limitations to rapid vaccine development, including the planning and executing of preclinical studies, clinical trial design and completion, establishing clinical endpoints, determining who and when to vaccinate, and vaccine production and licensure.[86]

Management

There is no current treatment for ZIKV infection in pregnancy. Per the CDC, important keys to management of confirmed or presumptive recent ZIKV infection during pregnancy include the following[68];

- Consideration of amniocentesis for ZIKV NAT, decision to proceed with amniocentesis should be individualized and testing limitations should be discussed.
- Serial ultrasound examinations every 3 to 4 weeks to assess fetal anatomy and growth.
- Notification of the pediatric team of risk of congenital ZIKV syndrome.
- Women with a fetal loss or stillbirth may be offered pathology testing for ZIKV infection with NAT and immunohistochemical staining of fetal tissues.
- In cases of a live birth with subsequent infant death, testing of placental and infant autopsy tissues with NAT and immunohistochemical staining of fetal tissues should be considered to aid in infant and maternal diagnosis.

It is important to note that ZIKV research is ongoing and there is much to learn regarding the virus and outcomes after infection in pregnancy; new information is continuously available. Practitioners are encouraged to stay up to date on the most current guidelines and recommendations. The CDC has multiple resources regarding testing, transmission and risks, prevention, pregnancy, and patient education tools, which are regularly updated. These resources can be found at https://cdc.gov/Zika.

REFERENCES

1. Kenneson A, Cannon MJ. Review and meta-analysis of the epidemiology of congenital cytomegalovirus (CMV) infection. Rev Med Virol 2007;17:253–76.
2. Dollard SC, Grosse SD, Ross DS. New estimates of the prevalence of neurological and sensory sequelae and mortality associated with congenital cytomegalovirus infection. Rev Med Virol 2007;17:355–63.
3. Fowler KB, Stagno S, Pass RF. Maternal age and congenital cytomegalovirus infection: screening of two diverse newborn populations, 1980-1990. J Infect Dis 1993;168:552–6.
4. Colugnati FA, Staras SA, Dollard SC, et al. Incidence of cytomegalovirus infection among the general population and pregnant women in the United States. BMC Infect Dis 2007;7:71.
5. Cannon MJ. Congenital cytomegalovirus (CMV) epidemiology and awareness. J Clin Virol 2009;46(Suppl 4):S6–10.
6. Stagno S, Pass RF, Cloud G, et al. Primary cytomegalovirus infection in pregnancy. Incidence, transmission to fetus, and clinical outcome. JAMA 1986;256:1904–8.
7. Johnson J, Anderson B. Screening, prevention, and treatment of congenital cytomegalovirus. Obstet Gynecol Clin North Am 2014;41:593–9.
8. Fowler KB, Stagno S, Pass RF. Maternal immunity and prevention of congenital cytomegalovirus infection. JAMA 2003;289:1008–11.
9. Lazzarotto T, Guerra B, Gabrielli L, et al. Update on the prevention, diagnosis and management of cytomegalovirus infection during pregnancy. Clin Microbiol Infect 2011;17:1285–93.
10. American College of Obstetricians and Gynecologists. ACOG practice bulletin no.142: cerclage for the management of cervical insufficiency. Obstet Gynecol 2014;123:372–9.
11. Enders G, Daiminger A, Bader U, et al. Intrauterine transmission and clinical outcome of 248 pregnancies with primary cytomegalovirus infection in relation to gestational age. J Clin Virol 2011;52:244–6.
12. Picone O, Vauloup-Fellous C, Cordier AG, et al. A series of 238 cytomegalovirus primary infections during pregnancy: description and outcome. Prenat Diagn 2013;33:751–8.
13. Pass RF, Fowler KB, Boppana SB, et al. Congenital cytomegalovirus infection following first trimester maternal infection: symptoms at birth and outcome. J Clin Virol 2006;35:216–20.
14. Fowler KB, Stagno S, Pass RF, et al. The outcome of congenital cytomegalovirus infection in relation to maternal antibody status. N Engl J Med 1992;326:663–7.
15. American College of Obstetricians and Gynecologists. Practice bulletin no. 151: cytomegalovirus, parvovirus B19, varicella zoster, and toxoplasmosis in pregnancy. Obstet Gynecol 2015;125:1510–25.
16. Centers for Disease Control and Prevention (CDC). Cytomegalovirus (CMV) and Congenital CMV infection. 2017. Available at: https://www.cdc.gov/cmv/clinical/features.html. Accessed April 15, 2017.
17. De Paschale M, Agrappi C, Manco MT, et al. Positive predictive value of anti-HCMV IgM as an index of primary infection. J Virol Methods 2010;168:121–5.

18. De Carolis S, Santucci S, Botta A, et al. False-positive IgM for CMV in pregnant women with autoimmune disease: a novel prognostic factor for poor pregnancy outcome. Lupus 2010;19:844–9.
19. Saldan A, Forner G, Mengoli C, et al. Testing for cytomegalovirus in pregnancy. J Clin Microbiol 2017;55:693–702.
20. Lazzarotto T, Guerra B, Lanari M, et al. New advances in the diagnosis of congenital cytomegalovirus infection. J Clin Virol 2008;41:192–7.
21. Hughes BL, Gyamfi-Bannerman C. Diagnosis and antenatal management of congenital cytomegalovirus infection. Am J Obstet Gynecol 2016;214:B5–11.
22. Revello MG, Zavattoni M, Baldanti F, et al. Diagnostic and prognostic value of human cytomegalovirus load and IgM antibody in blood of congenitally infected newborns. J Clin Virol 1999;14:57–66.
23. Picone O, Costa JM, Leruez-Ville M, et al. Cytomegalovirus (CMV) glycoprotein B genotype and CMV DNA load in the amniotic fluid of infected fetuses. Prenat Diagn 2004;24:1001–6.
24. Gouarin S, Gault E, Vabret A, et al. Real-time PCR quantification of human cytomegalovirus DNA in amniotic fluid samples from mothers with primary infection. J Clin Microbiol 2002;40:1767–72.
25. Hohlfeld P, Vial Y, Maillard-Brignon C, et al. Cytomegalovirus fetal infection: prenatal diagnosis. Obstet Gynecol 1991;78:615–8.
26. Lamy ME, Mulongo KN, Gadisseux JF, et al. Prenatal diagnosis of fetal cytomegalovirus infection. Am J Obstet Gynecol 1992;166:91–4.
27. Donner C, Liesnard C, Content J, et al. Prenatal diagnosis of 52 pregnancies at risk for congenital cytomegalovirus infection. Obstet Gynecol 1993;82:481–6.
28. Nicolini U, Kustermann A, Tassis B, et al. Prenatal diagnosis of congenital human cytomegalovirus infection. Prenat Diagn 1994;14:903–6.
29. Revello MG, Baldanti F, Furione M, et al. Polymerase chain reaction for prenatal diagnosis of congenital human cytomegalovirus infection. J Med Virol 1995;47:462–6.
30. Lipitz S, Yagel S, Shalev E, et al. Prenatal diagnosis of fetal primary cytomegalovirus infection. Obstet Gynecol 1997;89:763–7.
31. Liesnard C, Donner C, Brancart F, et al. Prenatal diagnosis of congenital cytomegalovirus infection: prospective study of 237 pregnancies at risk. Obstet Gynecol 2000;95:881–8.
32. Guerra B, Simonazzi G, Puccetti C, et al. Ultrasound prediction of symptomatic congenital cytomegalovirus infection. Am J Obstet Gynecol 2008;198(380): e381–7.
33. Benoist G, Salomon LJ, Jacquemard F, et al. The prognostic value of ultrasound abnormalities and biological parameters in blood of fetuses infected with cytomegalovirus. BJOG 2008;115:823–9.
34. Pass RF, Zhang C, Evans A, et al. Vaccine prevention of maternal cytomegalovirus infection. N Engl J Med 2009;360:1191–9.
35. Krause PR, Bialek SR, Boppana SB, et al. Priorities for CMV vaccine development. Vaccine 2013;32:4–10.
36. Cannon MJ, Westbrook K, Levis D, et al. Awareness of and behaviors related to child-to-mother transmission of cytomegalovirus. Prev Med 2012;54:351–7.
37. Ross DS, Rasmussen SA, Cannon MJ, et al. Obstetrician/gynecologists' knowledge, attitudes, and practices regarding prevention of infections in pregnancy. J Womens Health (Larchmt) 2009;18:1187–93.
38. Revello MG, Tibaldi C, Masuelli G, et al. Prevention of primary cytomegalovirus infection in pregnancy. EBioMedicine 2015;2:1205–10.

39. Hughes BL, Gans KM, Raker C, et al. A brief prenatal intervention of behavioral change to reduce the risk of maternal cytomegalovirus: a randomized controlled trial. Obstet Gynecol 2017;130(4):726–34.
40. Kimberlin DW, Jester PM, Sanchez PJ, et al. Valganciclovir for symptomatic congenital cytomegalovirus disease. N Engl J Med 2015;372:933–43.
41. Leruez-Ville M, Ghout I, Bussieres L, et al. In utero treatment of congenital cytomegalovirus infection with valacyclovir in a multicenter, open-label, phase II study. Am J Obstet Gynecol 2016;215:462.e1-e10.
42. Nigro G, Adler SP, La Torre R, et al. Passive immunization during pregnancy for congenital cytomegalovirus infection. N Engl J Med 2005;353:1350–62.
43. Revello MG, Lazzarotto T, Guerra B, et al. A randomized trial of hyperimmune globulin to prevent congenital cytomegalovirus. N Engl J Med 2014;370:1316–26.
44. Weaver SC, Costa F, Garcia-Blanco MA, et al. Zika virus: history, emergence, biology, and prospects for control. Antivir Res 2016;130:69–80.
45. Centers for Disease Control and Prevention (CDC). Areas with Zika. 2017. Available at: https://www.cdc.gov/zika/geo/index.html. Accessed April 18, 2017.
46. Citil Dogan A, Wayne S, Bauer S, et al. The Zika virus and pregnancy: evidence, management, and prevention. J Matern Fetal Neonatal Med 2017;30:386–96.
47. Rasmussen SA, Jamieson DJ, Honein MA, et al. Zika virus and birth defects–reviewing the evidence for causality. N Engl J Med 2016;374:1981–7.
48. Melo AS, Aguiar RS, Amorim MM, et al. Congenital Zika virus infection: beyond neonatal microcephaly. JAMA Neurol 2016;73:1407–16.
49. Adhikari EH, Nelson DB, Johnson KA, et al. Infant outcomes among women with Zika virus infection during pregnancy: results of a large prenatal Zika screening program. Am J Obstet Gynecol 2017;216:292.e1-e8.
50. Brasil P, Pereira JP Jr, Moreira ME, et al. Zika virus infection in pregnant women in Rio de Janeiro. N Engl J Med 2016;375:2321–34.
51. Honein MA, Dawson AL, Petersen EE, et al. Birth defects among fetuses and infants of US women with evidence of possible Zika virus infection during pregnancy. JAMA 2017;317:59–68.
52. Moura da Silva AA, Ganz JS, Sousa PD, et al. Early growth and neurologic outcomes of infants with probable congenital Zika virus syndrome. Emerg Infect Dis 2016;22:1953–6.
53. van der Linden V, Pessoa A, Dobyns W, et al. Description of 13 infants born during October 2015-January 2016 with congenital Zika virus infection without microcephaly at birth - Brazil. MMWR Morb Mortal Wkly Rep 2016;65:1343–8.
54. Del Campo M, Feitosa IM, Ribeiro EM, et al. The phenotypic spectrum of congenital Zika syndrome. Am J Med Genet A 2017;173:841–57.
55. Reynolds MR, Jones AM, Petersen EE, et al. Vital signs: update on Zika virus-associated birth defects and evaluation of all U.S. infants with congenital Zika virus exposure - U.S. Zika Pregnancy Registry, 2016. MMWR Morb Mortal Wkly Rep 2017;66:366–73.
56. Moore CA, Staples JE, Dobyns WB, et al. Characterizing the pattern of anomalies in congenital Zika syndrome for pediatric clinicians. JAMA Pediatr 2017;171:288–95.
57. Miranda-Filho Dde B, Martelli CM, Ximenes RA, et al. Initial description of the presumed congenital Zika syndrome. Am J Public Health 2016;106:598–600.
58. Bhatnagar J, Rabeneck DB, Martines RB, et al. Zika virus RNA replication and persistence in brain and placental tissue. Emerg Infect Dis 2017;23:405–14.
59. Atkinson B, Hearn P, Afrough B, et al. Detection of Zika virus in semen. Emerg Infect Dis 2016;22:940.

60. Cabral-Castro MJ, Cavalcanti MG, Peralta RH, et al. Molecular and serological techniques to detect co-circulation of DENV, ZIKV and CHIKV in suspected dengue-like syndrome patients. J Clin Virol 2016;82:108–11.

61. Paz-Bailey G, Rosenberg ES, Doyle K, et al. Persistence of Zika virus in body fluids - preliminary report. N Engl J Med 2017. [Epub ahead of print].

62. Murray KO, Gorchakov R, Carlson AR, et al. Prolonged detection of Zika virus in vaginal secretions and whole blood. Emerg Infect Dis 2017;23:99–101.

63. Osuna CE, Lim SY, Deleage C, et al. Zika viral dynamics and shedding in rhesus and cynomolgus macaques. Nat Med 2016;22:1448–55.

64. Faye O, Freire CC, Iamarino A, et al. Molecular evolution of Zika virus during its emergence in the 20(th) century. PLoS Negl Trop Dis 2014;8:e2636.

65. Ioos S, Mallet HP, Leparc Goffart I, et al. Current Zika virus epidemiology and recent epidemics. Med Mal Infect 2014;44:302–7.

66. Besnard M, Lastere S, Teissier A, et al. Evidence of perinatal transmission of Zika virus, French Polynesia, December 2013 and February 2014. Euro Surveill 2014; 19(13) [pii: 20751].

67. Duffy MR, Chen TH, Hancock WT, et al. Zika virus outbreak on Yap Island, Federated States OF Micronesia. N Engl J Med 2009;360:2536–43.

68. Oduyebo T, Polen KD, Walke HT, et al. Update: interim guidance for health care providers caring for pregnant women with possible Zika virus exposure - United States (including U.S. Territories), July 2017. MMWR Morb Mortal Wkly Rep 2017; 66:781–93.

69. Prince HE, Tobler LH, Yeh C, et al. Persistence of West Nile virus-specific antibodies in viremic blood donors. Clin Vaccine Immunol 2007;14:1228–30.

70. Roehrig JT, Nash D, Maldin B, et al. Persistence of virus-reactive serum immunoglobulin m antibody in confirmed West Nile virus encephalitis cases. Emerg Infect Dis 2003;9:376–9.

71. Rabe IB, Staples JE, Villanueva J, et al. Interim guidance for interpretation of Zika virus antibody test results. MMWR Morb Mortal Wkly Rep 2016;65:543–6.

72. Bingham AM, Cone M, Mock V, et al. Comparison of test results for Zika virus RNA in urine, serum, and saliva specimens from persons with travel-associated Zika virus disease - Florida, 2016. MMWR Morb Mortal Wkly Rep 2016;65:475–8.

73. Schaub B, Vouga M, Najioullah F, et al. Analysis of blood from Zika virus-infected fetuses: a prospective case series. Lancet Infect Dis 2017;17:520–7.

74. Cauchemez S, Besnard M, Bompard P, et al. Association between Zika virus and microcephaly in French Polynesia, 2013-15: a retrospective study. Lancet 2016; 387:2125–32.

75. Johansson MA, Mier-y-Teran-Romero L, Reefhuis J, et al. Zika and the risk of microcephaly. N Engl J Med 2016;375:1–4.

76. Meaney-Delman D, Rasmussen SA, Staples JE, et al. Zika virus and pregnancy: what obstetric health care providers need to know. Obstet Gynecol 2016;127: 642–8.

77. Papageorghiou AT, Thilaganathan B, Bilardo CM, et al. ISUOG Interim Guidance on ultrasound for Zika virus infection in pregnancy: information for healthcare professionals. Ultrasound Obstet Gynecol 2016;47:530–2.

78. Society for Maternal-Fetal Medicine (SMFM). Ultrasound screening for fetal microcephaly following Zika virus exposure. Am J Obstet Gynecol 2016;214: B2–4.

79. Leibovitz Z, Daniel-Spiegel E, Malinger G, et al. Prediction of microcephaly at birth using three reference ranges for fetal head circumference: can we improve prenatal diagnosis? Ultrasound Obstet Gynecol 2016;47:586–92.

80. International Society of Ultrasound in Obstetrics & Gynecology Education Committee. Sonographic examination of the fetal central nervous system: guidelines for performing the 'basic examination' and the 'fetal neurosonogram'. Ultrasound Obstet Gynecol 2007;29:109–16.
81. Carvalho FH, Cordeiro KM, Peixoto AB, et al. Associated ultrasonographic findings in fetuses with microcephaly because of suspected Zika virus (ZIKV) infection during pregnancy. Prenat Diagn 2016;36:882–7.
82. Vesnaver TV, Tul N, Mehrabi S, et al. Zika virus associated microcephaly/microencephaly-fetal brain imaging in comparison with neuropathology. BJOG 2017;124:521–5.
83. Mlakar J, Korva M, Tul N, et al. Zika virus associated with microcephaly. N Engl J Med 2016;374:951–8.
84. Centers for Disease Control and Prevention (CDC). Zika virus prevention. Available at: https://www.cdc.gov/zika/prevention/index.html. Accessed April 24, 2017.
85. Wylie BJ, Hauptman M, Woolf AD, et al. Insect repellants during pregnancy in the era of the Zika virus. Obstet Gynecol 2016;128:1111–5.
86. Thomas SJ, L'Azou M, Barrett AD, et al. Fast-track Zika vaccine development - is it possible? N Engl J Med 2016;375:1212–6.

Current Strategies to Prevent Maternal-to-Child Transmission of Human Immunodeficiency Virus

Leilah Zahedi-Spung, MD*, Martina L. Badell, MD

KEYWORDS

- HIV • Maternal-to-child transmission • Prevention • Perinatal transmission

KEY POINTS

- Early diagnosis and treatment of human immunodeficiency virus (HIV) is the most effective prevention strategy to reduce maternal-to-child transmission.
- Combined antiretroviral therapy should ideally be initiated before pregnancy or as early as tolerated in pregnancy to achieve maximal suppression of viral load.
- Prevention of maternal-to-child transmission of HIV requires a multidisciplinary approach.

EPIDEMIC

The Centers for Disease Control and Prevention (CDC) estimates that more than 1.2 million people are living with human immunodeficiency virus (HIV) in the United States today. Of these 1.2 million, an estimated 19% to 24% are women.[1] In 2010, it was estimated that 9500 women were newly infected with HIV; most (84%) were infected through heterosexual sex. Approximately 64% of women living with HIV are African American, making them disproportionately affected.[1] Advances in antepartum care and combined antiretroviral treatment (cART) have led to a dramatic reduction in the maternal-to-child transmission of HIV. By the end of 2014, there were 1995 children in the United States living with perinatal HIV.[1] In the United States between 2009 and 2014, almost 22,000 cases of potential perinatally acquired HIV infections were prevented.[1] In contrast, globally in 2009, 370,000 children became newly infected with HIV.[2] *The cumulative in utero, intrapartum, and postpartum HIV transmission rate without intervention is estimated to be 35% to 40%.*[3] Advances in

Disclosure Statement: There are no financial conflicts of interests or sources of funding to disclose for either author.
Department of Gynecology and Obstetrics, Emory University, Emory University Hospital, Midtown Perinatal Center, 550 Peachtree Street, 8th Floor, Atlanta, GA 30308, USA
* Corresponding author.
E-mail address: lzahedi@emory.edu

antiretroviral therapy have led to a great reduction in mortality attributed to HIV and a dramatic reduction in maternal-to-child transmission of HIV in resource-rich settings. *Utilization of* the *current recommendations for the management of HIV-positive pregnant women has led to an average maternal-to-child transmission rate of less than 1% in many US states.*[3] However, we still have work to do in improving maternal-to-child transmission rates. The CDC developed a new framework with the goal of eliminating maternal-to-child transmission in the United States. The key components of the framework include comprehensive care; case review to identify and address missed opportunities for prevention; research and long-term monitoring, which allows for the development of safe and efficacious interventions; and data reporting for HIV surveillance and evaluation of elimination of maternal-to-child transmission treatment programs.[4]

Prevention of maternal-to-child transmission is a multifaceted, multidisciplinary approach that encompasses the entirety of a woman's reproductive life. Given the many needs in resource-limited settings, the scope of this review focuses on the prevention of maternal-to-child transmission in resource-rich settings. A study in 2015 analyzed missed opportunities for prevention of maternal-to-child transmission between the years of 2005 and 2012 in the state of Georgia. This study identified 27 perinatally infected infants. They found that in 24 of the 27 cases, limitations in health care delivery and uptake were significant risk factors for the HIV-infected women. They also noted that 74% of women knew their HIV status before pregnancy, but only 50% received prenatal care. This study identified several risk factors to a lack of adherence to maternal-to-child transmission of HIV, including illicit drug use, lack of prenatal care, and lack of antepartum cART.[5]

PRECONCEPTION COUNSELING

Preconception counseling is an important aspect of women's health and is especially important for HIV-infected women. *One of the most important components of preconception counseling is* the *prevention of unintended pregnancies.* For HIV-infected women, this discussion should include initiation or continuation of cART; compliance with medication and prenatal appointments antepartum and post partum; addressing potential barriers to care and treatment throughout pregnancy and post partum; and, ultimately, prevention of maternal-to-child transmission.[3] Women infected with HIV should be optimized on their cART to ensure maximal viral suppression. In addition, any other medical comorbidities should be optimized. A thorough review of her prior obstetric history should be performed, and any previous poor obstetric outcomes should be addressed and appropriate referrals to maternal-fetal medicine colleagues should be placed. They should also receive any indicated vaccinations and appropriate prophylaxis or treatment of opportunistic infections. Women should undergo screening and treatment of any concomitant sexually transmitted infections. Importantly, screening for psychosocial factors that may impact pregnancy outcomes (eg, psychological and substance use disorders) should be completed and treatment initiated as appropriate. Lastly, couples should be counseled on the how to optimize conception while minimizing the risk of transmission of HIV to an uninfected male partner or transmission of a more resistant strain to an HIV-infected partner.[3,6,7]

DIAGNOSIS

The first step in preventing maternal-to-child transmission is establishing the diagnosis of HIV. *The earlier the diagnosis is known in a pregnancy, the sooner treatment can be started to prevent transmission to the fetus.* It was found that almost a quarter of the perinatal HIV transmissions reported by the CDC between 2008 and 2012 were due to maternal HIV infections that remained undiagnosed until the intrapartum or postpartum periods.[8] In order to achieve the goal of elimination of maternal-to-child transmission, the World Health Organization (WHO), the American Academy of Pediatrics, and the American College of Obstetricians and Gynecologists (ACOG) recommend using a universal opt-out approach for HIV testing as early as possible during pregnancy. Rapid HIV testing should be performed on labor and delivery for those whose status is undocumented and if positive antiretroviral prophylaxis should be started immediately without waiting for confirmatory testing results.[8,9] To date, all but 2 states, Nebraska and New York, have laws that are consistent with the CDC's opt-out HIV testing recommendations.[10] Studies have shown an opt-out approach can increase testing rates among pregnant women and, therefore, increase the number of pregnant women who know their status and can ultimately increase the number of HIV-infected women who are offered treatment and, thus, reduce maternal-to-child transmission.[10,11]

The CDC and ACOG also recommend repeat testing in the third trimester in certain geographic areas or for women who are known to be at high risk of becoming infected while pregnant. This population includes injection-drug users, women who have sex partners that are injection-drug users, women who exchange sex for money or drugs, women who are sex partners of HIV-infected persons, and women who have had a new or more than one sex partner throughout the pregnancy.[8-11] The geographic areas include settings where there is an elevated HIV incidence, more than 17 cases per 1000,000 person-years, or where prenatal screening identified at least 1 pregnant woman infected with HIV per 1000 women screened.[8-11] Universal opt-out HIV retesting for all pregnant women is recommended based on a 2005 CDC-sponsored study that reported *all women who seroconverted* during pregnancy denied new sexual partners, alcohol, or illicit drug use.[8]

Rapid HIV testing has a sensitivity and specificity close to 100%; however, the positive predictive value depends on the prevalence of the disease. After a positive screening test, either a positive HIV 1/2 antigen/antibody fourth-generation test or detectable HIV viral load establishes an HIV diagnosis. The window period for diagnosis for fourth-generation tests and the antigen tests is 11 days to 1 month, and they take 2 days to 2 weeks to get results. In comparison, the rapid test has a window period of 3 months, and the results are available within 20 minutes.[3] Once an established diagnosis of HIV is made during pregnancy, the focus is prevention of maternal-to-child transmission and treatment of the woman in a multidisciplinary fashion. Please see **Box 1** for key features of care of HIV-infected pregnant patients.

Box 1
Key principles when considering screening for human immunodeficiency virus during pregnancy

1. Universal screening for HIV is recommended at the first prenatal visit for all women.

2. Opt-out HIV screening is recommended.

3. Repeat HIV screening in the third trimester is recommended for all high-risk women.

4. For women who present in active labor with unknown HIV status, a rapid HIV test should be performed on arrival.

ANTEPARTUM TREATMENT

Once a diagnosis of HIV infection is established in a pregnant woman, multidisciplinary care should begin immediately. There should be close collaboration between HIV care providers, obstetric providers, pediatric providers, and social service providers. *The goal of treatment of HIV in pregnancy is to maximally suppress viral replication and viral load as well as providing pre-exposure prophylaxis to the fetus*[6,7,12] (**Box 2**).

Aneuploidy screening should be routinely offered to all HIV-infected pregnant women. Invasive testing, such as an amniocentesis, chorionic villus sampling, and cordocentesis, may place the fetus at increased risk of transmission of HIV.[6,7,13] However, to date no transmission of HIV has been reported after amniocentesis in women taking cART with suppressed viral loads. If an amniocentesis is determined to be necessary, then it should be ideally performed after initiation of cART and when the viral load is undetectable.[7]

In addition, case managers and social workers should be readily available for HIV-infected women throughout their pregnancy in order to enhance compliance

---

Box 2
Initial prenatal evaluation

Complete medical, obstetric, and gynecologic history

Evaluation for symptoms of AIDS

- Fever, night sweats, weight loss, a new and persistent cough, diarrhea, refractory vaginal candidiasis, oral candidiasis, and new outbreaks of herpes

Complete physical examination, including evaluation for disease progression

- In women with CD4 count <200 cells/mm³, should include evaluation of thrush, herpes simplex virus, lymphadenopathy, or rash

Detailed HIV history, including suspected transmission route, previous antiretroviral use, previous AIDS-defining illnesses, current prophylaxis regimen

Assessment of need for prophylaxis against opportunistic infections

Assess psychosocial supportive care needs, mental health services, substance abuse treatment, and smoking cessation

Baseline laboratory evaluation

CD4 cell count

- Initial visit & every 3 mo throughout pregnancy

Resistance testing before starting cART

- HLA-B5701 if abacavir use is anticipated

Complete blood count with differential, complete metabolic panel

- Repeat each trimester

Tuberculosis screening

Early diabetes screening of patients with a history of gestational diabetes, family history of diabetes, or those with prolonged use of protease inhibitor exposure

Plasma HIV RNA levels (viral load)

- Initial visit, 2–4 wk after initiating or changing cART regimen, monthly, and then again at 34–36 wk gestation
- Recommendations regardless of starting viral load

Hepatitis B surface antigen and antibody

Hepatitis C antibody

Concomitant sexually transmitted disease testing, including syphilis, gonorrhea, chlamydia, trichomoniasis

Evaluation of immunization status of rubella, varicella, hepatitis B, and pneumococci

Papanicolaou test and high-risk HPV testing

with medical visits and cART adherence. Women should be educated about HIV and prevention of maternal-to-child transmission and the importance of cART.[12] This discussion should include the risk of transmission and factors that modify that risk, the risks and benefits of cART, and safe sex practices with condoms.[7]

Given the gravity of the diagnosis of HIV, there is a significant risk of development of depression in these women. When left untreated, depression can lead to poor cART adherence and ultimately a shortened life span and increased risk of maternal-to-child transmission. Many HIV-infected women are also victims of trauma and intimate-partner violence, which contributes to the increased risk of posttraumatic stress disorder, depression, anxiety, and substance use disorder.[14]

ANTIRETROVIRAL DRUGS DURING PREGNANCY

Current recommendations are that antiretroviral treatment should be initiated for all HIV-infected pregnant women at their initial prenatal visit or as early as possible in pregnancy. The earlier a women can be started on a highly effective cART regimen that will decrease her HIV viral load to undetectable levels, the sooner the risk of perinatal transmission can be reduced and the likelihood of cesarean delivery can be reduced.[6,13] Antepartum and intrapartum antiretroviral treatment and prophylaxis, as well as infant prophylaxis, are recommended in combination because antiretroviral medications reduce perinatal transmission by several mechanisms, including lowering the viral load and providing pre-exposure and postexposure prophylaxis to the infant.[13]

The importance of adherence to the cART regimen needs to be discussed at length and emphasized when counseling HIV-infected pregnant women.[13] A recent series of systematic reviews identified individual and contextual factors and health system barriers affecting cART initiation, adherence, and retention in HIV-infected pregnant women. They identified lower age, lower education level, HIV denial, concern cART will harm the child, misplacing/forgetting medication, use of drugs or alcohol, transportation problems, and negative attitudes of health workers as barriers to cART adherence. They also identified that lack of knowledge regarding prevention of maternal-to-child transmission was a barrier to initiation of cART.[15]

When selecting medications, the known benefits and known and unknown risks of antiretroviral medications in pregnancy should be discussed and considered carefully. The regimens in pregnancy typically contain at least 3 medications and are individualized to patients based on comorbidities, convenience, side effects, drug interactions, resistance testing, and potential teratogenic effects.[6,13] The goal of cART is to produce at least a 1-log drop in viral load over 4 to 8 weeks. If such a response is not seen, then initial or repeat resistance testing should be performed as well as a thorough investigation of medication adherence and a search for potential drug interactions.[13,16] cART regimens in pregnancy typically consist of 2 nucleoside reverse transcriptase inhibitors and either a non-nucleoside reverse transcriptase inhibitor (NNRTI) or a protease inhibitor.[6] The US Department of Health and Human Services (HHS) has a multidisciplinary panel of experts in HIV care who are responsible for updating the HIV guidelines. The HHS Panel on Treatment of Pregnant Women with HIV Infection and Prevention of Perinatal Transmission publishes: *Recommendations for Use of Antiretroviral Drugs in Pregnant Women with HIV Infection and Interventions to Reduce Perinatal HIV Transmission in The United States.*[13]

The Panel categorizes antiretroviral medications for use in pregnancy as follows: preferred, alternative, use in special circumstances, not recommended, or insufficient data to recommend. Please see **Table 1** for the antiretroviral regimens recommended in pregnancy.

Table 1
Antiretroviral regimen recommendations in pregnancy

Drug	Comments	Dosing
Preferred 2-NRTI backbones		
ABC/3TC Epzicom	• Available as FDC • ABC not used in women who test positive for HLA-B*5701 because of risk of hypersensitivity reaction • High placental transfer	ABC (Ziagen): 300 mg twice daily or 600 mg once daily ABC/3TC: 1 tablet twice daily (600 mg ABC, 300 mg 3TC)

TDF/FTC
  Truvada
Or
TDF/3TC
  Viread & Epivir
	• TDF/FTC available as FDC
	• TDF/FTC or TDF with separate 3TC can be administered once daily
	• TDF has potential renal toxicity, take caution in patients with renal insufficiency
		TDF/FTC: 1 tablet once daily
		TDF & 3TC: 2 tablets once daily (300 mg each)

Preferred PI regimens		

ATV/RTV
  Reyataz + Norvir
    + 2-NRTI preferred backbone
	• Once-daily administration
	• Extensively used in pregnancy
	• Can lead to maternal hyperbilirubinemia, no reports of clinically significant neonatal hyperbilirubinemia
	• RTV boosting in pregnancy recommended
		ATV: 300 mg daily +
		RTV: 100 mg daily

Preferred integrase inhibitor regimen		

RAL
  Isentress
    + 2-NRTI preferred backbone
	• Rapid viral load reduction
	• Potential role in treatment of women who present late to care for initial therapy
	• Twice-daily dosing
	• If concerns of compliance, a PI regimen preferred to minimize risk of resistance
		RAL: 400 mg twice daily

Alternative initial regimens in pregnancy: regimens with efficacy in adults but with limited use in pregnancy, incomplete teratogenicity data, or associated with dosing, formulation, toxicity, or interaction issues		
Alternative 2-NRTI backbones		
ZDV/3TC Combivir	• Available as FDC • Most experience with use in pregnancy • Twice-daily dosing • Increased potential for hematologic toxicity	ZDV/3TC: 1 tablet twice daily
PI regimens		
LPV/RTV Kaletra	• Abundant use in pregnancy • More nausea than with preferred regimens • Twice-daily dosing • Recommend dose increase in third trimester	LPV/RTV: 400 mg LPV and 100 mg RTV twice daily Recommend increasing to 600 mg LPV plus 150 mg RTV twice daily during third trimester

(continued on next page)

Table 1 (continued)		
Drug	Comments	Dosing
NNRTI regimen		
EFV Sustiva OR (EFV/FTC/TDF) Atripla + preferred 2-NRTI backbone	• Concern regarding possible increase in birth defects in primate studies • Recommended in women who require drugs with significant interactions with PIs • Screen carefully for antenatal and postpartum depression • To be continued in women who begin pregnancy with good viral suppression on EFV	EFV: 600-mg tablet once daily at bedtime EFV/FTC/TDF: 1 tablet once daily at bedtime

The preferred regimens and drug combinations are designated as such for initiation of ART in ART-naïve pregnant women based on clinical data that show optimal safety and efficacy profiles in adults and are not associated with teratogenicity.

Abbreviations: ABC, abacavir; ART, antiretroviral treatment; EFV, efavirenz; FDC, fixed-drug combination; FTC, emtricitabine; LPV, lopinavir; NRTI, nucleoside reverse transcriptase inhibitor; PI, protease inhibitor; RAL, Raltegravir; RTV, ritonavir; TDF, tenofovir disoproxil fumarate; 3TC, lamivudine; ZDV, zidovudine.

Data from Refs.[6,13,17]

An example of a preferred cART regimen to initiate in HIV-infected pregnant women is emtricitabine/tenofovir, atazanavir, and ritonavir.[13] The main difference in cART regimens in pregnant women compared with nonpregnant women is the lack of recommendation for integrase inhibitor–based regimens for pregnant women. There is increasing literature about the safety of raltegravir in pregnancy, especially in women with a high viral load because of its ability to rapidly suppress viremia.[6] Because of the increasing body of literature and safety profile, raltegravir is the preferred integrase inhibitor for use in antiretroviral-naïve pregnant women. In addition, recent case series have reported rapid declines in viral load with the use of raltegravir late in pregnancy to achieve viral suppression and reduce the risk of perinatal transmission.[13] More data on the use of newer integrase inhibitors (many of which are administered once daily and/or part of a single combination pill) in pregnancy are needed. Lamivudine/zidovudine was the mainstay for nucleoside reverse transcriptase inhibitor regimens in pregnancy; although it is still highly efficacious, especially in antiretroviral-naïve women, it requires twice-daily dosing and has higher rates of side effects (nausea, headache, and neutropenia) and, therefore, is now considered an alternative regimen.[13,17]

Because of an ongoing debate regarding efavirenz, it is still categorized as an alternative NNRTI medication. There was significant concern regarding the potential teratogenicity of efavirenz. Previous studies linked efavirenz use with increased risks of neural tube defects. A recent large meta-analysis did not find an increased risk of neural tube defects in women who used efavirenz in the first trimester. Therefore, the current perinatal guidelines, as written by the panel, do not include a restriction of use of this medication before 8 weeks' gestation, despite the insert in the packaging saying otherwise.[18] Both the British HIV Association and the WHO support the use of efavirenz throughout pregnancy.[13,17]

The newest recommendations are that cART should be initiated as soon as possible in pregnant women even if the antiretroviral resistance testing results are not yet available.[13] Clinicians may consider starting a protease inhibitor–based cART regimen when resistance-testing results are not available because resistance to protease inhibitors is less common than resistance to NNRTIs in antiretroviral-naïve women.[6,13]

In general, HIV-infected women who enter pregnancy on a stable cART regimen should continue the cART regimen without adjustment. Discontinuation or disruption of cART can lead to viremia and increase the risk of HIV transmission.[6] With the advent of new antiretroviral medications, women may enter pregnancy on cART regimens that include antiretroviral medication with a paucity of data with regard to use in pregnancy. Viral suppression in pregnancy is of the utmost importance for both maternal health and prevention of perinatal transmission; therefore, continuation of these regimens is generally recommended. Consultation with an HIV perinatal specialist is recommended when considering altering cART regimens in pregnancy.[13]

Lastly, clinicians should inform HIV-infected pregnant women that there may be a small increased risk of preterm birth in those women who receive cART.[13] However, HIV treatment should not be withheld because of this possible complication. In addition, recent studies have found that certain cART regimens may be associated with low-birth-weight and small-for-gestational-age infants.[13] The panel compiled 27 studies from around the world that investigated the associated preterm delivery risk with cART regimens. They found that 13 of the 27 studies found an association between preterm delivery and protease inhibitor–based cART regimens. Specifically, the use of ritonavir to boost a protease inhibitor–based cART regimen was associated with preterm delivery.[13] Although clinicians and women should be aware of these possible increased risks, the benefits of cART regimens in pregnancy far outweigh these risks and, therefore, should be initiated and continued as recommended earlier.

INTRAPARTUM TREATMENT
Antiretroviral Management

It is well established that intravenous zidovudine given intrapartum significantly prevents the transmission of HIV to the fetus during delivery in a women with HIV viremia.[13] However, newer guidelines suggest that intravenous zidovudine may not be required for all HIV-infected women. The most recent guidelines published by the Panel on Treatment of HIV-Infected Pregnant Women and Prevention of Perinatal Transmission reports that intravenous zidovudine is not required for HIV-infected women with a viral load less than 1000 copies per milliliter in late pregnancy or near delivery (typically between 34–36 weeks) and for whom there are no concerns about adherence to their cART, as further reduction in perinatal transmission is unlikely.[13] However, intravenous zidovudine should be administered to HIV-infected women with a viral load greater than 1000 copies per milliliter regardless of adherence to cART.[13] Irrespective of viral load, a clinician may elect to use intravenous zidovudine intrapartum based on their clinical judgment. In addition, the most recent viral load should drive the decision for mode of delivery. Despite whether an HIV-infected woman has been shown to have resistance to zidovudine, it should still be used intrapartum, as it has unique properties that prevent perinatal transmission.[7,13]

Route of Delivery

Women with a viral load greater than 1000 copies per milliliter should be counseled on the benefit of a scheduled cesarean delivery to prevent transmission. In this case, intravenous zidovudine should be started 3 hours before cesarean delivery. The ACOG recommends that scheduled cesarean delivery for viral load greater than 1000 should be performed at 38 weeks' gestation to reduce the risk of onset of labor before delivery.[19] In women with a viral load less than 1000 copies per milliliter, the trial of labor and vaginal delivery do not significantly increase the risk of transmission. All antepartum cART should be continued on schedule throughout labor and delivery.[7,13]

In contrast, induction and scheduled cesarean delivery for obstetric reasons should be performed at standard times for these obstetric indications in women with a viral load less than 1000 copies per milliliter. In women with a known viral load greater than 1000 copies per milliliter or unknown viral load who present in active labor or with ruptured membranes, there is not enough evidence to determine whether cesarean delivery reduces perinatal HIV transmission; thus, the management of these patients should be individualized. In a woman who presents in active labor with unknown HIV status and then is found to be positive on rapid HIV testing, intravenous zidovudine should be promptly started and cesarean delivery should be considered.[6,7,13] Please see **Table 2** for a summary of these recommendations.

During labor or induction of labor, it is recommended to avoid any interventions that may increase maternal-to-fetal blood exchange unless there is a clear obstetric indication, including the use of a fetal scalp electrode, assisted delivery with forceps or vacuum extractor, and/or episiotomy.[6] New data suggest that the duration of rupture of membranes in women with a viral load less than 1000 copies per milliliter may not be associated with an increased risk of perinatal transmission. Therefore, in women on cART with viral suppression at term with ruptured membranes, obstetric care should be normalized. This recommendation also applies to artificial rupture of membranes, as new studies have determined that in the setting of cART and viral suppression, there is no increased risk of perinatal transmission. Therefore, artificial rupture of membranes can be safely performed for obstetric indications in those women with a viral load less than 1000 copies per milliliter who have been adherent with cART.[13] *When the infant is delivered, the infant should immediately be bulb suctioned and all maternal secretions should we washed off as soon as possible.*[7]

Table 2
Summary of intrapartum antiretroviral recommendations

Clinical Situation	Mode of Delivery	IV AZT	Timing of Delivery	cART
VL <1000, no obstetric indication for cesarean delivery, no antepartum cART adherence concerns	Vaginal delivery	Not required	Spontaneous or earlier for maternal/fetal indications	Continue oral cART during labor and delivery
VL <1000, no antepartum cART adherence concerns, obstetric indication for cesarean delivery	Cesarean delivery	Not required	≥39 wk or earlier for maternal/fetal indications	Continue oral cART during delivery
VL >1000	Cesarean delivery	Required	38 wk or earlier for maternal/fetal indications	Continue cART during delivery
VL unknown	Cesarean delivery	Required	38 wk or earlier for maternal/fetal indications	Continue cART during delivery if previously started

Abbreviations: ARV, antiretroviral; AZT, zidovudine; IV, intravenous; VL, viral load.

In challenging clinical scenarios regarding the perinatal care of HIV-infected women, such as preterm premature rupture of membranes, the National Perinatal HIV Hotline is available to provide evidence-based expert advice.[7,13] The National Perinatal HIV Hotline (888-448-8765) is a federally funded service and provides free clinical consultations to providers caring for HIV-infected pregnant women and their infants, especially for difficult cases.[13]

NEONATAL AND POSTPARTUM TREATMENT

The postpartum period is crucial for maternal and infant health, especially the ongoing prevention of HIV transmission to the infant. It is recommended that all HIV-exposed infants should receive postpartum antiretroviral prophylaxis to further reduce the risk of HIV transmission. *Infants should begin antiretroviral prophylaxis as soon as possible following delivery, ideally within 6 to 12 hours of birth.*[6,7,13] The standard of care for term infants born to mothers who received cART during pregnancy and maintained a viral suppression includes 4 weeks of oral zidovudine.[13] In all other situations, a 6-week course of oral zidovudine is recommended.[6,13] Based on several maternal and infant factors, some infants are at higher risk of HIV transmission after birth; in these cases, combination prophylaxis is recommended for at least 6 weeks. These risk factors include a lack of maternal antepartum or intrapartum antiretroviral treatment, only intrapartum zidovudine treatment received, or in women who received both antepartum and intrapartum antiretroviral treatment but had a detectable viral load, especially in those who underwent a vaginal delivery, women with known antiretroviral-drug resistance, or unknown HIV status at delivery.[6,13] Currently, there is no consensus on the ideal antiretroviral regimen for high-risk infants; however, several clinical trials are currently underway to address this issue. *The current recommendations for high-risk infants are as follows: 6 weeks of oral zidovudine plus 3 doses of nevirapine at prophylactic doses given during the first week of life, first dose at birth to 48 hours, the second dose at 48 hours after the first dose, and the third dose 96 hours after the second dose.* Additionally, some providers recommend a 3-drug infant antiretroviral regimen using a treatment dose of zidovudine, lamivudine, and nevirapine. This regimen is currently under investigation.[13] In infants born to mothers who were adherent to their cART regimen but did not achieve viral suppression, a discussion with the family and a pediatric HIV specialist to decide whether combination antiretroviral prophylaxis is appropriate. Additionally, in infants born to women with an unknown HIV status, if rapid testing is positive, antiretroviral prophylaxis should be started until the results of confirmatory testing are obtained.[13] *Again, the National Perinatal HIV Hotline (888-448-8765) can provide free clinical consultations to providers caring for at-risk HIV-exposed infants, especially for difficult cases.* They can also provide referrals to local or regional pediatric HIV specialists.[13] See **Table 3** for a summary of these recommendations. Please see the recommendations produced by the Panel on Treatment of HIV-Infected Pregnant Women and Prevention of Perinatal Transmission for additional dosing regimens based on weight and gestational age.[13]

Breastfeeding is contraindicated in women with HIV in the United States because of the high potential for HIV transmission through breast milk.[3,7,13] However, in resource-limited settings where a safe alternative to breastfeeding is not available to sufficiently replace breastfeeding, exclusive breastfeeding is preferable.[7] In resource-rich settings, such as the United States, exclusive formula feeding is the recommendation for all HIV-infected women and infants. Choosing not to breastfeed can be met with social, familial, and cultural barriers for many women; therefore, clinicians should be cognizant of this and be sure to provide adequate support to these women. It is

Table 3
Recommendations for antiretroviral prophylaxis for high-risk infants

Clinical Scenario	Recommendations
Infant born to a woman who did not receive antepartum cART or only received intrapartum AZT prophylaxis	6-wk oral AZT + 3 doses of nevirapine (at birth, 48 h after first dose, and 96 h after second dose), consultation with pediatric HIV specialist
Infant born to a woman who received antepartum cART but did not achieve optimal viral suppression	6-wk oral AZT + consider combination prophylaxis after consultation with parents and pediatric HIV specialist
Infant born to a woman with ARV-resistant virus	Unknown optimal prophylactic regimen, consult pediatric HIV specialist, 6-wk oral AZT + consider combination prophylaxis based on maternal ARV-resistance pattern

Abbreviations: ARV, antiretroviral; AZT, zidovudine.

also important to address recommendations against breastfeeding antenatally so that any possible barriers to formula feeding can be addressed at that time.[13]

CONTRACEPTION

Following delivery, women infected with HIV should be connected with an HIV specialist for ongoing care. In addition, these women need to receive counseling regarding contraception and how to effectively prevent unintended pregnancies and ongoing transmission to sexual partners. The CDC and ACOG recommend that all women with HIV be offered effective and appropriate contraception to prevent undesired pregnancies. Long-acting reversible contraceptives (LARCs), including implants and intrauterine devices, serve as excellent contraceptive options for HIV-infected women. LARC devices should be offered in the immediate postpartum period or in conjunction with a bridge to their postpartum visit. LARC devices can aid in pregnancy spacing and optimization of maternal health and cART adherence.[13] No contraceptive methods are contraindicated in HIV-positive women; however, special considerations about drug interactions with antiretroviral regimens should be discussed. For specific safety profiles and additional information, please reference the CDC's medical eligibility criteria.[20] Additionally, patients should be counseled regarding the importance of dual protection, concomitant use of condoms, and additional contraception methods.[21]

SUMMARY

Eliminating maternal-to-child transmission of HIV is a top priority for the WHO, CDC, ACOG and many other humanitarian and medical associations. Current recommendations for treatment of pregnant women who are HIV infected can reduce the rate of maternal-to-child transmission to less than 1%. Continued research is needed to optimize cART during pregnancy and to reach a goal of zero maternal-to-child HIV transmissions.

REFERENCES

1. Centers for Disease Control and Prevention. HIV among women. Available at: https://www.cdc.gov/hiv/group/gender/women/index.html. Accessed March 15, 2017.

2. Sidibe M, Goosby M. Countdown to zero: global plan towards the elimination of new HIV infections among children by 2015 and keeping their mothers alive, vol. 1. Switzerland: Joint United Nations Programme on HIV/AIDS; 2011. p. 6–10.

3. Rimawi B, Haddad L, Badell L, et al. Management of HIV infection during pregnancy in the United States: updated evidence-based recommendations and future potential practices. Infect Dis Obstet Gynecol 2016;2016:7594306.

4. Centers for Disease Control and Prevention. Elimination of mother-to-child HIV transmission (EMCT) in the United States. 2017. Available at: http://www.cdc.gov/hiv/group/gender/pregnantwomen/emct.html. Accessed March 15, 2017.

5. Camacho-Gonzales A, Kingbo M, Boylan A, et al. Missed opportunities for prevention of mother-to-child transmission in the United States: a review of cases from the state of Georgia, 2005-2012. AIDS 2015;29(12):1511–5.

6. Chappell C, Cohn SE. Prevention of perinatal transmission of human immunodeficiency virus. Infect Dis Clin North Am 2014;28(4):529–47.

7. Short AC. HIV. In: Berghella V, editor. Maternal-fetal evidence based guidelines. 2nd edition. London: Informa Healthcare; 2012. p. 236–44.

8. Liao C, Golden C, Anderson J, et al. Missed opportunities for repeat HIV testing in pregnancy: implications for elimination of mother-to-child transmission in the United States. AIDS Patient Care STDs 2017;31(1):20–6.

9. Committee opinion no: 635: prenatal and perinatal human immunodeficiency virus testing: expanded recommendations. Obstet Gynecol 2015;125(6):1544–7.

10. Centers for Disease Control and Prevention. State HIV testing laws: consent and counseling requirements. 2013. Available at: http://www.cdc.gov/hiv/policies/law/states/testing.html. Accessed March 22, 2017.

11. Centers for Disease Control and Prevention. An opt-out approach to HIV screening. 2016. Available at: http://www.cdc.gov/hiv/group/gender/pregnantwomen/opt-out.html. Accessed March 22, 2017.

12. Scott G, Brogly S, Muenz D, et al. Missed opportunities for prevention of mother-to-child transmission of human immunodeficiency virus. Obstet Gynecol 2017; 129(4):621–8.

13. Panel on treatment of HIV-infected pregnant women and prevention of perinatal transmission. Recommendations for use of antiretroviral drugs in pregnant HIV-1-infected women for maternal health and interventions to reduce perinatal HIV transmission in the United States. 2016. Available at: http://aidsinfo.nih.gov/contentfiles/lvguidelines/PerinatalGL.pdf. Accessed March 22, 2017.

14. Rimawi B, Smith S, Badell M, et al. HIV and reproductive healthcare in pregnant and postpartum HIV-infected women: adapting successful strategies. Future Virol 2016;11(8):577–81.

15. Hodgson I, Plummer M, Konopka S, et al. A systematic review of individual and contextual factors affecting ART initiation, adherence, and retention for HIV-infected pregnant and postpartum women. PLoS One 2014;9(11):e111421.

16. Mandelbrot L, Tubiana R, Le Chenadec J, et al. No perinatal HIV-1 transmission from women with effective antiretroviral therapy starting before conception. Clin Infect Dis 2015;61(11):1715–25.

17. Antiretroviral Pregnancy Registry Steering Committee. Antiretroviral pregnancy registry international interim report for 1 January 1989 through 31 July 2016. Wilmington (NC): Registry Coordinating Center; 2016. Available at: http://www.APRegistry.com.

18. Ford N, Calmy A, Mofenson L. Safety of efavirenz in the first trimester of pregnancy: an updated systematic review and meta-analysis. AIDS 2011;25(18): 2301–4.

19. Committee on Obstetric Practice. ACOG committee opinion 234: scheduled cesarean delivery and the prevention of vertical transmission of HIV Fnfection. Obstet Gynecol 2000;73(3):279–81.

20. Centers for Disease Control and Prevention. US medical eligibility criteria (US MEC) for contraceptive use. 2016. Available at: http://www.cdc.gov/reproductivehealth/contraception/mmwr/mec/summary.html. Accessed June 8, 2017.

21. Practice bulletin no. 167 summary: gynecologic care for women and adolescents with human immunodeficiency virus. Obstet Gynecol 2016;128(4):920–2.

Relationships Between Perinatal Interventions, Maternal-Infant Microbiomes, and Neonatal Outcomes

Gregory Valentine, MD[a,b], Derrick M. Chu, BSc[c,d,e], Christopher J. Stewart, PhD[f], Kjersti M. Aagaard, MD, PhD[c,d,e,f,g,h],*

KEYWORDS

- Microbiome • Perinatal • Pregnancy • Preterm birth • Prematurity • Neonate

KEY POINTS

- Premature neonates have a delay in the colonization of "healthy" commensal bacteria and a propensity toward harboring pathogenic bacteria, an attribute that may be a key etiology for the premature neonate's increased susceptibility to develop necrotizing enterocolitis or other infections.
- Mode of delivery does not seem to substantially alter the infant microbiome. Instead, only formula feeding and maternal diet have lasting impacts on the infant microbiome.
- The fetus does not lie in a sterile environment. It is likely that in utero exposure to microbes and/or a microbe's free DNA leads to fetal immune system priming and regulation.
- The maternal diet is a potent modifier of both the mother's and the infant's microbiome. Further studies are needed to evaluate the effects of the maternal diet on the breast milk microbiome.
- Dysbiosis of the maternal microbiome is currently a leading hypothesis underlying the etiology of preterm birth. Therefore, further studies evaluating the microbiome can help elucidate potential treatments for preventing preterm birth—the leading cause of death throughout the world in children under 5 years of age.

Potential Conflicts of Interest: None.
Funding: None.
[a] Department of Pediatrics, Baylor College of Medicine, 1 Baylor Plaza, Houston, TX 77030, USA; [b] Division of Neonatology, Texas Children's Hospital, West Tower, Suite B.06177, Mail Stop: BCM320, Houston, TX 77030, USA; [c] Department of Obstetrics and Gynecology, Division of Maternal-Fetal Medicine, Baylor College of Medicine, Texas Children's Hospital, 1 Baylor Plaza, Houston, TX 77401, USA; [d] Translational Biology and Molecular Medicine, Baylor College of Medicine, 1 Baylor Plaza, Houston, TX 77030, USA; [e] Medical Scientist Training Program, Baylor College of Medicine, Houston, TX, USA; [f] Alkek Center for Metagenomics and Microbiome Research, Baylor College of Medicine, 1 Baylor Plaza, Houston, TX 77030, USA; [g] Department of Molecular and Human Genetics, Baylor College of Medicine, 1 Baylor Plaza, Houston, TX 77030, USA; [h] Department of Molecular and Cell Biology, Baylor College of Medicine, 1 Baylor Plaza, Houston, TX 77030, USA
* Corresponding author. Department of Obstetrics and Gynecology, Division of Maternal-Fetal Medicine, Baylor College of Medicine, Texas Children's Hospital, 1 Baylor Plaza, Houston, TX 77401.
E-mail address: aagaardt@bcm.edu

Clin Perinatol 45 (2018) 339–355
https://doi.org/10.1016/j.clp.2018.01.008
0095-5108/18/© 2018 The Authors. Published by Elsevier Inc. This is an open access article under the CC BY-NC-ND license (http://creativecommons.org/licenses/by-nc-nd/4.0/).

INTRODUCTION

The human body is host to a diverse array of largely commensal bacteria, which collectively across all body niches comprise an individual's personal microbiome. The Human Microbiome Project, completed in 2012, sought to define reference "healthy" microbiomes by evaluating and characterizing the microbiome across multiple body sites in healthy individuals of different races and ethnicities in the United States. Overall, this robust, multicenter study found that niche specificity, bacterial diversity, and microbial gene carriage patterns far surpassed what was previously thought.[1–4] Importantly, commensal microbiota are more than simple bystanders because their presence and unique metabolic processes are essential components of our own physiology. Moreover, it is thought that the nature, state, and composition of the microbiome are related to (and likely contribute to) the development of several common human diseases. Dysbiosis of the human microbiome, defined as an aberrant microbial community, has been associated with the development of diabetes,[5–8] inflammatory bowel disease,[9–13] obesity,[14,15] metabolic syndrome,[16] and autoimmune disorders,[15,17,18–29] although causation has yet to be established.

In keeping with the developmental origins of health and disease hypothesis,[30–37] it is thought that the role of the microbiome in disease pathogenesis likely initiates in early life during key developmental windows, predisposing an individual to develop disease later in life when and if exposed to the right environmental triggers. Mice raised in the relative or complete absence of bacteria (gnotobiotic and germ-free mice) have immune deficits that cannot be restored completely unless the infant and mother are exposed to bacteria in pregnancy and early life.[38,39] For these reasons, understanding when and how the neonatal microbiome is first established, how it develops in the immediate postnatal period, and what external factors (eg, mode of delivery and breastfeeding) modify its trajectory has been a recent focus of the field.

Recent literature surrounding the perinatal microbiome has seen increased attention and focus. This article seeks to consolidate and evaluate the medical literature assessing common perinatal interventions, their effects on the infant microbiome, and their potential benefit to neonatal outcomes. First, pregnancy and the potential contribution of the maternal microbiome to preterm risk as well as the neonate's microbiome are discussed. Second, common perinatal interventions are explored, such as intrapartum antibiotic prophylaxis, mode of delivery, timing of delivery (premature vs term), hospitalization, and use of probiotics in both the mother and neonate. Finally, breastfeeding versus formula feeding is discussed and the impact each may have on neonatal outcomes.

PERINATAL AND POSTNATAL INTERVENTIONS AND THEIR IMPACT ON THE NEONATAL MICROBIOME

Although many perinatal interventions occur daily among the more than 4 million US births annually, including the use of probiotics or intrapartum antibiotic prophylaxis for group B streptococcus, and may seem relatively benign, the broad-reaching and longer-term impacts are unknown (**Fig. 1**). By contrast, broad-spectrum microbial interventions or manipulations have been studied a bit deeper and there is a bit more known about their impact on microbial communities, their structure, and their function. This article discusses the impact of preterm birth, common perinatal interventions, their influence on the fetal and neonatal microbiome, and the potential short-term and long-term neonatal outcomes.

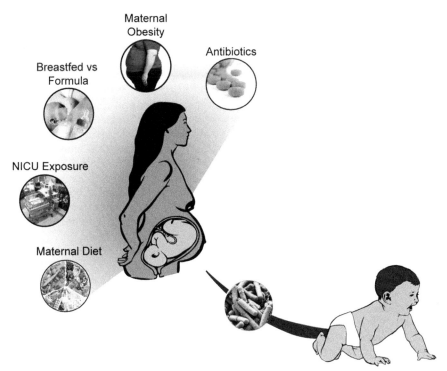

Fig. 1. Potential influences of the developing microbiome during pregnancy and early neonatal and infant life.

Preterm Delivery

Prematurity and the reasons leading to a preterm birth have lasting effects on both the neonatal microbiome and both the short-term and long-term outcomes in those neonates compared with delivery at term. As discussed previously, the maternal microbiome is essential in immune system priming of the fetus. Premature neonates are at higher risk for infection and intestinal problems, among other illnesses, owing to the lack of sufficient development of host tissues and immaturity of immune regulation at birth. Further issues may relate to a lack of time for the full effects of the in utero interactions with the maternal microbiome and/or a difference in the premature neonate's microbiome compared with the term neonate.

Thus, one key question to evaluate is, Does the microbiome differ between neonates born at term compared with those born preterm? One group of investigators from Spain evaluated 21 premature neonates' intestinal microbiota during the first 3 months of life and compared them to term, exclusively breastfed, vaginally delivered neonates. Premature neonates had increased levels of facultative anaerobic microorganisms and decreased levels of strict anaerobes, such as *Bifidobacterium*, *Bacteroides*, and *Atopobium*.[40] It is difficult, however, to assess if the changes they found are due to varying levels of gut maturity, lack of exclusive human milk feeding (all preterm infants included in this study received mixed feeding), or other associations with hospitalization and/or premature birth itself, for example, antibiotics. Furthering the idea that the microbiome is different among premature neonates compared with term neonates, other investigators have shown that very-low-birthweight neonates have decreased diversity of their microbiota, which may be due to living in a hospital environment itself.[24,41–43]

Not only do premature neonates have a delay in the colonization of "healthy" commensal bacteria, such as *Bifidobacterium*, but also the premature neonate's microbiome contains higher quantities of pathogenic bacteria and readily loses the richness and abundance first seen at birth. *Klebsiella, Weissella, Clostridium, Enterobacteriaceae, Enterococcaceae, Streptococcaceae*, and *Staphylococcaceae* have all been found more commonly in premature neonates' microbiota than in neonates born at term.[44] Concurrent with these results, other investigators found increased levels of *K pneumonia* in the preterm infant microbiota, and *C difficile* was detected exclusively in the preterm infants.[40]

Thus, premature neonates are more prone to foster and harbor pathogenic bacteria rather than beneficial commensals, and the diversity and richness of their microbial communities first seen at birth simplifies days to weeks later and after periods of often intense interventions and isolation as well as antimicrobial therapy. This characteristic of prematurity (or its necessary interventions) may be one key reason why this age group has a higher likelihood of necrotizing enterocolitis (NEC) and other infectious maladies than term neonates.

The microbiome of preterm infants (eg, gestational age of 23–30 weeks) varies during the initial weeks of life, with dominance by *Escherichia, Klebsiella, Enterococcus*, and *Staphylococcus* dominant in the gut.[45] The presence of certain taxa do correlate, however, with increased gestational and postnatal age, for instance *Bifidobacterium*.[46] Colonization by *Bifidobacterium* is during the initial weeks of life in preterm infants is associated with protection from NEC[47] and late-onset sepsis.[48] Additional research is needed, however, to determine is this association is causal to the prevention of these diseases (eg, promotes gut maturation) or rather that colonization by *Bifidobacterium* simply reflects a more mature gut. Nonetheless, the potential to modify the preterm infant gut microbiome with probiotics is an area of active investigation. The most widely used probiotics in preterm infants are single or combination products consisting of *Lactobacillus* and *Bifidobacterium*. Overall, trials and meta-analyses in this area have shown conflicting findings in terms of NEC and sepsis diagnosis. Importantly, the receipt of probiotics results in shifts to both the gut microbiome and metabolome, with *Bifidobacterium* (but not *Lactobacillus*) able to colonize the gut of preterm infants long-term (even after discharge from the neonatal intensive care unit [NICU]).[49]

Mode of Delivery

Reported use of cesarean deliveries has been documented as early as the 1500s although its modern usage was not pioneered and promulgated until the mid-twentieth century after the discovery of penicillin.[50] Although 40 years ago, 1 in 20 births were delivered by cesarean, to date, that figure has climbed to nearly 1 in 3 in the United States. Obstetric guidelines put forth by the *American Journal of Obstetrics and Gynecology* (*AJOG*) outline specific indications for cesarean deliveries to ensure the health of the mother and her infant.[51,52] Although the risks to the mother in the immediate postoperative period and in future pregnancies are well documented, the long-term impact of a cesarean delivery on infant health and disease is not well understood. Numerous epidemiologic studies have inconsistently linked cesarean delivery with increased risk of allergy, metabolic syndrome, and obesity later in life,[53,54] although given their likely multifactorial and heterogeneous nature, it has been difficult to discern correlation versus causation.

The reported impact of cesarean delivery on the infant microbiome has been touted as the missing link between cesarean and future disease burden, resulting from a lack of exposure to the microbial inhabitants of the maternal vagina. As such, investigators have already begun piloting vaginal swabbing of cesarean-born infants as means of correcting microbial community deficits. It is unclear, however, if these efforts are as yet justifiable without clear evidence of mechanism or direct benefit in relevant animal models.[53] Furthermore, the data supporting an association between cesarean delivery and an altered infant microbiome may be confounded by several clinical confounders, including prematurity, antibiotic usage, and maternal diabetes status, among others. In a large clinical cohort of longitudinally sampled mothers and infants, the authors found that the infant microbiome at 6 weeks of age did not vary by virtue of mode of delivery when controlling for various clinical factors. Only formula feeding and maternal diet seemed to have a lasting impact on the infant microbiome at this age. Therefore, although the question of whether or not cesarean delivery has a substantial long-term impact on the infant microbiome and ultimately in disease pathogenesis is uncertain, it nevertheless remains advisable to limit the use of cesarean deliveries by adhering to the official guidelines put forth by *AJOG* and other equivalent professional societies.

HUMAN BREASTMILK AND FORMULA FEEDING

The capacity to exclusive breastfeed or formula feed can have extensive effects on the neonatal microbiome. Breast milk and formula contain different bioactive components. For instance, formula contains macronutrients, vitamins, and a few oligosaccharides but is absent of the highly diverse human milk oligosaccharides (HMOs). Breast milk, however, contains macronutrients, vitamins, numerous HMOs and other oligosaccharides, growth factors, immune cells, immunoglobulins, hormones, cytokines, and a microbiome. The question becomes, Which components of human milk alter the neonatal enteric microbiome?

At the end of the nineteenth century, the overall infant mortality in the first year of life was as high as 30%. Medical providers noticed that breastfed infants had a higher chance of survival and lower incidence of infectious diarrhea than formula-fed infants.[55] Researchers began looking at what in breast milk may be protecting these neonates from increased mortality. Investigators soon found that the feces of breastfed infants contained different bacteria from those of the bottle-fed cohort.[56] In 1926, Schonfeld[57] published findings of a growth-promoting factor for *Bifidobacterium bifidus,* a protective commensal, contained in breast milk. This "bifidus factor" was later confirmed to be HMOs.[58–62] Now, more than 100 different HMOs have been identified, and not every woman has the same production of HMOs.

HMOs, besides being the bifidus factor, have numerous health benefits for the neonate. Because HMOs are resistant to the acidity of the infant stomach, they reach the distal small intestine and colon intact and at high concentrations. *Bifidobacterium longum* subsp *infantis (B infantis)* grows especially well when HMOs are present in the neonatal intestine. The proliferation of *B infantis* helps prevent pathogenic bacteria replicating as they compete for a limited nutrient supply. Also, *B infantis* is known to produce short-chain fatty acids that favor the growth of commensals in niches that might otherwise be colonized by potentially pathogenic bacteria.[55,63] Moreover, HMOs prevent the adhesion of viral, bacterial, and protozoan pathogens from attaching to the enteric epithelium, and, thus, prevent enteric infections in the neonate.[64,65] Another protective attribute of HMOs is that they serve as decoy attachment receptors for pathogens, which can reduce infection rates.[66,67] In fact, HMOs may even block HIV entry via preventing the attachment of the virus to its entry receptor DC-SIGN, and it may explain why mother-to-child transmission of HIV through breastfeeding is inefficient, with up to 90% of infants not acquiring infections despite continuous exposure to the virus through the breastmilk.[68]

A MOMS MATERNAL DIET, HER MICROBIOME, AND ITS POTENTIAL IMPACT ON LONG-TERM INFANT HEALTH

The prevailing dogma indicates that the neonate is born sterile and only after delivery is the neonate populated by bacteria. Under this belief, the French pediatrician Henry Tissier professed in 1900, "The fetus lies in a sterile environment."[69] Both historical evidence and more contemporary evidence, however, have challenged the notion of a completely sterile intrauterine environment. In 1982, bacteria were found present in the placenta, which began the pursuit of other researchers to determine if this was accurate.[70] More recently, numerous groups using both conventional culturing techniques and contemporary 16S rRNA gene and/or metagenomic sequencing, have found evidence of bacteria in association with presumed "sterile" tissues of healthy term pregnancies, such as the placenta and amniotic fluid.[71–81] Therefore, not only may the developing fetus be exposed to bacteria earlier than believed but also detection of microbial DNA has been well established in neonates at birth as well as fetuses and placentae prior to birth. Presumably, these microbes originate from the mother, although the route through which these organisms can enter the intrauterine space is not clearly established.[82,83] The authors and other investigators leading this field, however, remain uncertain if the organisms are viable or if free DNA is being detected. Still, the observation of a nonsterile intrauterine environment by metagenomic and other measures indicates that the contribution of the maternal microbiome in pregnancy may be as important to the neonatal microbiome as the immediate postnatal period.

Evidence of the Maternal Microbiome Influencing Neonatal Development

The role of maternal exposures and the maternal microbiome in the community and functional establishment of the infant microbiome may also influence immune repertoire and functional development. To test this hypothesis, one study evaluated the impact of the maternal microbiome on the intestinal immune system development of the offspring. Gomez de Aguero and colleagues[84] devised an experiment in which germ-free pregnant mice were transiently colonized with a genetically engineered form of Escherichia coli, which does not persist in the murine intestine. The pregnant mice that were transiently colonized gave birth to pups who had increased intestinal innate lymphoid cells and mononuclear cells compared with controls. In addition, these same researchers further looked into the effects of maternal antibodies and maternal microbial molecular transfer on the priming of the fetal immune system. They found that the maternal microbiome and maternal antibodies promote transfer of noninfective microbial molecules to the fetus. These microbial molecules are believed to prime the neonatal innate immune system and prepare the fetus for the postnatal inundation of microbes that eventually colonize the neonatal intestine.[84] Thus, microbes are essential in priming the fetal immune system and preparing the fetus against the plethora of pathogens it will soon encounter after birth (**Fig. 2**).

The Impact of the Maternal Diet and Health on the Early Neonatal Microbiome

The maternal microbiome fluctuates throughout gestation and is associated with obesity, altered caloric density, and content of diet, and comorbidities, such as gestational diabetes. Emerging evidence suggests that many of these factors are associated with differences in the early neonatal microbiome, suggesting that the state of

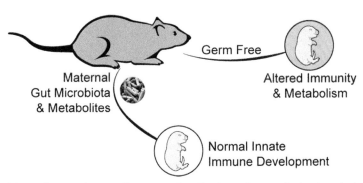

Fig. 2. Evidence from rodent studies suggesting the importance of microbes during gestational development for metabolic and immune health among offspring.

the maternal microbiome in pregnancy can have a considerable impact on what is transmitted to the neonate and how a microbiome ultimately develops. Diet is a potent modifying factor of the adult gut microbiome and consequently, in both animal models and human cohorts, the composition of the maternal diet in pregnancy is associated with distinct changes in the immediate neonatal gut microbiome as well.[83,85–87] In the Japanese macaque, a neonate born to a mother consuming a relatively high-fat diet in pregnancy was associated with a depletion of commensal species like *Campylobacter*, whereas in humans a maternal high-fat diet was associated with lower levels of *Bacteroides* species.[83,87] Work in animal models has demonstrated that commensal enteric species, in particular *Bacteroides*, are vital for normal gut immune development; therefore, lacking these beneficial microbes during this early developmental window is hypothesized to have a lasting effect on the neonate, ultimately predisposing the infant to atopy and other autoimmune disorders later on in life.[88–90]

The effect of maternal diet seems to extend beyond gestation. Research has shown that a high-fat diet leads to increased milk fat concentration and content compared with a high-carbohydrate diet.[91] No differences in milk production or quantity of milk, however, were observed. Therefore, neonates consuming breast milk from mothers with a high-fat diet consume higher energy intake, which can have potential effects on the development of their microbiome. Although it has not been studied, differences in the properties of the breastmilk likely affect which bacteria flourish in the neonatal microbiome, but further studies are needed to confirm this hypothesis. Along these same lines, the maternal diet may be associated with alterations in the breast milk microbiome. Unfortunately, there currently are no studies published evaluating this association. Investigations are currently exploring this hypothesis and will help understand any substantial impact the diet has on the breastmilk microbiome.

Maternal chronic conditions, such as gestational diabetes, overweight status, and obesity, are now known to have associated changes in the maternal microbiome. Bassols and colleagues[92] showed that women with gestational diabetes have a distinct placental microbiota profile, which includes a lower abundance of *Acinetobacter*, which was associated with higher glucose concentrations and a more proinflammatory maternal phenotype. In another study, Gomez-Arango and colleagues[93] evaluated the relationship between the enteric microbiome and metabolic hormones in overweight and obese pregnant women. Elevations of specific hormones, such as insulin, adipokine, and glucose-dependent insulinotropic polypeptide, were associated with elevations or reductions of specific bacteria. These results suggest that the enteric microbiome may have the potential to influence metabolism of the pregnant woman. The impact that these chronic conditions have on the fetus and neonate has not been extensively studied and is still open for investigation.

Antibiotic Administration

As discussed previously, the maternal microbiome potentially helps maintain pregnancy. Antibiotics disrupt and alter the microbiome. Thus, it is a natural progression of this thought that antibiotics and their effects on the microbiome can affect not only the mother but also the fetus. Antibiotics account for a majority of prescribed medications during pregnancy. One large Danish study showed that 51% of women had received 3 or more courses of antibiotics in the 4 years before, during, and after pregnancy.[94] In another study, maternal antibiotic administration was associated with a 30% increased risk of the offspring developing asthma.[94] Also, antibiotic usage in the pregnant woman has been linked to higher rates of neonatal illnesses, such as NEC, and increased rates of cerebral palsy and developmental delay.[95,96]

Further investigating the role of antibiotics on the maternal microbiome and neonatal outcomes, a murine model was devised. Pregnant, nonobese diabetic mice were given antibiotics. The offspring were observed to have immunologic changes in their intestines compared with those that did not receive antibiotics prenatally.[97] Furthermore, in humans, antibiotics during pregnancy alter the vaginal microbiome, which then lead to changes in the colonization and development of the neonatal microbiome[98] as well as an association with increased childhood obesity[99] and asthma.[94,100,101]

A systematic review published in 2013 showed that prophylactic antibiotics during the second or third trimesters in mothers with intact membranes do not decrease adverse outcomes and morbidity in pregnancy.[102] Also, even short-term antibiotic administration can have long-standing effects on the microbiome with possible associated changes in the immune system. In another study of 198 healthy term infants, maternal intrapartum antibiotic prophylaxis and birth method were documented. The infant gut microbiota was significantly different with intrapartum antibiotic prophylaxis exposure with persistence of the differences up to 12 months of age, with the findings found in both caesarean and vaginal deliveries.[103] An increase in pathogenic bacteria, such as *Enterococcus* and *Clostridium*, were over-represented at 3 months after the maternal intrapartum antibiotic prophylaxis. These findings support that antibiotics, even if for a short course, such as with intrapartum antibiotic prophylaxis, do have long-lasting effects on not only on the mother but also the neonate.

What, however, is the impact of antibiotics given directly to the neonates directly after birth, such as for early onset sepsis, on the neonatal microbiome? Premature neonates almost universally receive antibiotics at some point in their stay in the NICU, many in the first days of life. Gibson and colleagues[104] evaluated the impact of neonatal antibiotics on the development of antibiotic resistance, species diversity, and the prevalence of pathogenic bacteria predominating the neonatal microbiome. They found that antibiotics significantly decreased species richness and diversity in the intestinal microbiome.[104] In addition, multidrug-resistant bacterial members of the genera *Escherichia*, *Klebsiella*, and *Enterobacter* predominated the premature neonatal gastrointestinal microbiota.[104]

Brooks and colleagues[105] found in a separate study that bacteria from the neonate's surroundings in the NICU may be directly inoculated into the neonate and be the source of the pathogenic bacteria. For example, one infant had *K pneumonia* detected in the room on day of life 3, and it was then detected in the neonate's gut on day of life 9.[105] *Staphylococcus epidermidis*, *K pneumoniae*, *Bacteroides fragilis*, and *E coli* were found widely distributed throughout the rooms of the neonates, and they are all well-known pathogenic gastrointestinal colonizers.[105] Does the premature gut have a predisposition for these pathogenic colonizers due to the lack of time in utero, which helps facilitate the gut immune priming and development? Could early use of antibiotics predispose these neonates to these pathogens? Or, is it just simply living in the hospital environment? Likely, it is a combination of these factors, but further research is currently exploring these and other questions. Regardless, antibiotics given intrapartum as well as postpartum have direct effects on the neonatal microbiome.

THE MICROBIOME AND PRETERM BIRTH: FRIEND OR FOE?

Preterm birth is the leading cause of death among children under the age of 5 years old throughout the world, although its etiology is poorly understood and effective prevention and treatment options are lacking.[106] Although heterogeneous in nature, preterm birth is hypothesized to have an infectious etiology. A pathogenic organism, however, has yet to be attributed to preterm birth whereas antibiotic usage for a presumptive infection has not been shown to provide benefit.[107,108] The emergence of microbiome science applied to human health has led to the hypothesis that community level changes to the maternal microbiome is contributory to premature labor, rather than by infection of a specific microbe.[109] As such, efforts to characterize the "healthy" maternal microbiome of the vagina and other body sites has been prioritized, with the intent of identifying patterns of deviation associated with preterm birth risk.

During pregnancy, a woman's body undergoes both physical and hormonal changes across nearly every organ system to support fetal development, ready for parturition, and prepare for lactation in the postnatal period. Similarly, the maternal microbiome undergoes complementary rearrangements that are believed beneficial (a more thorough review of these changes can be found by Chu and colleagues[110]). The most notable of these changes with respect to preterm birth risk is the observation that in healthy pregnancies, the overall diversity of the vaginal microbiome tends to decrease into the third trimester, with *Lactobacillus* species tending to become the dominant member.[111] Within the vaginal milieu, lactobacillus species are believed to provide a natural defense against pathogenic overgrow within the vaginal canal by maintaining a low vaginal pH and may potentially explain the longstanding association of bacterial vaginosis with preterm birth.[112–115]

For these reasons, aberrant microbial communities, otherwise known as dysbiosis, in the vaginal microbiome has been hypothesized to contribute to premature labor, potentially by promoting proinflammatory cytokines that can be stimulated by such a derangement of the microbial milieu. There are conflicting data, however, on whether the vaginal microbiome has a characteristic profile that reliably predicts preterm birth.[116,117] Romero and colleagues[117] reported that the bacterial composition and abundance did not differ between mothers who delivered preterm compared with those who delivered at term whereas, conversely, DiGiulio and colleagues[116] reported that reduced *Lactobacillus* and increased *Gardnerella* or *Ureaplasma* were associated with increased risk of preterm birth. The discrepancy between these studies may be in part confounded by the known variation of the vaginal microbiome throughout pregnancy, which is characterized by enrichment of *Lactobacillus* with increasing gestational age, reduced overall richness and diversity, and greater overall stability.[116,117] Alternatively, ethnic and racial differences between the 2 cohorts may account for the differences seen between these studies, but this has yet to be accounted for in the current literature.

The uncertain association between the vaginal microbiome and preterm birth has spurred investigation into the microbial communities of other body sites, including the mouth, the gut, the placenta, and the intrauterine environment. Within the gut, Shiozaki and colleagues[118] found that the fecal microbiota had significantly higher levels of *Clostridium* and reduced levels of *Bacteroides* in women who had a preterm birth, although the impact of such changes to preterm labor is unknown.[118] Other intriguing studies have shown that the placental microbiome, which most closely resembles the oral microbiome, is altered in cases of preterm birth, whereas amniotic fluid collected in women who have preterm birth harbor bacteria from the oral cavity. These observations have been intriguing considering that periodontal disease is associated with a 7-fold increased risk of preterm birth.[119] Periodontal disease may lead to hematogenous spread of bacterial pathogens to the placenta and the fetus, disrupting the placental microbiome and ultimately leading to premature labor, although further studies in controlled animal models are needed evaluate this potential mechanism.

A microbiome-centric perspective has the potential to innovate the way in which interventions for preterm birth prevention are developed and administered. Traditionally, for microbe-related disorders, antibiotic regimens are given to kill the pathogenic organisms. In the context of preterm birth, however, such efforts have shown ineffective or even increase risk of preterm birth. Treatments targeting bacterial vaginosis during pregnancy did not prevent preterm birth in multiple studies and increased risk in others.[120–122] A 2012 Cochrane review demonstrated that treatment can eradicate

Table 1
Table of key topics in relationship to neonatal microbiome research and key associated articles

Topic	Key References Pertaining to Topic
Preterm delivery and effects on neonatal microbiome	Arboleya et al,[40] 2012; Schwiertz et al,[24] 2003; Magne et al,[41] 2006; Roudière et al,[42] 2009; Rougé et al,[43] 2010; Morowitz et al,[44] 2011; Stewart et al,[45] 2017; Butel et al,[46] 2007; Stewart et al,[47] 2016; Stewart et al,[48] 2017; Abdulkadir et al,[49] 2016
Mode of delivery and neonatal microbiome	Boley et al,[50] 1991; Aagaard et al,[53] 2016; Yuan et al,[54] 2016; American College of Obstetricians and Gynecologists,[51,52] 2014
Breastmilk and formula feeding and neonatal microbiome	Bode,[55] 2012; Gauhe et al,[58] 1954; Gyorgy et al,[59–61] 1954; Rose et al,[62] 1954; Gibson & Wang,[63] 1994; Kunz et al,[64] 2000; Newburg et al,[65] 2005; Simon et al,[66] 1997; Gustafsson et al,[67] 2006
Maternal diet and neonatal microbiome	Ma et al,[83] 2014; David et al,[85] 2014; Gohir et al,[86] 2015; Chu et al,[87] 2016; Troy & Kasper,[88] 2010; Round & Mazmanian,[89] 2010; Mazmanian et al,[90] 2005; Mohammad et al,[91] 2009; Bassols et al,[92] 2016; Gomez-Arango et al,[93] 2016
Antibiotics and neonatal microbiome	Stokholm et al,[94] 2014; Kenyon et al,[95] 2001; Kenyon et al,[96] 2008; Tormo-Badia et al,[97] 2014; Stokholm et al,[98] 2014; Mueller et al,[99] 2015; Vidal et al,[100] 2013; Jepsen et al,[101] 2003; Flenady et al,[102] 2013; Azad et al,[103] 2016; Gibson et al,[104] 2016; Brooks et al,[105] 2014
Microbiome and birth associations	Brocklehurst et al,[107] 2013; Oliver & Lamont,[108] 2013; Baldwin et al,[109] 2015; Chu et al,[110] 2016; Aagaard et al,[111] 2012; Litich et al,[112] 2003; McDonald et al,[113] 1991; Romero et al,[114] 2002; Hay et al,[115] 1994; Offenbacher et al,[116] 1996; Nygren et al,[117] 2008; McDonald et al,[118] 2007; Thinkhamrop et al,[119] 2015; Schwiertz et al,[15] 2010; Koren et al,[16] 2012

bacterial vaginosis but does not have any significant impact on the prevention of pre-term birth or preterm prelabor rupture of membranes. Therefore, it is not recommended to screen and treat all pregnant women with bacterial vaginosis to prevent preterm birth or preterm premature rupture of membranes.[107]

Ultimately, therapies aimed at preventing preterm birth may focus on maintaining healthy communities, rather than treating for specific pathogens. Before such treatment approaches are realized, however, additional work is needed to evaluate the impact of the maternal microbiome across different body niches, inclusive of the mouth, the vagina, and the intrauterine environment.

SUMMARY

Overall, perinatal interventions have significant impact on both the maternal and neonatal microbiomes (**Table 1** lists references per topic). Some key questions, however, are still left unanswered. Does dysbiosis of the enteric microbiome play a larger role in the development of preterm birth? If so, are there any therapies that can be targeted to ameliorate this dysbiosis and protect against preterm birth? There is limited research evaluating the impact of antenatal steroids on the fetal and/or neonatal microbiome. How do antenatal steroids affect the maternal, fetal, and neonatal microbiomes? Finally, it is known that microbial contact begins in utero, but is this true colonization or just transient seeding? Because it is virtually impossible to ascertain this fact in human experiments, future investigations in animal models are imperative to help determine if it is truly colonization or simply a transient seeding that has an impact on the fetus. These and other questions are now imperative for researchers to address, to evaluate and further the understanding of the microbiome, its development, and its potential interactions on the development of disease states in the host. Through this understanding, potential directed therapies can be initiated, which could lead to improvements in neonatal outcomes throughout the world.

REFERENCES

1. Aagaard K, Petrosino J, Keitel W, et al. The Human Microbiome Project strategy for comprehensive sampling of the human microbiome and why it matters. FASEB J 2013;27(3):1012–22.
2. Human Microbiome Project Consortium. Structure, function and diversity of the healthy human microbiome. Nature 2012;486(7402):207–14.
3. Human Microbiome Project Consortium. A framework for human microbiome research. Nature 2012;486(7402):215–21.
4. Jumpstart Consortium Human Microbiome Project Data Generation Working Group. Evaluation of 16S rDNA-based community profiling for human microbiome research. PLoS One 2012;7(6):e39315.
5. Tilg H, Moschen AR. Microbiota and diabetes: an evolving relationship. Gut 2014;63(9):1513–21.
6. Larsen N, Vogensen FK, van den Berg FW, et al. Gut microbiota in human adults with type 2 diabetes differs from non-diabetic adults. PLoS One 2010;5(2): e9085.
7. Wu X, Ma C, Han L, et al. Molecular characterisation of the faecal microbiota in patients with type II diabetes. Curr Microbiol 2010;61(1):69–78.
8. Qin J, Li Y, Cai Z, et al. A metagenome-wide association study of gut microbiota in type 2 diabetes. Nature 2012;490(7418):55–60.
9. Mangin I, Bonnet R, Seksik P, et al. Molecular inventory of faecal microflora in patients with Crohn's disease. FEMS Microbiol Ecol 2004;50(1):25–36.

10. Gophna U, Sommerfeld K, Gophna S, et al. Differences between tissue-associated intestinal microfloras of patients with Crohn's disease and ulcerative colitis. J Clin Microbiol 2006;44(11):4136–41.

11. Manichanh C, Rigottier-Gois L, Bonnaud E, et al. Reduced diversity of faecal microbiota in Crohn's disease revealed by a metagenomic approach. Gut 2006; 55(2):205–11.

12. Joossens M, Huys G, Cnockaert M, et al. Dysbiosis of the faecal microbiota in patients with Crohn's disease and their unaffected relatives. Gut 2011;60(5): 631–7.

13. Lepage P, Häsler R, Spehlmann ME, et al. Twin study indicates loss of interaction between microbiota and mucosa of patients with ulcerative colitis. Gastroenterology 2011;141(1):227–36.

14. Ley RE. Obesity and the human microbiome. Curr Opin Gastroenterol 2010; 26(1):5–11.

15. Schwiertz A, Taras D, Schäfer K, et al. Microbiota and SCFA in lean and overweight healthy subjects. Obesity (Silver Spring) 2010;18(1):190–5.

16. Koren O, Goodrich JK, Cullender TC, et al. Host remodeling of the gut microbiome and metabolic changes during pregnancy. Cell 2012;150(3):470–80.

17. Markle JG, Frank DN, Mortin-Toth S, et al. Sex differences in the gut microbiome drive hormone-dependent regulation of autoimmunity. Science 2013;339(6123): 1084–8.

18. Turnbaugh PJ, Bäckhed F, Fulton L, et al. Diet-induced obesity is linked to marked but reversible alterations in the mouse distal gut microbiome. Cell Host Microbe 2008;3(4):213–23.

19. Turnbaugh PJ, Hamady M, Yatsunenko T, et al. A core gut microbiome in obese and lean twins. Nature 2009;457(7228):480–4.

20. Turnbaugh PJ, Ley RE, Mahowald MA, et al. An obesity-associated gut microbiome with increased capacity for energy harvest. Nature 2006;444(7122): 1027–31.

21. Backhed F, Manchester JK, Semenkovich CF, et al. Mechanisms underlying the resistance to diet-induced obesity in germ-free mice. Proc Natl Acad Sci U S A 2007;104(3):979–84.

22. Cani PD, Neyrinck AM, Fava F, et al. Selective increases of bifidobacteria in gut microflora improve high-fat-diet-induced diabetes in mice through a mechanism associated with endotoxaemia. Diabetologia 2007;50(11):2374–83.

23. Willing B, Halfvarson J, Dicksved J, et al. Twin studies reveal specific imbalances in the mucosa-associated microbiota of patients with ileal Crohn's disease. Inflamm Bowel Dis 2009;15(5):653–60.

24. Schwiertz A, Gruhl B, Löbnitz M, et al. Development of the intestinal bacterial composition in hospitalized preterm infants in comparison with breast-fed, full-term infants. Pediatr Res 2003;54(3):393–9.

25. Marchesi JR, Dutilh BE, Hall N, et al. Towards the human colorectal cancer microbiome. PLoS One 2011;6(5):e20447.

26. Sobhani I, Amiot A, Le Baleur Y, et al. Microbial dysbiosis and colon carcinogenesis: could colon cancer be considered a bacteria-related disease? Therap Adv Gastroenterol 2013;6(3):215–29.

27. Sobhani I, Tap J, Roudot-Thoraval F, et al. Microbial dysbiosis in colorectal cancer (CRC) patients. PLoS One 2011;6(1):e16393.

28. Wang T, Cai G, Qiu Y, et al. Structural segregation of gut microbiota between colorectal cancer patients and healthy volunteers. ISME J 2012;6(2):320–9.

29. Devaraj S, Hemarajata P, Versalovic J. The human gut microbiome and body metabolism: implications for obesity and diabetes. Clin Chem 2013;59(4): 617–28.
30. Barker DJ. The origins of the developmental origins theory. J Intern Med 2007; 261(5):412–7.
31. Barker DJ, Gluckman PD, Godfrey KM, et al. Fetal nutrition and cardiovascular disease in adult life. Lancet 1993;341(8850):938–41.
32. Barker DJ, Osmond C. Infant mortality, childhood nutrition, and ischaemic heart disease in England and Wales. Lancet 1986;1(8489):1077–81.
33. Barker DJ, Winter PD, Osmond C, et al. Weight in infancy and death from ischaemic heart disease. Lancet 1989;2(8663):577–80.
34. Aagaard-Tillery KM, Grove K, Bishop J, et al. Developmental origins of disease and determinants of chromatin structure: maternal diet modifies the primate fetal epigenome. J Mol Endocrinol 2008;41(2):91–102.
35. Suter M, Bocock P, Showalter L, et al. Epigenomics: maternal high-fat diet exposure in utero disrupts peripheral circadian gene expression in nonhuman primates. FASEB J 2011;25(2):714–26.
36. Suter MA, Takahashi D, Grove KL, et al. Postweaning exposure to a high-fat diet is associated with alterations to the hepatic histone code in Japanese macaques. Pediatr Res 2013;74(3):252–8.
37. Suter MA, Chen A, Burdine MS, et al. A maternal high-fat diet modulates fetal SIRT1 histone and protein deacetylase activity in nonhuman primates. FASEB J 2012;26(12):5106–14.
38. Macpherson AJ, Harris NL. Interactions between commensal intestinal bacteria and the immune system. Nat Rev Immunol 2004;4(6):478–85.
39. Round JL, Mazmanian SK. The gut microbiota shapes intestinal immune responses during health and disease. Nat Rev Immunol 2009;9(5):313–23.
40. Arboleya S, Binetti A, Salazar N, et al. Establishment and development of intestinal microbiota in preterm neonates. FEMS Microbiol Ecol 2012;79(3):763–72.
41. Magne F, Abély M, Boyer F, et al. Low species diversity and high interindividual variability in faeces of preterm infants as revealed by sequences of 16S rRNA genes and PCR-temporal temperature gradient gel electrophoresis profiles. FEMS Microbiol Ecol 2006;57(1):128–38.
42. Roudière L, Jacquot A, Marchandin H, et al. Optimized PCR-Temporal Temperature Gel Electrophoresis compared to cultivation to assess diversity of gut microbiota in neonates. J Microbiol Methods 2009;79(2):156–65.
43. Rougé C, Goldenberg O, Ferraris L, et al. Investigation of the intestinal microbiota in preterm infants using different methods. Anaerobe 2010;16(4):362–70.
44. Morowitz MJ, Denef VJ, Costello EK, et al. Strain-resolved community genomic analysis of gut microbial colonization in a premature infant. Proc Natl Acad Sci U S A 2011;108(3):1128–33.
45. Stewart CJ, Embleton ND, Clements E, et al. Cesarean or vaginal birth does not impact the longitudinal development of the gut microbiome in a cohort of exclusively preterm infants. Front Microbiol 2017;8:1008.
46. Butel MJ, Suau A, Campeotto F, et al. Conditions of bifidobacterial colonization in preterm infants: a prospective analysis. J Pediatr Gastroenterol Nutr 2007; 44(5):577–82.
47. Stewart CJ, Embleton ND, Marrs EC, et al. Temporal bacterial and metabolic development of the preterm gut reveals specific signatures in health and disease. Microbiome 2016;4(1):67.

48. Stewart CJ, Embleton ND, Marrs ECL, et al. Longitudinal development of the gut microbiome and metabolome in preterm neonates with late onset sepsis and healthy controls. Microbiome 2017;5(1):75.
49. Abdulkadir B, Nelson A, Skeath T, et al. Routine use of probiotics in preterm infants: longitudinal impact on the microbiome and metabolome. Neonatology 2016;109(4):239–47.
50. Boley JP. The history of caesarean section. 1935. CMAJ 1991;145(4):319–22.
51. American College of Obstetricians and Gynecologists, Society for Maternal-Fetal. Obstetric care consensus no. 1: safe prevention of the primary cesarean delivery. Obstet Gynecol 2014;123(3):693–711.
52. American College of Obstetricians and Gynecologists (College), Society for Maternal-Fetal Medicine, Caughey AB, et al. Safe prevention of the primary cesarean delivery. Am J Obstet Gynecol 2014;210(3):179–93.
53. Aagaard K, Stewart CJ, Chu D. Una destinatio, viae diversae: does exposure to the vaginal microbiota confer health benefits to the infant, and does lack of exposure confer disease risk? EMBO Rep 2016;17(12):1679–84.
54. Yuan C, Gaskins AJ, Blaine AI, et al. Association between cesarean birth and risk of obesity in offspring in childhood, adolescence, and early adulthood. JAMA Pediatr 2016;170(11):e162385.
55. Bode L. Human milk oligosaccharides: every baby needs a sugar mama. Glycobiology 2012;22(9):1147–62.
56. Moro E. Morphologie und bakteriologische Untersuchungen uber die Darmbakterien des Sauglings: Die bakterien-flora des normalen Frauenmilchstuchls. Jahrbuch Kinderh 1900;61:686–734.
57. Schonfeld H. Uber die Beziehung der einzelnen Bestandteile der Frauenmilch zur Bifidusflora. Jahrbuch Kinderh 1926;113:19–60.
58. Gauhe A, Gyorgy P, Hoover JR, et al. Bifidus factor. IV. Preparations obtained from human milk. Arch Biochem Biophys 1954;48(1):214–24.
59. Gyorgy P, Hoover JR, Kuhn R, et al. Bifidus factor. III. The rate of dialysis. Arch Biochem Biophys 1954;48(1):209–13.
60. Gyorgy P, Kuhn R, Rose CS, et al. Bifidus factor. II. Its occurrence in milk from different species and in other natural products. Arch Biochem Biophys 1954;48(1):202–8.
61. Gyorgy P, Norris RF, Rose CS. Bifidus factor. I. A variant of Lactobacillus bifidus requiring a special growth factor. Arch Biochem Biophys 1954;48(1):193–201.
62. Rose CS, Kuhn R, Zilliken F, et al. Bifidus factor. V. The activity of alpha- and beta-methyl-N-acetyl-D-glucosaminides. Arch Biochem Biophys 1954;49(1):123–9.
63. Gibson GR, Wang X. Regulatory effects of bifidobacteria on the growth of other colonic bacteria. J Appl Bacteriol 1994;77(4):412–20.
64. Kunz C, Rudloff S, Baier W, et al. Oligosaccharides in human milk: structural, functional, and metabolic aspects. Annu Rev Nutr 2000;20:699–722.
65. Newburg DS, Ruiz-Palacios GM, Morrow AL. Human milk glycans protect infants against enteric pathogens. Annu Rev Nutr 2005;25:37–58.
66. Simon PM, Goode PL, Mobasseri A, et al. Inhibition of Helicobacter pylori binding to gastrointestinal epithelial cells by sialic acid-containing oligosaccharides. Infect Immun 1997;65(2):750–7.
67. Gustafsson A, Hultberg A, Sjöström R, et al. Carbohydrate-dependent inhibition of Helicobacter pylori colonization using porcine milk. Glycobiology 2006;16(1):1–10.

68. Breastfeeding and HIV International Transmission Study Group, Coutsoudis A, Dabis F, Fawzi W, et al. Late postnatal transmission of HIV-1 in breast-fed children: an individual patient data meta-analysis. J Infect Dis 2004;189(12): 2154–66.
69. Tissier H. Recherches sur la flore intestinale des nourrissons (e'tat normal et pathologique). G Carre and C Naud 1900;1–253.
70. Kovalovszki L, Villányi Z, Pataki I, et al. Isolation of aerobic bacteria from the placenta. Acta Paediatr Acad Sci Hung 1982;23(3):357–60.
71. Jiménez E, Marín ML, Martín R, et al. Is meconium from healthy newborns actually sterile? Res Microbiol 2008;159(3):187–93.
72. Cowling P, McCoy DR, Marshall RJ, et al. Bacterial colonization of the non-pregnant uterus: a study of pre-menopausal abdominal hysterectomy specimens. Eur J Clin Microbiol Infect Dis 1992;11(2):204–5.
73. Møller BR, Kristiansen FV, Thorsen P, et al. Sterility of the uterine cavity. Acta Obstet Gynecol Scand 1995;74(3):216–9.
74. Stout MJ, Conlon B, Landeau M, et al. Identification of intracellular bacteria in the basal plate of the human placenta in term and preterm gestations. Am J Obstet Gynecol 2013;208(3):226.e1–7.
75. Dong XD, Li XR, Luan JJ, et al. Bacterial communities in neonatal feces are similar to mothers' placentae. Can J Infect Dis Med Microbiol 2015;26(2):90–4.
76. Aagaard K, Ma J, Antony KM, et al. The placenta harbors a unique microbiome. Sci Transl Med 2014;6(237):237ra65.
77. Antony KM, Ma J, Mitchell KB, et al. The preterm placental microbiome varies in association with excess maternal gestational weight gain. Am J Obstet Gynecol 2015;212(5):653.e1–16.
78. Prince AL, Ma J, Kannan PS, et al. The placental membrane microbiome is altered among subjects with spontaneous preterm birth with and without chorioamnionitis. Am J Obstet Gynecol 2016;214(5):627.e1–16.
79. Collado MC, Rautava S, Aakko J, et al. Human gut colonisation may be initiated in utero by distinct microbial communities in the placenta and amniotic fluid. Sci Rep 2016;6:23129.
80. Doyle RM, Alber DG, Jones HE, et al. Term and preterm labour are associated with distinct microbial community structures in placental membranes which are independent of mode of delivery. Placenta 2014;35(12):1099–101.
81. Steel JH, Malatos S, Kennea N, et al. Bacteria and inflammatory cells in fetal membranes do not always cause preterm labor. Pediatr Res 2005;57(3):404–11.
82. Chu DM, Ma J, Prince AL, et al. Maturation of the infant microbiome community structure and function across multiple body sites and in relation to mode of delivery. Nat Med 2017;23(3):314–26.
83. Ma J, Prince AL, Bader D, et al. High-fat maternal diet during pregnancy persistently alters the offspring microbiome in a primate model. Nat Commun 2014;5: 3889.
84. Gomez de Aguero M, Ganal-Vonarburg SC, Fuhrer T, et al. The maternal microbiota drives early postnatal innate immune development. Science 2016; 351(6279):1296–302.
85. David LA, Maurice CF, Carmody RN, et al. Diet rapidly and reproducibly alters the human gut microbiome. Nature 2014;505(7484):559–63.
86. Gohir W, Whelan FJ, Surette MG, et al. Pregnancy-related changes in the maternal gut microbiota are dependent upon the mother's periconceptional diet. Gut Microbes 2015;6(5):310–20.

87. Chu DM, Antony KM, Ma J, et al. The early infant gut microbiome varies in association with a maternal high-fat diet. Genome Med 2016;8(1):77.

88. Troy EB, Kasper DL. Beneficial effects of Bacteroides fragilis polysaccharides on the immune system. Front Biosci (Landmark Ed) 2010;15:25–34.

89. Round JL, Mazmanian SK. Inducible Foxp3+ regulatory T-cell development by a commensal bacterium of the intestinal microbiota. Proc Natl Acad Sci U S A 2010;107(27):12204–9.

90. Mazmanian SK, Liu CH, Tzianabos AO, et al. An immunomodulatory molecule of symbiotic bacteria directs maturation of the host immune system. Cell 2005; 122(1):107–18.

91. Mohammad MA, Sunehag AL, Haymond MW. Effect of dietary macronutrient composition under moderate hypocaloric intake on maternal adaptation during lactation. Am J Clin Nutr 2009;89(6):1821–7.

92. Bassols J, Serino M, Carreras-Badosa G, et al. Gestational diabetes is associated with changes in placental microbiota and microbiome. Pediatr Res 2016; 80(6):777–84.

93. Gomez-Arango LF, Barrett HL, McIntyre HD, et al. Connections between the gut microbiome and metabolic hormones in early pregnancy in overweight and obese women. Diabetes 2016;65(8):2214–23.

94. Stokholm J, Sevelsted A, Bønnelykke K, et al. Maternal propensity for infections and risk of childhood asthma: a registry-based cohort study. Lancet Respir Med 2014;2(8):631–7.

95. Kenyon SL, Taylor DJ, Tarnow-Mordi W, et al. Broad-spectrum antibiotics for preterm, prelabour rupture of fetal membranes: the ORACLE I randomised trial. ORACLE Collaborative Group. Lancet 2001;357(9261):979–88.

96. Kenyon S, Pike K, Jones DR, et al. Childhood outcomes after prescription of antibiotics to pregnant women with spontaneous preterm labour: 7-year follow-up of the ORACLE II trial. Lancet 2008;372(9646):1319–27.

97. Tormo-Badia N, Håkansson Å, Vasudevan K, et al. Antibiotic treatment of pregnant non-obese diabetic mice leads to altered gut microbiota and intestinal immunological changes in the offspring. Scand J Immunol 2014;80(4):250–60.

98. Stokholm J, Schjørring S, Eskildsen CE, et al. Antibiotic use during pregnancy alters the commensal vaginal microbiota. Clin Microbiol Infect 2014;20(7): 629–35.

99. Mueller NT, Whyatt R, Hoepner L, et al. Prenatal exposure to antibiotics, cesarean section and risk of childhood obesity. Int J Obes (Lond) 2015;39(4):665–70.

100. Vidal AC, Murphy SK, Murtha AP, et al. Associations between antibiotic exposure during pregnancy, birth weight and aberrant methylation at imprinted genes among offspring. Int J Obes (Lond) 2013;37(7):907–13.

101. Jepsen P, Skriver MV, Floyd A, et al. A population-based study of maternal use of amoxicillin and pregnancy outcome in Denmark. Br J Clin Pharmacol 2003; 55(2):216–21.

102. Flenady V, Hawley G, Stock OM, et al. Prophylactic antibiotics for inhibiting preterm labour with intact membranes. Cochrane Database Syst Rev 2013;(12):CD000246.

103. Azad MB, Konya T, Persaud RR, et al. Impact of maternal intrapartum antibiotics, method of birth and breastfeeding on gut microbiota during the first year of life: a prospective cohort study. BJOG 2016;123(6):983–93.

104. Gibson MK, Wang B, Ahmadi S, et al. Developmental dynamics of the preterm infant gut microbiota and antibiotic resistome. Nat Microbiol 2016;1:16024.

105. Brooks B, Firek BA, Miller CS, et al. Microbes in the neonatal intensive care unit resemble those found in the gut of premature infants. Microbiome 2014;2(1):1.
106. Liu L, Oza S, Hogan D, et al. Global, regional, and national cuases of under-5 mortality in 2000-15: an updated systematic analysis with implications for the sustainable development goals. Lancet 2016;388(10063):3027–35.
107. Brocklehurst P, Gordon A, Heatley E, et al. Antibiotics for treating bacterial vaginosis in pregnancy. Cochrane Database Syst Rev 2013;(1):CD000262.
108. Oliver RS, Lamont RF. Infection and antibiotics in the aetiology, prediction and prevention of preterm birth. J Obstet Gynaecol 2013;33(8):768–75.
109. Baldwin EA, Walther-Antonio M, MacLean AM, et al. Persistent microbial dysbiosis in preterm premature rupture of membranes from onset until delivery. PeerJ 2015;3:e1398.
110. Chu DM, Meyer KM, Prince AL, et al. Impact of maternal nutrition in pregnancy and lactation on offspring gut microbial composition and function. Gut Microbes 2016;7(6):459–70.
111. Aagaard K, Riehle K, Ma J, et al. A metagenomic approach to characterization of the vaginal microbiome signature in pregnancy. PLoS One 2012;7(6):e36466.
112. Leitich H, Bodner-Adler B, Brunbauer M, et al. Bacterial vaginosis as a risk factor for preterm delivery: a meta-analysis. Am J Obstet Gynecol 2003;189(1):139–47.
113. McDonald HM, O'Loughlin JA, Jolley P, et al. Vaginal infection and preterm labour. Br J Obstet Gynaecol 1991;98(5):427–35.
114. Romero R, Espinoza J, Chaiworapongsa T, et al. Infection and prematurity and the role of preventive strategies. Semin Neonatol 2002;7(4):259–74.
115. Hay PE, Lamont RF, Taylor-Robinson D, et al. Abnormal bacterial colonisation of the genital tract and subsequent preterm delivery and late miscarriage. BMJ 1994;308(6924):295–8.
116. DiGiulio DB, Callahan BJ, McMurdie PJ, et al. Temporal and spatial variation of the human microbiota during pregnancy. Proc Natl Acad Sci USA 2015;112(35):11060–5. https://doi.org/10.1073/pnas.1502875112.
117. Romero R, Hassan SS, Gajer P, et al. The vaginal microbiota of pregnant women who subsequently have spontaneous preterm labor and delivery and those with a normal delivery at term. Microbiome 2014;2:18. https://doi.org/10.1186/2049-2618-2-18.
118. Shiozaki A, Yoneda S, Yoneda N, et al. Intestional micobiota is different in women with preterm birth: results from terminal restriction fragment length polymorphism analysis. PLoS one 2014;9(11):e111374.
119. Offenbacher S, Katz V, Fertik G, et al. Periodontal infection as a possible risk factor for preterm low birth weight. J Periodontol 1996;67(10 Suppl):1103–13.
120. Nygren P, Fu R, Freeman M, et al. Evidence on the benefits and harms of screening and treating pregnant women who are asymptomatic for bacterial vaginosis: an update review for the U.S. Preventive Services Task Force. Ann Intern Med 2008;148(3):220–33.
121. McDonald HM, Brocklehurst P, Gordon A. Antibiotics for treating bacterial vaginosis in pregnancy. Cochrane Database Syst Rev 2007;(1):CD000262.
122. Thinkhamrop J, Hofmeyr GJ, Adetoro O, et al. Antibiotic prophylaxis during the second and third trimester to reduce adverse pregnancy outcomes and morbidity. Cochrane Database Syst Rev 2015;(6):CD002250.

Perinatal Brain Injury
Mechanisms, Prevention, and Outcomes

Christopher M. Novak, MD[a], Maide Ozen, MD[b,c], Irina Burd, MD, PhD[c,d,e],*

KEYWORDS

- Perinatal brain injury • Encephalopathy • Intraventricular hemorrhage
- Periventricular leukomalacia • Perinatal arterial ischemic stroke • Cerebral palsy
- Hypothermia • Prevention

KEY POINTS

- Highlight the mechanism contributing to the development of common etiologies of perinatal brain injury in preterm and term neonates.
- Review the most up-to-date research and recommendations regarding preventive strategies aimed at improving outcomes for those neonates with or at risk for common etiologies of perinatal brain injury.
- Highlight the outcomes of neonates diagnosed with common etiologies of perinatal brain injury and the impact of preventive strategies currently used to improve outcomes.

INTRODUCTION

Perinatal brain injury may lead to significant long-term neurodevelopmental impairment, including cognitive, neurologic, motor, and sensory disability. Perinatal brain injury affects infants born at all gestational ages, but its incidence and morbidity increases with decreasing gestational age.[1]

Disclosure Statement: The authors declare that this article was created in the absence of any commercial or financial relationships that could be construed as potential conflicts of interest.
[a] Department of Gynecology and Obstetrics, Division of Maternal-Fetal Medicine, Johns Hopkins University School of Medicine, 600 North Wolfe Street, Phipps 214, Baltimore, MD 21287-4922, USA; [b] Department of Pediatrics, Division of Neonatal-Perinatal Medicine, Johns Hopkins University School of Medicine, 1800 Orleans Street, Baltimore, MD 21287-4922, USA; [c] Integrated Research Center for Fetal Medicine, Department of Gynecology and Obstetrics, Johns Hopkins University School of Medicine, 600 North Wolfe Street, Phipps 228, Baltimore, MD 21287-4922, USA; [d] Neuroscience Intensive Care Nursery Program, Department of Pediatrics, Division of Neonatal-Perinatal Medicine, Johns Hopkins University School of Medicine, 1800 Orleans Street, Baltimore, MD 21287-4922, USA; [e] Department of Neurology, Johns Hopkins University School of Medicine, 1800 Orleans Street, Baltimore, MD 21287-4922, USA
* Corresponding author. Division of Maternal Fetal Medicine, Department of Gynecology and Obstetrics, Integrated Research Center for Fetal Medicine, 600 North Wolfe Street, Phipps 228, Baltimore, MD 21287-4922.
E-mail address: iburd@jhmi.edu

Improved perinatal care of the very preterm and low birth weight infant, and neuro-protective preventive strategies aimed at reducing the risk and severity of perinatal brain injury, have resulted in a greater number of affected infants surviving later in life with less severe neurodevelopmental disability.[2,3] Increased administration of antenatal corticosteroids is a possible explanation for the observed increases in sur-vival, and decrease in cerebral palsy (CP) and neurodevelopmental impairment in extremely low birth weight infants from 1982 to 2002.[2] A single-center study of 536 very preterm infants born before 33 weeks of gestation with a 2-year follow-up, revealed a significant improvement in motor outcomes and decreased rate of CP from 12% in 2000 to 1% in 2010 that was, in part, attributed to the increased admin-istration of magnesium sulfate to women at risk of preterm birth over the study pe-riods.[3] More recently, improved outcomes are now being recognized for those neonates born at cusp of viability. Data from 4274 infants born between 22 and 24 weeks spanning 3 epochs (2000–2003, 2004–2007, and 2008–2011) at National Institute of Child Health and Human Development (NICHD) Neonatal Research Network centers showed an increase in overall survival from 30% to 36%, and survival without neurodevelopmental impairment from 16% to 20%, between epoch 1 and epoch 3, although the incidence of moderate to severe CP did not decrease signifi-cantly across epochs (15% in epoch 1 and 11% in epochs 2 and 3).[4]

In these sections, common etiologies of perinatal brain injury will be reviewed, including hypoxic–ischemic encephalopathy (HIE), intraventricular hemorrhage (IVH), periventricular leukomalacia (PVL), perinatal stroke, and CP (**Table 1**). Although these causes of perinatal brain injury are separate clinical entities, they remain interrelated by their risk factors and pathogenesis. The underlying mechanism of injury involves an initial insult to the vulnerable, developing fetal brain that is usually either of hypox-ic–ischemic, hemorrhagic, or infectious in nature, and sets off a cascade of events leading to further brain injury.[18]

COMMON MECHANISM OF INJURY

Perinatal brain injury can affect infants born at any gestational age; however, very pre-term fetuses (born <32 weeks of gestation) are less equipped to adapt to perinatal in-sults as term infants, making them more prone to brain injury.[1] In most cases, a common pathway of injury is elicited by an initial hypoxic–ischemic or inflammatory insult that incites a cascade of events that potentiates perinatal brain injury.[18]

An excellent review by Giussani[19] highlights the adaptive physiologic mechanisms that are present in the term fetus that enables it to respond to a period of impaired oxygenation or systemic hypotension. When oxygenated blood supply is limited, the fetus meets its metabolic needs by binding a greater concentration of oxygen to hemoglobin, preferentially shunting oxygenated blood to tissues at greatest risk of hypoxic injury, and limiting oxygen consumption. In response to hypoxia, the fetal heart rate slows, permitting increased cardiac myocardial oxygen extraction, and increasing end-diastolic filling time and ventricular end-diastolic volume. This in-creases stroke volume, arterial blood pressure, and circulatory redistribution of blood flow secondary to peripheral vasoconstriction with vasodilation of the blood vessels that perfuse the brain, heart, and adrenal glands.

In contrast with the adaptive mechanisms of the term fetus, the preterm fetus has an immature cerebrovascular autoregulation system and exhibits a pressure-passive circu-lation. When faced with a period of hypoxia or systemic hypotension, preterm fetuses are unable to sustain increased cerebral perfusion, which makes them more prone to hypoxia–ischemia and neurologic injury. The initial hypoxic–ischemic insult is the primary

Table 1
Aspects of common etiologies of perinatal brain injury

Perinatal Brain Injury Type	Gestational Age	Mechanism of Injury	Neuropathologic Findings	Preventive Measures	References
Hypoxic–ischemic encephalopathy	Late preterm, term (>35 wk)	Hypoxia–ischemia leading to common pathway of injury	Diffuse gray and white matter injury affecting most vulnerable regions of brain	Therapeutic hypothermia Postnatal erythropoietin	5–8
Intraventricular hemorrhage	Preterm (primarily <32 wk)	Injury to fragile premature vessels of germinal matrix	Germinal matrix bleeding with extension into ventricular system	Antenatal corticosteroids Delayed umbilical cord clamping	9–11
Periventricular leukomalacia	Preterm (primarily <32 wk)	Hypoperfusion to border zone regions of brain	Periventricular focal necrosis, cystic formation, or diffuse white matter injury	None	18
Perinatal stroke	Preterm, term	Regional ischemia owing to arterial or sinovenous occlusion or hemorrhagic infarction	Regional infarction owing to vascular occlusion or hemorrhage	None	12–14
Cerebral palsy	Preterm, term	Multifactorial, only 10%–20% of cases owing to an intrapartum hypoxic–ischemic event	Clinical syndrome with variable findings depending on underlying etiology	Magnesium sulfate	6,15–17

mechanism of neuronal injury in which cells are unable to meet their metabolic demands.[18] Those regions of the brain with the greatest metabolic demands—the sensorimotor cortex, thalamus, cerebellum, and brain stem—are most vulnerable to injury.[5] After the initial insult and upon reperfusion of cerebral tissues, there is a transient restoration of cellular metabolic function. This period is followed by a secondary decrease in glucose metabolism and deficiency in high-energy phosphates that results in a secondary injury from excitatory amino acids, apoptosis, reactive oxygen species, and inflammation that causes most of the cerebral injury over time.[20–24]

In response to cellular injury, the excitatory amino acids glutamate and aspartate are released in the brain and exert an excitotoxic effect on the susceptible developing brain.[21] Activation of the N-methyl-D-aspartate and α-amino-3-hydroxy-5-methyl-4-isoxazole-propionic acid receptors found on neurons and oligodendroglial precursors results in the accumulation of toxic intracellular calcium, impaired cellular recovery, cellular death, and microglial activation with the release of toxic factors detrimental to the health of neighboring neural cells.[22] Mitochondrial impairment ensues with the release of proapoptotic proteins resulting in cellular apoptosis.[23] The generation of reactive oxygen species further disrupts cellular structure and function, contributing to neuronal damage.[24] Last, inflammation induced by the activation of microglia and macrophages with the production and release of proinflammatory cytokines, chemokines, proteases, complement factors, excitotoxic amino acids, reactive oxygen species, and nitric oxide further exacerbates secondary brain injury[25] (Fig. 1).

In addition to the inciting hypoxic–ischemic event, intrauterine infection or inflammation has been shown to potentiate perinatal brain injury by altering the cerebral response to hypoxia.[25] In humans, chorioamnionitis is a known risk factor for the development of several types of perinatal brain injury. In these cases, the activation of microglia and macrophages secondary to infection leads to an inflammatory milieu in the fetal brain, resulting in brain injury.[18]

HYPOXIC–ISCHEMIC ENCEPHALOPATHY
Definition

HIE, a subtype of neonatal encephalopathy, is a clinical syndrome of central nervous system dysfunction resulting from impaired cerebral blood flow secondary to persistent, interrupted blood flow to the fetus. The impaired placental gas exchange leads to fetal acidemia and neurologic morbidity that is manifested as depressed consciousness, abnormal muscle tone and reflexes, seizures, and respiratory difficulties.[6] The diagnosis of moderate to severe HIE is linked to the later development of CP, which often is attributed to an acute intrapartum event. The majority of CP cases occur before the onset of labor, but approximately 10% to 20% are from acute intrapartum hypoxia–ischemia.[6,26]

Unlike perinatal brain injury in very preterm infants, neonatal encephalopathy and HIE have typically been defined in infants born at or beyond 35 weeks of gestation. The criteria for definite and probable preterm HIE that includes infants born at 33 weeks and younger have been proposed,[27] based on the recognition that biochemical screening and encephalopathy scoring criteria currently in use for infants born at 35 weeks of gestation or greater are also applicable to preterm infants born between 33 and 35 weeks of gestation.[28]

Incidence

Neonatal encephalopathy from all causes affects approximately 3 in 1000 live births, whereas the incidence of HIE ranges from 1 to 2 per 1000 term births.[29] The incidence

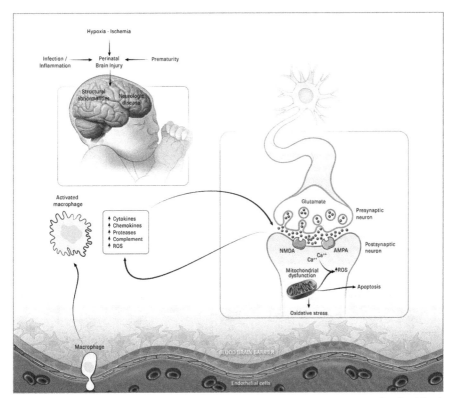

Fig. 1. The effects of hypoxia–ischemia, inflammation, and prematurity on the fetal brain may lead to a common pathway of perinatal brain injury marked by neuronal excitotoxicity, mitochondrial impairment with cellular apoptosis and generation of reactive oxygen species (ROS), and inflammation induced by microglial activation. AMPA, α-amino-3-hydroxy-5-methyl-4-isoxazole-propionic acid; NMDA, N-methyl-D-aspartate.

of preterm HIE varies from 1.3 in 1000 to 5 to 9 in 1000 live births.[27] In a retrospective study of 586 infants from 2000 to 2005, HIE developed in 10% of infants exposed to an intrapartum sentinel event and 2.5% of infants with isolated nonreassuring fetal heart monitoring during labor.[30] The presence of an isolated intrapartum maternal fever or chorioamnionitis increased the risk of neonatal encephalopathy 3-fold and 5-fold,[31] respectively, likely from potentiation of inflammation induced by a hypoxic–ischemic event.

Mechanism

The underlying cause of HIE is the interruption of fetal cerebral blood flow that can be of a maternal, placental, or fetal etiology.[6,30] Maternal conditions resulting in inadequate placental perfusion can be either acute or chronic, and include cardiopulmonary arrest, acute hypotension, pulmonary embolism, or vascular disease. Placental factors that result in HIE are usually acute disturbances in placental perfusion and include abruptio placentae, uterine rupture, umbilical cord prolapse, or shoulder dystocia. Fetal factors include fetal thrombosis, embolism, or fetomaternal hemorrhage. Regardless of the etiology, hypoxia–ischemia in the term neonate results in acute neuronal injury in the deep gray matter, as described.

Prevention

The prevention of long-term sequelae from HIE is focused primarily on neonatal care because preventive obstetric interventions have largely proven to be unsuccessful. Additionally, most HIE is not from an acute peripartum event, but likely developed at some time before the onset of labor. In the 10% to 20% of cases caused by an acute peripartum event,[6,26] avoidance of the etiologic disturbance of placental perfusion is not always possible, because many cases result from an acute disruption in placental perfusion.[6,30] Continuous fetal heart monitoring, although common in the United States, is not associated with a decrease in the perinatal death rate (relative risk [RR]; 0.86; 95% confidence interval [CI], 0.59–1.23) or CP rate (RR, 1.75; 95% CI, 0.84–3.63) and is associated with an increased cesarean section rate (RR, 1.63; 95% CI, 1.29–2.07) and an increased operative vaginal delivery rate (RR, 1.15; 95% CI, 1.01–1.33); the only benefit reported is a reduction in neonatal seizures (RR, 0.50; 95% CI, 0.31–0.80).[32] Neonatal interventions that may improve outcomes in infants diagnosed with or at risk for HIE include therapeutic hypothermia and erythropoietin (Epo) administration.

Therapeutic hypothermia

Therapeutic hypothermia for infants with moderate to severe HIE is currently the standard of care and increases long-term survival without disability. Options include either whole body hypothermia[33] or selective head cooling.[34] Currently, therapeutic hypothermia is limited to infants with moderate or severe encephalopathy and initiated within 6 hours for a treatment duration of 72 hours at a goal temperature of 33.5°C.[7] The original NICHD trial of whole body hypothermia showed a decrease in death or moderate or severe disability at 24 months of age, from 62% to 44% (RR, 0.72; 95% CI, 0.54–0.95) for therapeutic hypothermia compared with controls.[33] A metaanalysis of 1214 neonates showed that therapeutic hypothermia, either from whole body or head cooling, decreased death or major neurodevelopmental disability (RR, 0.76; 95% CI, 0.69–0.84) and increased survival with normal neurologic function (RR, 1.63; 95% CI, 1.36–1.95) at 18 months of life.[35]

Erythropoietin

Epo has emerged as a possible neuroprotective agent for neonates with HIE. Animal models of hypoxic–ischemic injury have shown that Epo attenuates cytokine-mediated inflammation by reducing reactive astrocytosis and microglia activation, and supports the recovery of neuronal cells and limits the extent of injury.[36] A recent phase II trial to assess if multiple doses of Epo administered with therapeutic hypothermia to newborns with HIE improved neuroradiographic and short-term outcomes showed less moderate/severe and subcortical brain injury on MRI and some improved motor function at 1 year of age.[8] Currently, there is phase III, multicenter, randomized, double-blind, placebo-controlled trial enrolling infants born at 36 weeks of gestation or greater with HIE who are receiving standard therapy with therapeutic hypothermia to assess if the addition of high-dose Epo reduces the rate of death, motor, or cognitive deficits at 2 years of age.[37]

Outcomes

Long-term outcomes of HIE cases secondary to an acute intrapartum event are variable. A recent, 2017 secondary analysis of the original NICHD whole body hypothermia study[33] showed that of the 208 infants in the original study, 84 had an acute perinatal sentinel event, and 55% of those infants had an abnormal brain MRI that most often exhibited thalamic and basal ganglia lesions. At 18 to 22 months of follow-up and at 6 to 7 years of follow-up, there was no difference in the neurodevelopmental outcomes between neonates who did and did not experience a perinatal sentinel event.[38] In a 2008 retrospective review of 500 term infants diagnosed with encephalopathy, 41 cases identified were owing to an acute intrapartum event with at least 12 months of follow-up, and death, CP, developmental delay, and normal development were noted in 20%, 41%, 15%, and 24% of cases, respectively.[39] The occurrence of normal development in nearly one-quarter of cases highlights the possibility that neonatal brain plasticity and repair in response to an acute event likely plays a significant role in long-term neurodevelopmental outcomes.

INTRAVENTRICULAR HEMORRHAGE
Definition

IVH describes bleeding that originates in the subependymal germinal matrix and ruptures through the ependymal into the lateral ventricle. IVH is graded as 4 categories, can be unilateral or bilateral, and can be symmetric or asymmetric[40]:

- Grade I: Germinal matrix hemorrhage;
- Grade II: IVH without ventricular dilation;
- Grade III: IVH with acute ventricular dilation (clot fills >50% of the ventricle); and
- Intraparenchymal lesion (previously grade IV): Intraparenchymal hemorrhage.

Incidence

IVH incidence is indirectly proportional to gestational age.[41] The overall incidence of IVH from a NICHD study was 32% for infants born between 22 and 28 weeks of gestation with a birth weight between 401 and 1500 g.[42] Severe IVH (grade III and IV) occurred in 38%, 26%, and 7% of infants surviving more than 12 hours born at 22, 24, and 28 weeks of gestation, respectively. Similar to HIE, the presence of chorioamnionitis is another risk factor for IVH, and is associated with up to a 1.6-fold increased risk of severe IVH in preterm infants born before 33 weeks of gestation.[43]

Mechanism

The lack of supportive tissue surrounding thin-walled capillaries in the germinal matrix of the premature infant's brain increases the risk of IVH.[10] The structural integrity of these vessels is related to the presence of glial fibers emanating from astrocyte endfeet that is deficient along with pericytes, tight junctions, and the presence of an immature basal ganglia in preterm infants. The fragility of these vessels makes them more prone to rupture spontaneously or in response to stress, such as hypoxia–ischemia. In addition, the immature cerebrovascular autoregulation system of preterm infants increases the risk of cerebral ischemia in response to systemic hypotension, leading to a greater risk of injury to the fragile vessels of the germinal matrix.[18]

Prevention

Because IVH mostly affects preterm infants, primary prevention should be directed at the prevention of preterm birth. The incidence of IVH has been shown to decrease by 3.5% with each additional week of gestation achieved through 32 weeks.[41] If preterm birth cannot be prevented, the focus should be on optimizing peripartum care to reduce the risk, severity, and potential sequelae of IVH.

Antenatal corticosteroids
Antenatal corticosteroids are a key therapy to decrease the risk of IVH.[44] In a 2016 cross-sectional review of nearly 26,000 very low birth weight infants born 32 weeks or fewer of gestation, antenatal corticosteroid administration was associated with a

decreased incidence of any grade IVH (odds ratio [OR], 0.68; 95% CI, 0.62–0.75) and severe IVH (OR, 0.51; 95% CI, 0.45–0.58). Additionally, these benefits were seen with administration as early as 22 weeks of gestation.[9] In a 2017 metaanalysis of randomized controlled trials that included 6093 infants, antenatal corticosteroids was associated with a decreased incidence of IVH (OR, 0.55; 95% CI, 0.40–0.76).[45] Although the optimal timing of antenatal corticosteroids administration to maximize neonatal benefit, and reduce the risk of severe neonatal brain injury, is 1 to 7 days before delivery,[46,47] administration within 24 hours of delivery, and potentially as early as 3 hours before delivery may reduce infant in-hospital mortality rates by at least 26%.[47]

Maternal transport
For mothers expected to deliver preterm, antepartum transportation to a facility equipped to handle preterm and very low birth weight infants may reduce the incidence of IVH (13.2% vs 27.4%) and severe IVH (32.9% vs 44.1%) compared with infants transferred after birth.[48]

Delayed cord clamping
Several studies have shown a reduction in IVH from delayed umbilical cord clamping in preterm infants delivered at up to 35 weeks of gestation.[49,50] A 2012 systematic review of 10 trials containing 539 infants that defined delayed umbilical cord clamping as a delay of more than 30 seconds and up to 180 seconds found a lower incidence of IVH in the delayed umbilical cord clamping group compared with the immediate clamping group (RR, 0.59; 95% CI, 0.41–0.85).[11] In January 2017, the American College of Obstetricians and Gynecologists defined delayed umbilical cord clamping as a delay of at least 30 to 60 seconds and reaffirmed their position to delay umbilical cord clamping in preterm infants, citing the benefit of decreasing IVH.[51]

Outcomes

Identification of IVH and its complications is achieved by cranial ultrasound screening, with up to 50% of all cases being otherwise asymptomatic.[52] Nearly all cases of IVH in preterm infants occur within the first 5 days of postnatal life,[52] with approximately one-half of cases in very low birth weight infants occurring within 6 hours of postnatal life.[53] For these reasons, guidelines set forth by the American Academy of Neurology and the Pediatric Committee of the Child Neurology Society recommends that routine cranial ultrasound screening be performed on all infants born at less 30 weeks of gestation, or greater than 30 weeks of gestation with any clinical suspicion of IVH, be performed between 7 and 14 days of age, and repeated at 36 to 40 weeks postmenstrual age.[54]

IVH is a significant cause of morbidity and long-term neurodevelopmental impairment. There is no current therapy to limit the extent of injury once it has developed, and treatment is largely supportive, with the goals of preserving cerebral perfusion, minimizing further injury, and detecting complications. Posthemorrhagic hydrocephalus results from the obstruction of cerebrospinal fluid flow and inhibition of cerebrospinal fluid resorption secondary to intraventricular blood clots, and complicates 1%, 4%, 25%, and 28% of cases of grades I through IV IVH, respectively.[55] Obstruction ultimately can lead to scar formation, further ventricular dilatation with increased intracranial pressure and edema, and further periventricular white matter damage.[56] A large, cohort study of extremely low birth weight infants showed that those with severe IVH requiring shunt placement were at greatest risk for adverse neurodevelopmental and growth outcomes at 18 to 22 months compared with those with and without severe IVH and with no shunt.[57] In periviable infants born between 22 and 24 weeks of gestation, a statistically significant decreased incidence of posthemorrhagic hydrocephalus requiring shunt placement (*P*<.001) has been observed in infants born between 2004 to 2007 and 2008 to 2011, compared with those born between 2000 and 2003, despite the fact that the rates of severe IVH did not change during these times periods.[4]

Morbidity and mortality related to IVH is proportional to its severity. Some data suggest that grade I or II IVH may have a greater degree of neurologic handicap compared with infants without abnormalities on cranial ultrasound examination,[58] although this finding is not universally supported.[59] A single-center retrospective cohort study showed that extremely low birth weight infants with grades I and II IVH had higher rates of Mental Developmental Index scores of less than 70, major neurologic abnormality, and neurodevelopmental impairment at 20 months corrected age compared with infants with normal cranial ultrasound examinations.[60] In contrast, in a longitudinal multicenter NICHD study involving 1472 infants born at less than 27 weeks cranial ultrasound, grades I and II IVH were not associated with an increased risk of neurodevelopmental impairment at 2 years of age.[59] The prevalence of CP increases with IVH severity and is seen in 8%, 11%, 19%, and 50% for grades I through IV IVH, respectively.[61] Mortality rates are 4%, 10%, 18%, and 40% for IVH grades I through IV, respectively.[55]

PERIVENTRICULAR LEUKOMALACIA
Definition

PVL is defined as injury to the deep cerebral white matter that can be seen in 2 characteristic patterns: focal periventricular necrosis and diffuse cerebral white matter injury.[18] Focal periventricular necrosis is seen most commonly in the cerebral white matter at the level of the trigone of the lateral ventricles and near the foramen of Monro. These sites are located at the border zones of the immature penetrating cerebral vasculature, making them more susceptible to impaired perfusion at times of systemic hypotension. Diffuse cerebral white matter injury can be seen in conjunction with focal periventricular necrosis, and also occurs as a result of perturbations in cerebral blood flow secondary to vascular immaturity. The result is a loss of premyelinating oligodendrocytes and an increase in hypertrophic astrocytes leading to white matter volume loss and ventriculomegaly.

Incidence

Similar to IVH, PVL most often affects preterm infants born at less than 32 weeks of gestation, with an incidence that increases with decreasing gestational age.[62] White matter changes may not be appreciated on the initial ultrasound and may not be detected until the follow-up ultrasound examination or MRI is performed. PVL is detected by cranial ultrasound at 6 weeks of life in approximately 10% of very low birth weight infants.[62] In infants born at less than 28 weeks of gestation and surviving to near-term postmenstrual age, early cranial ultrasound examination obtained between 4 and 14 days of life has been shown to detect either grade III or IV IVH or cystic PVL in 9.7% of cases. A follow-up brain MRI obtained at 35 to 42 weeks postmenstrual age has been shown to detect moderate to severe white matter abnormalities in 19.3% of cases.[63] The incidence of PVL in periviable infants born between 22 and 24 weeks of gestation has remained stable at 6% to 7% from 2000 to 2011.[4]

Mechanism

The underlying cause of PVL, like IVH, is related to the immature cerebral vasculature and cerebrovascular autoregulation system.[18] In response to systemic hypotension, preterm infants cannot increase cerebral perfusion to border zone regions of the brain supplied by the immature penetrating cerebral vasculature. This condition sets off the cascade of events caused by hypoxia–ischemia resulting in brain injury that again is potentiated by chorioamnionitis and increases in the setting of positive neonatal cerebrospinal fluid cultures.[62]

Prevention

There are no current strategies that specifically target the prevention of PVL, and the current management of at-risk infants is aimed at maintenance of cerebral perfusion after delivery, although optimal blood pressure targets are unknown. Similar to IVH, the primary preventive strategy is prevention of preterm birth, transfer to an appropriate medical facility for those cases in which preterm delivery is likely,[48] and maternal administration of corticosteroids,[45] which have been shown to decrease the risk of grades III or IV IVH and PVL from 27.6% to 19.2% (adjusted, OR 0.67; 95% CI, 0.57–0.79) in periviable gestations from 22 to 25 weeks.[64]

Outcomes

Long-term neurodevelopmental outcomes correlate with the extent of white matter injury. Moderate to severe cerebral white matter abnormalities detected by MRI studies performed on very preterm infants born before 30 weeks of gestation were predictive of several adverse neurodevelopmental outcomes at 2 years of age, including cognitive delay (OR, 3.6; 95% CI, 1.5–8.7), motor delay (OR, 10.3; 95% CI, 3.5–30.8), neurosensory impairment (OR, 4.2; 95% CI, 1.6–11.3), and CP (OR, 9.6; 95% CI, 3.2–28.3).[65] In a separate study of 186 very preterm infants born at less than 30 weeks of gestation or weighing less than 1250 g who had a brain MRI at term equivalent age and again at the 7-year follow-up, cerebral white matter abnormality scores were normal, mildly abnormal, and moderately or severely abnormal in 45%, 36%, and 19% of cases, respectively. The increased severity of cerebral white matter abnormality scores strongly correlated with lower intelligence quotient scores and worse motor outcomes at 7 years of age.[66] Infants diagnosed with PVL are at risk for the development of spastic quadriplegia or diplegia, a form of CP that affects the lower extremities to a greater extent than the upper extremities, owing to the fact that the descending fibers of the motor cortex responsible for the function of the lower extremities transverse the periventricular area and are most likely to be injured. In a 2013 review of 25 children diagnosed by MRI with PVL, 24 of which were the product of a preterm delivery, 9 (36%) had spastic diplegia and 12 (48%) had spastic quadriplegia.[67]

PERINATAL STROKE
Definition

A perinatal stroke is a cerebrovascular event occurring between 20 weeks of fetal life and 28 postnatal days that is confirmed by neuropathologic studies or neuroimaging findings consistent with a focal cerebral infarction.[12] Perinatal ischemic stroke can be divided into perinatal arterial ischemic stroke (PAIS) and cerebral sinovenous thrombosis, which account for 70% and 10% of cases, respectively. The remaining 20% of perinatal strokes are from intracerebral hemorrhage.[13]

Incidence

The precise incidence of perinatal stroke is difficult to ascertain owing to variations in the definition, diagnosis, and case identification. The reported incidence of PAIS is 1 per 2800 to 5000 live births, whereas perinatal hemorrhagic stroke complicates 1 per

16,000 live births.[12,68,69] Most cases of PAIS occur in term infants,[70] and are identified by neuroimaging evaluation obtained for evaluation of a neurologic abnormality. Seizures are the presenting symptoms of a PAIS in up to 95% of cases,[70] with a delayed onset of seizure of more than 12 hours after birth or the presence of a focal motor seizure being predictors of stroke.[71] Other than seizures, nearly two-thirds of patients also present with diffuse neurologic signs, including abnormal tone or level of consciousness. Focal neurologic signs occur in 30% of patients, the majority of which are lateralizing hemiparesis.[70] Preterm infants with PAIS may present with more subtle signs, including respiratory distress or apnea and poor feeding.[72]

Mechanisms

There are several potential etiologies of a PAIS, all of which result in regional ischemia and hypoxia. In a single-center cohort study, embolism was the underlying cause in one-third of identified cases.[73] Potential sources of emboli in the neonatal circulation include right-to-left shunts in cases of congenital heart disease or the presence of a patent foramen ovale that can permit venous emboli to enter the arterial circulation. Other etiologies of PAIS account for 4% to 6% of cases each and include infection resulting in endothelial injury and meningitis (6%), trauma (5%), blood loss (4.5%), and asphyxia (4%).[73] Placental pathology has also been implicated as a potential cause with the possible release of emboli originating from thrombosed placental vessels into the fetal circulation as placental separation occurs at birth, or by the induction of a thromboinflammatory process in the fetus or neonate.[74]

Prevention

There are currently no strategies that decrease the risk of perinatal stroke. In a study of Epo therapy in neonates with PAIS, 21 neonates with MRI-confirmed PAIS received Epo at the time of diagnosis, and 24 and 48 hours after the first dose. There were no adverse effects on vital signs, or hematologic or coagulation parameters. In a subgroup analysis of 10 treated neonates, there were no differences in residual infarct volumes or neurodevelopmental outcomes compared with historical controls.[14] Once diagnosed, management is supportive and treatment is directed at the underlying condition and prevention of further injury. The American Heart Association[75] and CHEST[76] guidelines recommend anticoagulation for PAIS only in cases with a documented cardiac embolic source or prothrombotic state.

Outcomes

Neurodevelopmental outcomes are variable in survivors of perinatal arterial stroke and depend on the extent and distribution of injury. In 1 study of term infants with an average follow-up of 42 months, 33% had normal neurodevelopment.[77] CP and cognitive impairment were seen in 47% and 41% of children, respectively. In a second cohort of 36 infants diagnosed with perinatal stroke followed for at least 12 months after birth, 81% of children had abnormal outcomes, with CP, epilepsy, language delay, and behavioral abnormalities affecting 58%, 39%, 25%, and 22% of patients, respectively.[78] In a recent study, presumed PAIS, greater infarct volume, and the presence of comorbid epilepsy, but not infarct location or laterality, showed a strong negative correlation with attention and cognitive performance at school age.[79] In neonates with a PAIS, approximately 3% are at risk of having a recurrent symptomatic thromboembolic event that is associated with the presence of a prothrombotic state, cardiac malformation, or other underlying disease.[80]

CEREBRAL PALSY
Definition

CP is a clinical syndrome characterized by the presence of nonprogressive motor disturbances affecting muscle tone, posture, and movement that results from a cerebral abnormality of the developing brain and evolves within the first years of life.[15]

Incidence

Infants born at any gestational age can be affected with CP, but CP increases with decreasing gestational age. Although 58% of CP cases occur in infants born at or beyond 37 weeks of gestation, CP affects only 0.1% of this gestational age cohort. In comparison, very preterm births account for 25% of all CP cases, but 8.7% of those born at less than 32 weeks of gestation will develop CP. Infants born between 32 and 37 weeks of gestation account for 17% of all CP cases, and 3% of those born within this gestational age range will develop CP.[81] Efforts to decrease preterm births have reduced the rate of CP related to very preterm birth, but this measure has had little effect on the prevalence of CP because very preterm births account for only 2% of all births. As a result, the incidence of CP has remained unchanged at 1.5 to 2.5 cases per 1000 live births, despite improvements in perinatal care.[82]

Mechanisms

CP results from injury to the developing brain that can occur during the antepartum, intrapartum, or postnatal periods. An intrapartum hypoxic–ischemic insult is often associated with the development of CP, but only accounts for 10% to 20% of all cases.[6,26] The etiology of CP is multifactorial, and can result from any of the perinatal brain injuries previously discussed. In a cohort review of 235 children diagnosed with CP from 1986 to 2003, the most common clinical factors or pathologies associated with CP were prematurity (78%), intrauterine growth restriction (34%), intrauterine infection (28%), antepartum hemorrhage (27%), and multiple gestation (20%).[16]

Prevention

The prevention of preterm birth, antenatal administration of corticosteroids,[45] and delayed umbilical cord clamping[51] have variably been shown reduce the risk of prematurity, IVH, and PVL, which are all associated with an increased risk for the later development of CP. However, because only a small percentage of CP cases are seen in infants born at less than 32 weeks of gestation, these interventions have not decreased the overall incidence of CP.[15,82] Furthermore, interventions aimed at decreasing HIE and resulting CP, such as the use of continuous fetal heart rate monitoring, have not been shown to be beneficial.[32]

Magnesium sulfate

Magnesium sulfate can stabilize vascular tone, reduce reperfusion injury, reduce cytokine-mediated injury, and ameliorate neuronal injury in animal models.[83–85] Several randomized trials have shown that the administration of magnesium sulfate to mothers at risk of preterm delivery within 24 hours decreases gross motor dysfunction or CP among infants born prematurely.[74,86–88] The largest study by Rouse and colleagues[88] and the NICHD Maternal-Fetal Medicine Network showed a significant decrease in the rate of moderate or severe CP with the antenatal administration of magnesium sulfate to mothers at risk of preterm delivery before 32 weeks of gestation (RR, 0.55; 95% CI, 0.32–0.95). A 2009 metaanalysis of 5 randomized controlled trials found a statistically significant decrease in CP (RR, 0.70; 95% CI, 0.55–0.89) and moderate to severe CP (RR, 0.60; 95% CI, 0.43–0.84).[17] These findings are further supported by a 2016 metaanalysis of 6 randomized, controlled trials and 5 cohort studies that included 18,655 preterm infants and showed a statistically significant decrease in moderate to severe CP (OR, 0.61; 95% CI, 0.42–0.89).[89] In January 2016, the American College of Obstetricians and Gynecologists, supported by the Society for Maternal-Fetal Medicine, reaffirmed their recommendation on the use of magnesium sulfate as a fetal neuroprotective agent in cases of anticipated preterm birth before 32 weeks of gestation.[90]

Caffeine

The Caffeine for Apnea of Prematurity trial[91] established the efficacy and safety of caffeine for apnea of prematurity in neonates born weighing 500 to 1250 g. Follow-up at 18 to 21 months in this cohort showed that caffeine improved the rate of survival without neurodevelopmental disability (OR, 0.77; 95% CI, 0.64–0.93), and decreased the incidence of CP (OR, 0.58; 95% CI, 0.39–0.87) and cognitive delay (OR, 0.81; 95% CI, 0.66–0.99).[92] At the 11-year follow-up, caffeine reduced the risk of motor impairment (OR, 0.66; 95% CI, 0.48–0.9), although there was no significant decrease in the rate or severity of CP.[93]

Outcomes

In most children, depending on the type and severity of CP, the diagnosis of CP is made within the first 2 years of life.[94] Associated neurodevelopmental or sensory impairments such as pain, intellectual disability, epilepsy, behavioral disorders, bowel and bladder control problems, speech-language disorders, and hearing impairment affect approximately 75%, 49%, 35%, 26%, 24%, 23%, and 4% of patients, respectively, and are more likely to observed in patients with more severe motor disabilities.[95] The management of CP involves a multidisciplinary approach that is largely supportive and aimed at improving the quality of life of those affected by the condition. Although nearly 90% of patients will survive to adulthood,[96] those with severe handicaps may die in early childhood, most often from aspiration pneumonia and respiratory disease.[97]

SUMMARY

Over the last 2 decades, advances and changes in obstetric and pediatric care have resulted in improved survival and neurodevelopmental outcomes of very preterm infants.[2,3] More widespread use of antenatal corticosteroids, delayed cord clamping, and maternal magnesium sulfate administration have reduced the risk of IVH, PVL, and CP.[17,45,51] In term infants, postnatal interventions such as therapeutic hypothermia, changes in mechanical ventilation strategies, and Epo administration have further improved outcomes.[9,33,34]

Despite these improvements, perinatal brain injury continues to be a significant cause of long-term neurodevelopmental disability.[96] Research into novel therapeutic strategies targeting various aspects of the diverse mechanisms of perinatal brain injury is needed to continue improving long-term outcomes. Maternal administration of mesenchymal stem cells,[98] cytokine inhibitor therapy,[99] and maternal progesterone therapy[100] have all shown promise in animal models. The 2016 OPPTIMUM study (Vaginal Progesterone Prophylaxis for Preterm Birth),[101] a double-blind, randomized, placebo-controlled trial of vaginal progesterone for preterm birth prevention found a lower risk of brain injury on ultrasound examination in the progesterone group compared with placebo (OR, 0.50; 95% CI, 0.31–0.84). The understanding that perinatal brain injury is not only secondary to prematurity or hypoxia–ischemia, but involves a complex cascade of underlying cellular and immunologic factors often triggered by both antenatal and postnatal inflammation in response to these events, is paramount to advancing research for the discovery of novel therapeutic strategies.[102]

REFERENCES

1. Larroque B, Ancel PY, Marret S, et al. Neurodevelopmental disabilities and special care of 5-year-old children born before 33 weeks of gestation (the EPIPAGE study): a longitudinal cohort study. Lancet 2008;371:813–20.
2. Wilson-Costello D, Friedman H, Minich N, et al. Improved neurodevelopmental outcomes for extremely low birth weight infants in 2000-2002. Pediatrics 2007; 119:37–45.
3. Abily-Donval L, Pinto-Cardoso G, Chadie A, et al. Comparison in outcomes at two-years of age of very preterm infants born in 2000, 2005, and 2010. PLoS One 2015;10:e0114567.
4. Younge N, Goldstein RF, Bann CM, et al. Survival and neurodevelopmental outcomes among periviable infants. N Engl J Med 2017;376:617–28.
5. Chugani HT, Phelps ME. Maturational changes in cerebral function in infants determined by 18FDG positron emission tomography. Science 1986;231:840–3.
6. Executive summary: neonatal encephalopathy and neurologic outcome, second edition. Report of the American College of Obstetricians and Gynecologists' Task Force on Neonatal Encephalopathy. Obstet Gynecol 2014;123:896–901.
7. Papile LA, Baley JE, Benitz W, et al. Hypothermia and neonatal encephalopathy. Pediatrics 2014;133:1146–50.
8. Wu YW, Mathur AM, Chang T, et al. High-dose erythropoietin and hypothermia for hypoxic-ischemic encephalopathy: a phase II trial. Pediatrics 2016;137: e20160191.
9. Wei JC, Catalano R, Profit J, et al. Impact of antenatal steroids on intraventricular hemorrhage in very-low-birth-weight infants. J Perinatol 2016;36:352–6.
10. Ballabh P. Intraventricular hemorrhage in premature infants: mechanism of disease. Pediatr Res 2010;67:1–8.
11. Rabe H, Diaz-Rossello JL, Duley L, et al. Effect of timing of umbilical cord clamping and other strategies to influence placental transfusion at preterm birth on maternal and infant outcomes. Cochrane Database Syst Rev 2012;(8):CD003248.
12. Raju TN, Nelson KB, Ferriero D, et al. Ischemic perinatal stroke: summary of a workshop sponsored by the National Institute of Child Health and Human Development and the National Institute of Neurological Disorders and Stroke. Pediatrics 2007;120:609–16.
13. Govaert P, Ramenghi L, Taal R, et al. Diagnosis of perinatal stroke I: definitions, differential diagnosis and registration. Acta Paediatr 2009;98:1556–67.
14. Benders MJ, van der Aa NE, Roks M, et al. Feasibility and safety of erythropoietin for neuroprotection after perinatal arterial ischemic stroke. J Pediatr 2014; 164:481–6.
15. Blair E. Epidemiology of the cerebral palsies. Orthop Clin North Am 2010;41: 441–55.
16. Strijbis EM, Oudman I, van Essen P, et al. Cerebral palsy and the application of the international criteria for acute intrapartum hypoxia. Obstet Gynecol 2006; 107:1357–65.

17. Constantine MM, Weiner SJ. Effects of antenatal exposure to magnesium sulfate on neuroprotection and mortality in preterm infants: a meta-analysis. Obstet Gynecol 2009;114:354–64.

18. Khwaja O, Volpe JJ. Pathogenesis of cerebral white matter injury of prematurity. Arch Dis Child Fetal Neonatal Ed 2008;93:F153–61.

19. Giussani DA. The fetal brain sparing response to hypoxia: physiological mechanisms. J Physiol 2016;594:1215–30.

20. McDonald JW, Johnston MV. Physiological and pathophysiological roles of excitatory amino acids during central nervous system development. Brain Res Brain Res Rev 1990;15:41–70.

21. Burd I, Welling J, Kannan G, et al. Excitotoxicity as a common mechanism for fetal neuronal injury with hypoxia and intrauterine inflammation. Adv Pharmacol 2016;76:85–101.

22. Galluzzi L, Blomgren K, Kroemer G. Mitochondrial membrane permeabilization in neuronal injury. Nat Rev Neurosci 2009;10:481–94.

23. Halliwell B. Reactive oxygen species and the central nervous system. J Neurochem 1992;59:1609–23.

24. Giulian D, Vaca K. Inflammatory glia mediate delayed neuronal damage after ischemia in the central nervous system. Stroke 1993;24:l84–90.

25. Eklind S, Mallard C, Leverin AL, et al. Bacterial endotoxin sensitizes the immature brain to hypoxic-ischaemic injury. Eur J Neurosci 2001;13:1101–6.

26. Graham EM, Ruis KA, Hartman AL, et al. A systematic review of the role of intrapartum hypoxia-ischemia in the causation of neonatal encephalopathy. Am J Obstet Gynecol 2008;199:587–95.

27. Gopagondanahalli KR, Li J, Fahey MC, et al. Preterm hypoxic-ischemic encephalopathy. Front Pediatr 2016;4:114.

28. Chalak LF, Rollins N, Morriss MC, et al. Perinatal acidosis and hypoxic-ischemic encephalopathy in preterm infants of 33 to 35 weeks' gestation. J Pediatr 2012; 160:388–94.

29. Kurinczuk JJ, White-Koning M, Badawi N. Epidemiology of neonatal encephalopathy and hypoxic-ischemic encephalopathy. Early Hum Dev 2010;86:329–38.

30. Martinez-Biarge M, Madero R, Gonzalez A, et al. Perinatal morbidity and risk of hypoxic-ischemic encephalopathy associated with intrapartum sentinel events. Am J Obstet Gynecol 2012;206:148.e1-7.

31. Blume HK, Li CI, Loch CM, et al. Intrapartum fever and chorioamnionitis as risks for encephalopathy in term newborns: a case-control study. Dev Med Child Neurol 2008;50:19–24.

32. Alfirevic Z, Devane D, Gyte GM, et al. Continuous cardiotocography (CTG) as a form of electronic fetal monitoring (EFM) for fetal assessment during labour. Cochrane Database Syst Rev 2017;(2):CD006066.

33. Shankaran S, Laptook AR, Ehrenkranz RA, et al. Whole-body hypothermia for neonates with hypoxic-ischemic encephalopathy. N Engl J Med 2005;353: 1574–84.

34. Wyatt JS, Gluckman PD, Liu PY, et al. Determinants of outcomes after head cooling for neonatal encephalopathy. Pediatrics 2007;119:912–21.

35. Tagin MA, Woolcott CG, Vincer MJ, et al. Hypothermia for neonatal hypoxic ischemic encephalopathy: an updated systematic review and meta-analysis. Arch Pediatr Adolesc Med 2012;166:558–66.

36. Rangarajan V, Juul SE. Erythropoietin: emerging role of erythropoietin in neonatal neuroprotection. Pediatr Neurol 2014;51:481–8.

37. High-dose Erythropoietin for Asphyxia and Encephalopathy (HEAL). 2016. Available at: https://clinicaltrials.gov/ct2. (Identification No. NCT02811263). Accessed July 11, 2017.

38. Shankaran S, Laptook AR, McDonald SA, et al. Acute perinatal sentinel events, neonatal brain injury pattern, and outcome of infants undergoing a trial of hypothermia for neonatal hypoxic-ischemic encephalopathy. J Pediatr 2017;180: 275–8.

39. Okereafor A, Allsop J, Counsell SJ, et al. Patterns of brain injury in neonates exposed to perinatal sentinel events. Pediatrics 2008;121:906–14.

40. Martin RJ, Fanaroff AA, Walsh MC. Fanaroff and Martin's neonatal-perinatal medicine: diseases of the fetus and infant. 10th edition. Philadelphia: Saunders; 2015.

41. Bajwa NM, Berner M, Worley S, et al. Population based age stratified morbidities of premature infants in Switzerland. Swiss Med Wkly 2011;141:w13212.

42. Stoll BJ, Hansen NI, Bell EF, et al. Neonatal outcomes of extremely preterm infants from the NICHD Neonatal Research Network. Pediatrics 2010;126:443–56.

43. Soraisham AS, Singhal N, McMillan DD, et al. A multicenter study on the clinical outcome of chorioamnionitis in preterm infants. Am J Obstet Gynecol 2009;200: 372.e1-6.

44. Liggins GC, Howie RN. A controlled trial of antepartum glucocorticoid treatment for prevention of the respiratory distress syndrome in premature infants. Pediatrics 1972;50:515–25.

45. Roberts D, Brown J, Medley N, et al. Antenatal corticosteroids for accelerating fetal lung maturation for women at risk of preterm birth. Cochrane Database Syst Rev 2017;(3):CD004454.

46. Melamed N, Shah J, Soraisham A, et al. Association between antenatal corticosteroid administration-to-birth interval and outcomes of preterm neonates. Obstet Gynecol 2015;125:1377–84.

47. Norman M, Piedvache A, Borch K, et al. Association of short antenatal corticosteroid administration-to-birth intervals with survival and morbidity among very preterm infants: results from the EPICE cohort. JAMA Pediatr 2017;171(7): 678–86.

48. Mohamed MA, Aly H. Transport of premature infants is associated with increased risk for intraventricular hemorrhage. Arch Dis Child Fetal Neonatal Ed 2010;95:F403–7.

49. Jelin AC, Zlatnik MG, Kuppermann M, et al. Clamp late and maintain perfusion (CLAMP) policy: delayed cord clamping in preterm infants. J Matern Fetal Neonatal Med 2016;29:1705–9.

50. Mercer JS, Vohr BR, McGrath MM, et al. Delayed cord clamping in very preterm infants reduces the incidence of intraventricular hemorrhage and late-onset sepsis: a randomized, controlled trial. Pediatrics 2006;117:1235–42.

51. Committee on Obstetric Practice. Committee Opinion No. 684: delayed umbilical cord clamping after birth. Obstet Gynecol 2017;129:e5–10.

52. Intracranial hemorrhage: germinal matrix-intraventricular hemorrhage. In: Volpe JJ, editor. Neurology of the newborn. 5th edition. Philadelphia: Saunders; 2008. p. 517.

53. Al-Abdi SY, Al-Aamri MA. A systematic review and meta-analysis of the timing of early intraventricular hemorrhage in preterm neonates: clinical and research implications. J Clin Neonatal 2014;3:76–88.

54. Ment LR, Bada HS, Barnes P, et al. Practice parameter: neuroimaging of the neonate: report of the Quality Standards Subcommittee of the American

Academy of Neurology and the Practice Committee of the Child Neurology Society. Neurology 2002;58:1726–38.

55. Christian EA, Jin DL, Attenello F, et al. Trends in hospitalization of preterm infants with intraventricular hemorrhage and hydrocephalus in United States, 2000-2010. J Neurosurg Pediatr 2016;17:260–9.

56. Cherian S, Whitelaw A, Thoresen M, et al. The pathogenesis of neonatal post-hemorrhagic hydrocephalus. Brain Pathol 2004;14:305–11.

57. Adams-Chapman I, Hansen NI, Stoll BJ, et al. Neurodevelopmental outcome of extremely low birth weight infants with posthemorrhagic hydrocephalus requiring shunt insertion. Pediatrics 2008;121:e1167–77.

58. Mukerji A, Shah V, Shah PS. Periventricular/intraventricular hemorrhage and neurodevelopmental outcomes: a meta-analysis. Pediatrics 2015;136:1132–43.

59. Payne AH, Hintz SR, Hibbs AM, et al. Neurodevelopmental outcomes of extremely low-gestational-age neonates with low-grade periventricular-intraventricular hemorrhage. JAMA Pediatr 2013;167:451–9.

60. Patra K, Wilson-Costello D, Taylor HG, et al. Grades I-II intraventricular hemorrhage in extremely low birth weight infants: effects on neurodevelopment. J Pediatr 2006;149:169–73.

61. Beaino G, Khoshnood B, Kaminski M, et al. Predictors of cerebral palsy in very preterm infants: the EPIPAGE prospective population-based cohort study. Dev Med Child Neurol 2010;52:e119–25.

62. Tsimis ME, Johnson CT, Raghunathan RS, et al. Risk factors for periventricular white matter injury in very low birthweight neonates. Am J Obstet Gynecol 2016;214:380.e1-6.

63. Hintz SR, Barnes PD, Bulas D, et al. Neuroimaging and neurodevelopmental outcome in extremely preterm infants. Pediatrics 2015;135:e32–42.

64. Carlo WA, McDonald SA, Fanaroff AA, et al. Association of antenatal corticosteroids with mortality and neurodevelopmental outcomes among infants born at 22 to 25 weeks' gestation. JAMA 2011;306:2348–58.

65. Woodward LJ, Anderson PJ, Austin NC, et al. Neonatal MRI to predict neurodevelopmental outcomes in preterm infants. N Engl J Med 2006;355:685–94.

66. Anderson PJ, Treyvaud K, Neil JJ, et al. Associations of newborn brain magnetic resonance imaging with long-term neurodevelopmental impairments in very preterm children. J Pediatr 2017;187:58–65.e1.

67. Imamura T, Ariga H, Kaneko M, et al. Neurodevelopmental outcomes of children with periventricular leukomalacia. Pediatr Neonatol 2013;54:367–72.

68. Agrawal N, Johnston SC, Wu YW, et al. Imaging data reveal a higher pediatric stroke incidence than prior US estimates. Stroke 2009;40:3415–21.

69. Armstrong-Wells J, Johnston SC, Wu YW, et al. Prevalence and predictors of perinatal hemorrhagic stroke: results from the Kaiser pediatric stroke study. Pediatrics 2009;123:823–8.

70. Kirton A, Armstrong-Wells J, Chang T, et al. Symptomatic neonatal arterial stroke: the International Pediatric Stroke Study. Pediatrics 2011;128:e1402–10.

71. Rafay MF, Cortez MA, de Veber GA, et al. Predictive value of clinical and EEG features in the diagnosis of stroke and hypoxic ischemic encephalopathy in neonates with seizures. Stroke 2009;40:2402–7.

72. Golomb MR, Garg BP, Edwards-Brown M, et al. Very early arterial ischemic stroke in premature infants. Pediatr Neurol 2008;38:329–34.

73. Govaert P, Ramenghi L, Taal R, et al. Diagnosis of perinatal stroke II: mechanisms and clinical phenotypes. Acta Paediatr 2009;98:1720–6.

74. Elbers J, Viero S, MacGregor D, et al. Placental pathology in neonatal stroke. Pediatrics 2011;127:e722–9.

75. Roach ES, Golomb MR, Adams R, et al. Management of stroke in infants and children: a scientific statement from a Special Writing Group of the American Heart Association Stroke Council and the Council on Cardiovascular Disease in the Young. Stroke 2008;39:2644–91.

76. Monagle P, Chan AKC, Goldenberg NA, et al. Antithrombotic therapy in neonates and children: antithrombotic therapy and prevention of thrombosis, 9th ed: American College of Chest Physicians evidence-based clinical practice guidelines. Chest 2012;141:e737s–801.

77. Sreenan C, Bhargava R, Robertson CM. Cerebral infarction in the term newborn: clinical presentation an long-term outcome. J Pediatr 2000;137:351–5.

78. Lee J, Croen LA, Lindan C, et al. Predictors of outcome in perinatal arterial stroke: a population-based study. Ann Neurol 2005;58:303–8.

79. Bosenbark DD, Krivitzky L, Ichord R, et al. Clinical predictors of attention and executive functioning outcomes in children after perinatal arterial ischemic stroke. Pediatr Neurol 2017;69:79–86.

80. Kurnik K, Kosch A, Strater R, et al. Recurrent thromboembolism in infants and children suffering from symptomatic neonatal arterial stroke: a prospective follow-up study. Stroke 2003;34:2887–92.

81. Hirvonen M, Ojala R, Korhonen P, et al. Cerebral palsy among children born moderately and late preterm. Pediatrics 2014;134:e1584–93.

82. Oskoui M, Coutinho F, Dykeman J, et al. An update on the prevalence of cerebral palsy: a systematic review and meta-analysis. Dev Med Child Neurol 2013; 55:509–19.

83. McDonald JW, Silverstein FS, Johnston MV. Magnesium reduces N-methyl-D-aspartate (NMDA)-mediated brain injury in perinatal rats. Neurosci Lett 1990; 109:234–8.

84. Weglicki WB, Phillips TM, Freedman AM, et al. Magnesium-deficiency elevates circulating levels of inflammatory cytokines and endothelin. Mol Cell Biochem 1992;110:169–73.

85. Burd I, Breen K, Friedman A, et al. Magnesium sulfate reduces inflammation-associated brain injury in fetal mice. Am J Obstet Gynecol 2010;202:292.e1-9.

86. Crowther CA, Hiller JE, Doyle LW, et al. Effect of magnesium sulfate given for neuroprotection before preterm birth: a randomized controlled trial. JAMA 2003;290:2669–76.

87. Marret S, Marpeau L, Zupan-Simunek V, et al. Magnesium sulphate given before very-preterm birth to protect infant brain: the randomized controlled PREMAG trial. BJOG 2007;114:310–8.

88. Rouse DJ, Hirtz DG, Thom E, et al. A randomized, controlled trial of magnesium sulfate for the prevention of cerebral palsy. N Engl J Med 2008;359:895–905.

89. Zeng X, Xue Y, Tian Q, et al. Effects and safety of magnesium sulfate on neuroprotection: a meta-analysis based on PRISMA guidelines. Medicine (Baltimore) 2016;95:e2451.

90. American College of Obstetricians and Gynecologists Committee on Obstetric Practice, Society for Maternal-Fetal Medicine. Committee Opinion No. 455: Magnesium sulfate before anticipated preterm birth for neuroprotection. Obstet Gynecol 2010;115:669–71.

91. Schmidt B, Roberts RS, Davis P, et al. Caffeine therapy for apnea of prematurity. N Engl J Med 2006;354:2112–21.

92. Schmidt B, Roberts RS, Davis P, et al. Long-term effects of caffeine therapy for apnea of prematurity. N Engl J Med 2007;357:1893–902.

93. Schmidt B, Roberts RS, Anderson PJ, et al. Academic performance, motor function, and behavior 11 years after neonatal caffeine citrate therapy for apnea of prematurity: an 11-year follow-up of the CAP randomized clinical trial. JAMA Pediatr 2017;171:564–72.

94. Granild-Jensen JB, Rackauskaite G, Flachs EM, et al. Predictors for early diagnosis of cerebral palsy from national registry data. Dev Med Child Neurol 2015; 57:931–5.

95. Novak I, Hines M, Goldsmith S, et al. Clinical prognostic messages from a systematic review on cerebral palsy. Pediatrics 2012;130:e1285–312.

96. Hemming K, Hutton JL, Colver A, et al. Regional variation in survival of people with cerebral palsy in the United Kingdom. Pediatrics 2005;116:1383–90.

97. Eyman RK, Grossman HJ, Chaney RH, et al. Survival of profoundly disabled people with severe mental retardation. Am J Dis Child 1993;147:329–36.

98. Lei J, Firdaus W, Rosenzweig JM, et al. Murine model: maternal administration of stems cells for prevention of prematurity. Am J Obstet Gynecol 2015;212: 639.e1-10.

99. Leitner K, Al Shammary M, McLane M, et al. IL-1 receptor blockade prevents focal cortical brain injury but not preterm birth in a mouse model of inflammation-induced preterm birth and perinatal brain injury. Am J Reprod Immunol 2014;71:418–26.

100. Tronnes AA, Koschnitzky J, Daza R, et al. Effects of lipopolysaccharide and progesterone exposures on embryonic cerebral cortex development in mice. Reprod Sci 2016;23:771–8.

101. Norman JE, Marlow N, Messow CM, et al. Vaginal progesterone prophylaxis for preterm birth (the OPPTIMUM study): a multicentre, randomised, double-blind trial. Lancet 2016;387:2106–16.

102. Yanni D, Korzeniewski S, Allred EN, et al. Both antenatal and postnatal inflammation contribute information about the risk of brain damage in extremely preterm newborns. Pediatr Res 2017;82(4):691–6.

Moving?

Make sure your subscription moves with you!

To notify us of your new address, find your **Clinics Account Number** (located on your mailing label above your name), and contact customer service at:

Email: journalscustomerservice-usa@elsevier.com

800-654-2452 (subscribers in the U.S. & Canada)
314-447-8871 (subscribers outside of the U.S. & Canada)

Fax number: 314-447-8029

Elsevier Health Sciences Division
Subscription Customer Service
3251 Riverport Lane
Maryland Heights, MO 63043

*To ensure uninterrupted delivery of your subscription, please notify us at least 4 weeks in advance of move.

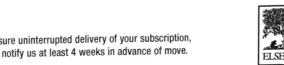

Printed and bound by CPI Group (UK) Ltd, Croydon, CR0 4YY

03/10/2024

01040392-0008